··························

Metabolic Consequences of Changing Dietary Patterns

Volume Editor

A.P. Simopoulos
The Center for Genetics, Nutrition and Health,
Washington, D.C.

8 figures and 49 tables, 1996

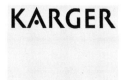

KARGER

Basel · Freiburg · Paris · London · New York ·
New Delhi · Bangkok · Singapore · Tokyo · Sydney

··················

World Review of Nutrition and Dietetics

Library of Congress Cataloging-in-Publication Data
Metabolic consequences of changing dietary patterns / volume editor, A.P. Simopoulos.
(World review of nutrition and dietetics; vol. 79)
Includes bibliographical references and index.
1. Nutritionally induced diseases – Cross-cultural studies. 2. Food habits.
3. Diet in disease. I. Simopoulos, Artemis P., 1933–. II. Series.
[DNLM: 1. Diet. 2. Food habits – ethnology. 3. Metabolism. W1 WO898 v.79 1996/
QT 235 M587 1996]
QP141.A1W59 vol. 79 [RA645.N87]
612.3 s--dc20 [612.3'9]
ISBN 3–8055–6296–9 (hardcover: alk. paper)

Bibliographic Indices. This publication is listed in bibliographic services, including Current Contents® and Index Medicus.

© Copyright 1996 by S. Karger AG, P.O. Box, CH–4009 Basel (Switzerland)
Printed in Switzerland on acid-free paper by Thür AG Offsetdruck, Pratteln
ISBN 3–8055–6296–9

Metabolic Consequences of Changing Dietary Patterns

··························

World Review of Nutrition and Dietetics

Vol. 79

Series Editor

Artemis P. Simopoulos
The Center for Genetics, Nutrition and Health,
Washington, D.C., USA

KARGER   Basel · Freiburg · Paris · London · New York ·
New Delhi · Bangkok · Singapore · Tokyo · Sydney

....
Contents

Bridget H.-H. Hsu-Hage, Mark L. Wahlqvist, Clayton, Melbourne, Vic.

Historical Development of Chinese Dietary Patterns and Nutrition from the Ancient to the Modern Society 133

J.D. Chen, Hong Xu, Beijing

Tea Consumption and Cancer 154

Santosh K. Katiyar, Hasan Mukhtar, Cleveland, Ohio

Coffee and Cancer: A Review of Human and Animal Data . . 185

Astrid Nehlig, Strasbourg; *Gérard Debry,* Nancy

Preface

Dietary patterns have varied over time, depending on agricultural practices, climatic, ecological, cultural and socioeconomic factors which determine the foods that are available to human beings. Looking at the evolutionary aspects of diet prior to the development of agriculture 10,000–12,000 years ago, it appears that human beings evolved on a diet that was higher in protein, complex carbohydrates, fiber, vitamin C, calcium, and nutrient density; and lower in simple carbohydrates, total fat, saturated fat, and trans fatty acids, than today's diet of the developed and developing countries, while maintaining a balance between the omega-6 and omega-3 polyunsaturated fatty acids. Paleolithic nutrition, or the nutrition of hunter-gatherer's is the diet for which our genetic profile was programmed. Health and normal development depend on the interaction of genetic and environmental factors. Diet, or nutrition, is an environmental factor of major importance along with physical activity. In fact, the sedentary lifestyle that is prominent in developed societies is an important factor in the development of increased food intake, obesity, insulin resistance, diabetes, hypertension, cardiovascular disease and even cancer.

Over the past 20 years, scientific advances and political interest have led to the development of national dietary recommendations for populations. Dietary recommendations are aimed for healthy people. But, many of the dietary guidelines include statements such as 'eat less saturated fat and cholesterol' or 'maintain healthy weight' or 'eat less sugar and salt'. Therefore, they also incorporate concepts for the prevention and development of diseases that are 'lifestyle' related, such as obesity, hypertension, cardiovascular disease, and possibly cancer.

There is already good evidence that specific dietary patterns may increase the likelihood of specific diseases or health outcomes, e.g., diets rich in fruits and vegetables may reduce lung cancer, and diets high in saturated fat and cholesterol are associated with cardiovascular disease. In addition to altered dietary patterns, decreases in meal frequency lead to metabolic changes. For example, serum total and low-density lipoprotein (LDL) cholesterol and apolipoprotein B (ApoB) levels may be lowered by increasing meal frequency alone, with no alteration in the nature or amount of the food eaten. Reductions in serum insulin levels and 24-hour urinary C-peptide excretion also occur. Studies have examined the response of cholesterol biosynthesis and circulating hormone concentrations to meal frequency to better understand processes of regulation of human cholesterol metabolism. The results showed parallel lowering of insulin and glucose-dependent insulinotropic polypeptide (GIP) concentrations and a lower rate of deuterium uptake into cholesterol with increased meal frequency. Thus, the data suggest that hormone-related mechanisms, secondary to the pattern of energy intake, are important in the regulation of human cholesterol synthesis.

It was considered timely to develop a volume in the series *World Review of Nutrition and Dietetics* that will examine dietary patterns and the metabolic consequences in populations undergoing dietary and other lifestyle changes. The Australian Aborigines are one of the most recently acculturated hunter-gatherer groups that have been extensively investigated in terms of the metabolic consequences of the altered dietary patterns. In the paper 'The Transition of Australian Aboriginal Diet and Nutritional Health', Amanda Lee clearly describes the dire consequences of the rapid change from a hunter-gatherer diet and lifestyle to the adoption of the Australian settlers' diet in 30 years. The contemporary lifestyle experienced by many 'westernized' Aboriginal people, which incorporates low physical activity and an energy-dense diet rich in rapidly absorbed carbohydrate and fat, is thought to produce hyperglycemia and stimulate a high postprandial insulin response. This produces increased glucose turnover in insulin-sensitive tissues and exacerbates selective insulin resistance, favoring those nonglucose regulatory metabolic pathways where insulin is functioning normally or near normally, that is, hepatic triglyceride and very-low-density lipoprotein (VLDL) synthesis and accumulation of fat in the adipose tissue. The consumption of long chain saturated fatty acids present in the Western diet have been shown to directly stimulate hepatic gluconeogenesis and raise the circulating levels of free fatty acids which reduce glucose utilization in peripheral tissues and produce insulin resistance. While physical inactivity and high intakes of refined carbohydrate and saturated fat are maintained, insulin resistance, hyperinsulinemia and glucose intolerance become more pronounced leading to obesity, NIDDM and hypertriglyceridemia.

Dr. Lee states that 'The main metabolic abnormalities of diabetes mellitus can be greatly improved, and also potentially prevented by reversion to a traditional hunter-gatherer lifestyle even for an experimental period as short as 7 weeks. During the study a small group of 14 Aboriginal diabetics travelled to ancestral coastal and inland territories where they existed entirely on traditional foods. Metabolic changes included decrease in fasting glucose, improved postprandial glucose clearance, improved insulin response, and reduction of fasting plasma triglyceride level. Additional improvements included a significant decrease in blood pressure, and increases in serum folate, vitamin B_{12} and vitamin E.' The implications of these findings to public health are enormous and indicate the importance of physical activity, low energy dense diet and weight control in the management and prevention of diabetes in Aboriginal people. Aboriginal people are demonstrating that the beneficial qualities of hunter-gatherer diet and meal patterns can be incorporated with increased physical activity into contemporary 'Western' lifestyle.

In a world of new foods, migrant populations are particularly sensitive to determinants such as traditional food, food availability and accessibility, food preparation skills and facilities and the household economy. In 'Food Variety of Adult Melbourne Chinese: A Case Study of a Population in Transition', Bridget H.-H. Hsu-Hage and Mark L. Wahlqvist postulated that an increase in food consumption is a key to secure dietary diversity. The results of their study, derived from recent Chinese immigrant groups in Australia, suggest that introduction of new foods is a way of increasing food variety. The most impressive finding is the generally low essential nutrient intakes in those with a low food variety.

Demetre Labadarios et al. in 'Traditional Diets and Meal Patterns in South Africa' described the changes in dietary patterns that have occurred among rural Africans in the various regions of South Africa. Traditionally their diet was based on hunting small and large animals, and eating a lot of wild plants and fruits. Their food supply protected them from deficiency diseases such as kwashiorkor and pellagra. When maize (corn) was increasingly introduced, being deficient in niacin and tryptophan, these diseases began to become common. Beginning in 1920–1930, new dietary habits were acquired resulting in a lower consumption of minerals and vitamins, and by 1959 the modern African was becoming a tea drinker, instead of drinking fermented milk, and ignored the very valuable and abundant supplies of indigenous spinaches rich in calcium, iron and magnesium. A tendency was developed to discredit indigenous foods and to sell vegetables to buy white bread and corn. Labadarios et al. summarize the changes that have occurred with transition as follows: 'Regarding the other South African populations, transitions in food consumption follow a common pattern. The changes which have taken place are similar to those which occurred in many western populations during the last two or three generations. In the white, Indian, and colored populations, there have been increases in intakes of energy, fat and protein, with varying falls in intakes of plant foods. The changes have been associated with rises in socio-economic status. Broadly, for all of the populations under discussion, on the one hand, mortality rates in the very young have lessened and average survival time has increased. On the other hand, there have been rises in the occurrence of chronic disorders/diseases linked with increase in socio-economic status. In our view, there would seem little hope, despite recommendations, of any of the population returning in measure to diets of lower energy and fat content and with greater representation of plant foods.'

The paper on 'Cultural and Nutritional Aspects of Traditional Korean Diet' by Sook Hee Kim and Se-Young Oh describes the factors that shaped traditional Korean dietary patterns. People had different table settings according to their social status. The number of side dishes increased as one's social status was elevated. Emphasis was given to serving a variety of foods. In royal court, more diverse and extravagant meals were provided. Two hundred and ten various dishes were found in the cookbooks used in the royal court in the 18th century. During royal families' birthday parties, 46–74 different kinds of foods were served to the king. The common people had three meals a day when there was enough food and two meals otherwise. Between meals, light meals were served which might be related to the type of work they were doing. Another characteristic of the Korean diet is the large number of vegetables – about 280 different kinds. Most Koreans had a vegetarian diet throughout their 5,000-year history, but rapid changes in both their food supply and eating behavior have occurred in the last 30 years.

In 'The Historical Development of Chinese Dietary Patterns and Nutrition from the Ancient to the Modern Society', J.D. Chen and Hong Xu describe the evolution of dietary patterns and medicinal foods over the past 3,500 years. Of interest is the fact that the number of meals per day increased with income, as was the case in Korea. Usually, there were three meals per day and snacks were offered to children, the elderly and the rich. Tradition emphasized that 'breakfast should be eaten well, lunch must be in one's fill, and food for dinner should be little', and this is followed today. However, because of changes at work, lunch is fast becoming a smaller meal than dinner, as is the case in Western countries. Despite this, the Chinese dietary guidelines continue to emphasize calorie distribution for three meals: breakfast 30%, lunch 40%, and dinner 30%.

Tea is extensively taken by many people around the world, and so is coffee. Next to water, tea is the most popular beverage consumed worldwide. In terms of evolution, both tea and coffee are newcomers to our diet. There has been increasing interest on the beneficial effects of tea and on the possible adverse effects of coffee. It was therefore considered appropriate to include two extensive reviews on these subjects. The paper on 'Tea Consumption and Cancer' by Santosh K. Katiyar and Hasan Mukhtar reviews the status of tea on cancer. The authors conclude that, 'the available epidemiologic information does not indicate that tea consumption has a statistically significant causative effect on human cancers . . .' and believe that 'tea consumption is likely to have beneficial effects in reducing certain cancers in certain populations'.

The impact of daily consumption of coffee on tumorigenesis has been the subject of extensive research both in animals and humans. Astrid Nehlig and Gérard Debry in their paper 'Coffee and Cancer: A Review of Human and Animal Data' review the differences of caffeine metabolism in animals and humans. Whereas no differences in the metabolic fate of caffeine is observed between men and women, the caffeine half-life is 25% longer (6.9 h) in the luteal phase of the menstrual cycle compared with the follicular phase (5.5 h). Pregnancy and oral contraceptives increase the half-life of caffeine. The authors conclude that most of the literature favors the hypothesis of coffee and caffeine not being human carcinogens. There is still some debate on the carcinogenic effect of coffee on pancreas, colon and bladder. Coffee could even be protective in breast cancer and fibrocystic breast disease. However, it appears that rigorous studies are still necessary to reach a real consensus about the possible carcinogenic effect of lifetime exposure to coffee and caffeine in humans.

This volume should be of interest to scientists studying the evolutionary aspects of diet, dietary patterns and their metabolic effects on human health and disease, and policy-makers involved in making dietary recommendations. Specifically, medical and social anthropologists, geneticists, physicians, nutritionists, dietitians, food technologists, public health specialists, and scientists involved in various aspects of agriculture will find this volume of great interest.

Artemis P. Simopoulos, MD

Simopoulos, AP (ed): Metabolic Consequences of Changing Dietary Patterns.
World Rev Nutr Diet. Basel, Karger, 1996, vol 79, pp 1–52

....

The Transition of Australian Aboriginal Diet and Nutritional Health

Amanda Lee[1]

Menzies School of Health Research, Darwin, N.T., Australia

Contents

[1] Thank you to Prof. John Mathews, Prof. Kerin O'Dea and Peter McCutcheon, who commented on an earlier form of this review.

Introduction

European settlement of the Australian continent only 200 years ago heralded major dietary and lifestyle changes for Aboriginal people. The transition from a nomadic hunter-gatherer lifestyle incorporating a varied, nutrient-dense diet to a settled existence and an energy-dense diet, high in fat and refined sugars, is widely believed to have contributed to the deterioration of Aboriginal health. This review covers the transition of Australian Aboriginal diet and meal patterns and the deleterious nutritional and metabolic consequences of dietary change. Contemporary food choices amongst urban Aborigines have rarely been studied. Consequently the review focuses on available data from remote regions.

Aboriginal Ancestors

The ancestors of Australian aborigines first migrated to Australia from South-East Asia 40,000–50,000 years ago and moved slowly south across the continent [1, 2]. This migration was probably the first time humans had been exposed to a 'new' environment in which they had not coevolved with competitive carnivores [3]. It has been argued that these people irreversibly changed the face of Australia by causing rapid extinction and dwarfing of large mammals, marsupials, monotremes, birds and reptiles [3]. People relied initially on plant foods which also grew in South-East Asia, and southern migration of Aboriginal ancestors would have necessitated dietary adaptations to unfamiliar species; the process of *'eat, die, and learn'* [4]. In fact, Aboriginal people in arid central Australia now eat indigenous foods that are ignored in the tropical north [5].

Traditional Aboriginal Lifestyle and the Quest for Food

Aborigines eventually adopted the lifestyle of nomadic hunter-gatherers in diverse geographical and climatic conditions, from the coastal, savanna and open woodland areas of the tropical north, to the arid inland regions, and the fertile temperate eastern and south-western seaboards (fig. 1). A large difference in local population densities and in tribal, linguistic and cultural patterns has been observed between these regions [6–11]. Despite striking environmental variation, Aboriginal hunter-gatherer lifestyle, production modes and meal patterns were remarkably similar across the continent [12]. However, actual dietary intake varied greatly between tribal groups and there was also marked seasonal dietary diversity within each region.

Ethnographic Sources and Methodological Issues
The fertile temperate seaboard areas of the continent were settled rapidly by Europeans from 1788, and little reliable information is available about the traditional lifestyle, diet and meal patterns of Aboriginals from these regions [13–15]. Conversely, traditional culture has been relatively maintained amongst Aboriginal groups in remote northern and desert regions. However, no Aboriginal group continues to pursue a wholly traditional lifestyle.

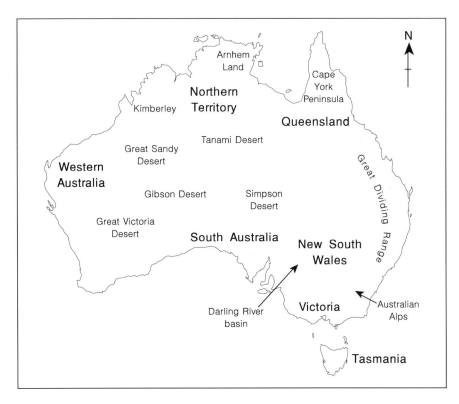

Fig. 1. Map of Australia showing areas mentioned in text.

The ethnographic literature providing information about traditional Aboriginal diet includes records of those Europeans who first contacted Aboriginal society, such as early explorers [16–23], mission and government representatives [24–26], anthropologists [13–15, 27–37] and a small number of medical observers [38–41]. Several early studies concentrated on Aboriginal food and dietary habits [42–51]. These early records should be viewed cautiously, because the degree of '*judgement, generalization or abstraction*' of facts is unknown [52, 53]. Moreover, early dietary observations were made for only a short period of time and did not generally consider the effect of seasons on the availability of food.

Much of the very limited quantitative dietary data available comes from studies of Aboriginal groups who had previous contact with Europeans, but temporarily reverted to traditionally-orientated lifestyle for a small number of days [54, 55]. Despite several methodological problems, these data have been used frequently to depict traditional nutritional intake [56, 57]. In particular, the data were extrapolated to develop the hypothesis that hunter-gatherers constitute '*the original affluent society*' spending less time (on average 3–5 h/day) to ensure their livelihood than agricultural or industrial populations [58].

Traditional Aboriginal Lifestyle

A brief description of traditional Aboriginal lifestyle is necessary to appreciate indigenous diet and meal patterns. Traditional Aboriginal groups lived a nomadic hunter-gatherer lifestyle imposed by the constant necessity to seek food and, in the drier regions of the continent, water. A varying number of family groups comprised the basic foraging group or band of 20–30 people including children. The tribe, or cluster of these bands, was divided into sections or moieties, which generally prescribed marriage and ceremonial obligations. Defined tribal estates, ranging from approximately 500 to 100,000 km², tended to be more confined in areas where both water and foods were plentiful [10, 11, 25, 59]. Strong religious beliefs were expressed through ritual practices, myths and deep spiritual and emotional attachment to the land. People lived in a communal state where cooperation and reciprocity was assured by traditional Law. Moieties extended beyond tribal boundaries which enabled access to resources in adjacent areas during time of environmental stress and fostered intertribal ceremonial gatherings when foods were plentiful [60]. Such gatherings occurred regularly in several regions, including the alpine areas of south-eastern Australia where the Bogong moth was a reliable food source during summer months [61].

Survival depended on the bands' intimate knowledge of their land, sources of water, and the detailed effects of the seasonal cycle on plant foods and game. Traditional knowledge and Law was transmitted from one generation to the next by an intensive and rigorous ritual system [62].

Generally, no substantial dwellings were built; windbreaks, brush shelters or caves provided shelter. There was a general reliance on improvisation and the few material possessions were multifunctional and portable. In the desert regions women used wooden scooped dishes and digging sticks, and men used simple weapons such as spears, spear throwers and boomerangs [63]. In the tropical coastal regions harpoons and specialized canoes were used to capture turtles and dugongs. Shells or paperbark containers were used or baskets were woven from pandanus or grasses. Throughout the continent grindstones were used to mill seeds [64].

Interband trade was widespread and associated with elaborate ceremonial exchange cycles. Such trading created '*chains of connection*' [65], which linked together people from different regions, resulting in the spread of information as well as material goods. In particular the leaves of 'native tobacco' (*Nicotiana gossei, N. excelsior* and *Dubosia hopwoodii*), were traded over wide areas [66]. Surprisingly, there is little evidence of extensive trade of food [67].

Agriculture

Horticulture and animal husbandry were not practiced formally, although the environment was modified by innovative methods to increase food production. In particular, regular mosaic burning or 'fire-stick farming' was common [68, 69]. Fire was used to trap animals, and the regeneration of new growth attracted game. The germination of many favoured food plants was also assisted by burning. On a wide scale, fire may have advanced the savanna grasslands of northern Australia and thus extended Aboriginal habitat [10].

Other examples of food production techniques include irrigation, dispersal of fruit seeds around camp sites, fertilization of plants, cultivation of grubs and the leaving of some fruits and 'growing points' of yams to aid cultivation of new plants. In the Darling River basin of western New South Wales, green native millet was harvested, stacked and then threshed when the seeds were dry [70]. In some northern areas nets were used to capture small marsupials. Various plants were soaked in water to stupefy emus and fish. Other fishing methods, including the construction of nets and elaborate traps, have also been described [71–73].

Traditional Storage of Food

Foraging parties generally gathered sufficient food for their immediate requirements and rarely stored food for later use [67, 69]. However, specific examples of food storage have been described [67, 74–76], particularly of seeds in marginal desert areas and the Darling River basin [70, 77–80]. The drying and storage of fruits, such as *Solanum* sp. and *Santalum* sp., in the Western Desert have also been noted [80–84].

The Sexual Division of Labour

Many anthropological models of Aboriginal subsistence have emphasized sexual separateness in the traditional division of labour; men were the 'hunters' of animal foods and women were the 'gatherers' of plant foods [85–87]. Recent evidence suggests however, that stereotyping of the sexual division of labour may have contributed to a de-emphasis of women's hunting of animal foods, such as small marsupials, shellfish, reptiles and insects, hence minimizing estimations of the animal component of the diet [88–90]. These studies tend to highlight the traditional interdependence of women and men in procuring food. Women provided the subsistence diet of highly reliable foods including those animal foods listed above in addition to honey, eggs and plant foods. They procured foods in groups, compatible with child-minding responsibilities, and their yields were directly proportional to the effort invested [88–90]. Men primarily hunted alone or in pairs for large game (mammals, birds, reptiles and fish), procuring fruits and other plant foods for themselves during the hunt. When hunting was successful their quarry provided prized feasts for the entire band.

Traditional Aboriginal Diet and Meal Patterns

Extensive lists of plant and animal foods have been produced [5, 46, 47, 91–99]. However, with two possible exceptions which attempted to rank foods by their nutritional significance and availability [100, 101], the relative contribution of individual food sources is difficult to determine from these records.

Meat Orientation of the Diet
For many years it was believed that the Aboriginal diet was predominately vegetarian, and a statement that the central Australian desert diet was comprised of '70–80% plant foods' [93] had been widely accepted [87, 101–103]. This is no longer believed to be the case. Meggitt [93] compared foods by estimated weight, which probably overassessed the nutritional significance of the vegetable component of the diet. Support for the vegetarian basis of the traditional desert diet had also been interpreted from botanical lists, observations illustrating the ripening of different plant food species throughout the year [96] and evidence of storage of plant foods. However, none of these sources attempted to quantify actual dietary intake, and the effects of climate, seasonality and specific location must also be considered [37, 70, 96]. For example, the often quoted estimation that in the extremely arid Western desert during the drought years of the 1960s, 95% of the primarily vegetarian diet was provided by women at least 90% of the time [104], was not supported by different observers who noted few plant staples in other arid areas at that time [80, 84].

There is increasing evidence that both tropical savanna/coastal [54, 105] and desert [86, 90] diets were meat-oriented; vegetable foods provided an important supplement, rather than an alternative to animal foods, with proportions changing throughout the seasons [10, 25, 36, 82, 84, 100]. For example, the coastal people of Cape York concentrated so much on the procurement of marine animals that vegetable foods were considered a luxury [7]. Desert Aborigines have described themselves specifically as meat eaters [106]. Early observers commented on the intake of the meat of smaller mammals as a 'mainstay' of the diet of central Australian tribes [80]. The dietary significance of lizard meat to the people of the western desert has particularly been noted [107]. It was stated that 'these Aborigines definitely show a strong preference for meat food' and '... unless in times of game scarcity or in a tribe whose natural territory is particularly deficient in animal food, meat appears to be their chief item of food' [45]. Other important animal sources in the diet, such as eggs, birds, frogs, honey ants and grubs of the family *Cossidae* have also been recorded [54, 84, 108].

Plant Foods

Of the many plant foods listed, most were eaten infrequently, with only a few staples contributing significantly to the diet [37, 96]. As an example, plant foods in desert regions included: yams (*Ipomoea costata, Vigna lanceolata*); fruits known as bush raisins and bush tomatoes (*Solanum chippendalei, S. centrale*); fruits of figs (*Ficus* sp.); fruits of the quandong (*Santalum acuminatum*), the related 'plum' (*S. lanceolatum*); corms of bush onion (*Cyperus rotundus*); the wild 'orange' (*Capparis* sp.), truffles (*Scleroderma* sp.), gall nuts ('mulga apple', 'bloodwood apple') and seeds from both trees (*Acacia* sp., *Eucalyptus* sp.) and grasses (*Portulaca* sp., *Eragrostis* sp., *Panicum* sp., *Fimbristylis* sp.).

Accounts of seed processing, the 'tedious game' [109], highlight the labour-intensive aspects of seed collecting, winnowing, threshing, yandying, parching, pounding, grinding and cooking [11, 27, 90]. The role of seeds in the diet is considered to have been most predominant in grassland areas associated with seasonal flooding of river systems such as the Darling River basin [56]. Archaeological evidence indicates that seed grinding had continued in this area for 15,000 years [61]. It has been argued that greater efficiency of the wet-milled grass seed processing, compared with dry-milled tree seeds, accounts for the larger populations which inhabited grassland regions [78]. Indeed, the importance of seeds in the diet in other areas may have been exaggerated, particularly in tropical regions where the availability of wild rice (*Oryza sativa*) may have removed the need to resort to the labour-intensive processing of seeds [5].

Dietary Diversity

The subsistence behaviour of bands across the continent achieved a varied omnivorous diet. Although the diet was primarily meat-oriented, the need for variety of vegetable and animal foods in the diet was seen to be important [101, 110–113].

The diversity of the food supply was affected by geographical landform, climate and season. Coastal territories, incorporating access to relatively stable and dependable estuarine and marine resources, generally provided greater habitat diversity. Although seasonal fluctuations in food supply greatly influenced foraging patterns, most observers describe a successively varied and ample range of both plant and animal foods, even in the arid zone [45, 81, 114, 115].

Most details are available from tropical coastal Australia where the seasonal variation of diet was particularly marked [29, 31, 32, 36, 54, 59, 98, 116–118]. Most Aboriginal groups in these regions identify six distinct seasons. The abundance of water during the wet season dictated not only the types of foods available, but, together with the heavy growth of tall grass, restricted people's movement and rendered many foods inaccessible. During the wet season people tended to band close to a reliable source of food such as the coast, particularly near a river mouth, open forest or monsoon forest, spreading out into lower lying areas as the flood waters subsided. The few wet season fruits available included the 'red apple' (*Syzigium suborbiculare*) and cheesefruit (*Morinda citrifolia*), but generally the height of the wet season was the 'hungry time' [119] when undependable game formed the basis of the diet.

Vegetable foods were most abundant during the early dry season (April–July), when a great variety of yams (*Dioscorea bulbifera, D. transversa, D. sativa, Ipomoea* sp., *Vigna vexillata*), waterlilies (*Nymphaea* sp.) and fruits (*Mimusops elengi, Tacca leontopetaloides, Pouteria sericea,* wild 'grape' *Ampelocissus acetosa,* wild figs *Ficus* sp.) were available. With calmer seas, salt-water turtles, dugongs and deep sea fish were again hunted from bark or dugout canoes [43] although there is evidence that only a small group of tribes used dugong as a major food source [7]. Immediately after the wet season large fish (barrammundi, saratoga and catfish) were easiest to catch in the wide, shallow flood waters, and, later, file snakes (*Achrochordus javanicus*) became stranded in pools on the flood plains.

By the end of the dry season (September–November) vegetable foods were scarce. The most common was the cycad (*Cycas media, C. angulata*), although wild rice (*Oryza* sp.), the nuts of the pandanas palm (*Pandanas spirilis*), the growing shoot of palms (*Livistonia* sp., *Hydriastele wendlandiana*), and the seeds of several species of kurrajong (*Brachychiton* sp. and *Sterulia caudata*) were also still available in small quantities in some regions. Honey and animal foods such as magpie geese, shellfish, long-necked turtles, goannas, wallabies, kangaroos and emus, were particularly important during this time. From October to December, groups became larger as people congregated close to remaining supplies of fresh water.

Therefore, the varied microenvironments of the tropical north ensured a consistent, though changing, supply of food. Open forest and woodland was the richest plant community, offering an abundance of fruits even in the wet season, root foods in the early dry season and seeds in the late dry [120–122].

Daily Meal Patterns

The quantity and quality of food intake also varied greatly on a day-to-day basis. The usual pattern was of subsistence intake supplemented by 'feasts' when large game were successfully hunted. Fruit, bulbs, nectar, gums, flowers and honey tended to be consumed as collected whilst hunting and foraging. Other plant foods, such as yams and seed-cake damper (a type of unleavened 'bread' cooked in coals), were prepared at either 'dinner' camps during the day, or at 'base' camps at the end of the day.

During 'feasts' people tended to rapidly consume extremely large quantities [45, 102, 123], and consumption of meat of up to 12.5 kg per capita per sitting have been observed [80]! Traditional desert people were also able to rapidly drink large quantities of fluid (up to 2 liters in 35 s) [84]. 'In the matter of food and water their appetites are gigantic, and the quantities of both which they will consume are almost incredible... whatever degree of repletion is reached, to refuse food is almost unheard of' [80]. It has been argued that these feasts provided excess energy which was stored as adipose tissue to cover periods of relative food shortage [124].

Food Preparation
Maximum nutritional value was retained from food preparation practices [45, 100]. 'There is no refinement of food, no storage, no overcooking, little waste and no leaching of vitamins and minerals in cooking water' [125].

Many plant foods were eaten raw, with fruits, bulbs, nectar and gums often eaten freshly after picking. Some vegetable foods were cooked to enhance palatability, either roasted on an open fire, buried in hot sand and ashes, or roasted in bark and/or leaves between layers of hot stones [45, 54]. Several foods required careful preparation to remove toxins prior to roasting [31, 54, 98]. For example *D. sativa, D. bulbifera* ('cheeky-yams') and *C. media* ('burrawong nut') were cut up or pounded and left in water for several days to remove 'bitterness'. Tree, grass and waterlily seeds and *C. media* were frequently made into a damper which was baked in hot sand and ashes.

Methods of cooking animals varied across the continent, and were usually prescribed by traditional Law [45, 80, 126, 127]. Smaller animals were baked in hot sand and ashes, either directly or wrapped in bark and leaves. Large animals were usually singed prior to removal of the stomach, intestines and liver. Offal was generally cooked separately and savoured. The animal was either dissected or baked whole in hot sand and ashes, ensuring the greatest possible retention of nutrients. Sometimes heated stones were placed in the body cavity. Meat was eaten rare, usually at one sitting. There was little wastage; the omental and mesenteric fat, internal organs, and blood and bone marrow of macropods were prized, as were the fat and blood 'soup' contents of the inverted turtle, and the liver of sharks and stingrays, which were mixed and consumed with the flesh [54, 128, 129]. Large bones were broken with stones and the marrow extracted, while smaller bones were chewed, or even pounded and eaten [45].

Food Distribution

There was no direct relationship between individual effort and reward in the right to consume produce [62]. Foods were proportioned and distributed according to traditional Law; strict cultural practices determined by kin obligations. Sharing of food had a social, as well as a physiological function, enabling the affirmation of relationships [130]. The distribution of some food items was also associated with particular conventions such as ceremonies and atonement [131]. In some areas older men received the choice cuts of an animal, and the remaining portions were distributed according to age and status [24, 41, 119, 127, 132]. In other areas the hunter was the last to receive a portion and would remain without if insufficient meat was provided [31]. There is evidence that the men generally had greater access to protein and delicacies such as liver and fat, while women tended to eat less in favour of their families, and old women received the smallest portions [24, 102, 119].

Children were breast-fed until approximately 3 years of age, the age of weaning depending on the arrival of another sibling [54, 133, 134]. Solids were not introduced until eruption of teeth [54, 133]. Responsibility for feeding tended to rest with the child, who was expected to indicate desire for food, and was fed on demand, deciding 'what and when to eat' [135]. Older children had priority over the feeding of small infants [133, 135].

Traditional Dietary Preferences

There is considerable evidence that dietary preferences affected traditional food-related attitudes, behaviour and diet, and that most individuals shared a preference for meat, fat, honey and fresh food [10, 90, 104]. Preferences for the large monitors (*Varanus gouldiiand, V. gigantus*), witchetty grubs (*Cossidae* sp.), emus and marine mammals are believed to be due to their relatively high fat content [27, 43, 80, 136]. It has been noted that '... people constantly discuss the best time to collect various foods so that the animals will be in the most desirable condition for eating, that is, when they are "fat" ' [137]. There have also been reports of game being left uneaten when it was considered to contain insufficient fat [90, 106].

A 'sweet tooth' has been described as a 'leading characteristic of both sexes at all ages' [80], and many early observers have commented on the dietary preference for sweet foods [45, 96, 138]. Traditional diet was generally low in sugars [139]. However, sweetness was provided by honey ants (*Melophorus inflatus*), the honey of the native bee, blossoms (*Grevillea* sp.), lerp (secretion from the insect *Psylla* living on the leaves of *Eucalyptus* sp.) and gums. A favoured sweet drink was produced from the blossoms of *Hakea* sp. soaked in water [84]. The enthusiastic pursuit of honey was noted to be out of all proportion to the small quantities obtained [54, 80]. For example there have been reports of Aboriginal women carrying branches of a scented flowering bush for 5 miles to attract honey bees [90].

Traditional Food Taboos

Various food-related taboos may have had the potential to influence nutritional status of some sections of traditional society, but the effect on variety or quality of the diet is difficult to gauge, due to lack of precise information about the nature and duration of such restrictions. There are several discrepancies in reports of taboos from the same area [54] which may be explained by seasonal or ceremonial differences or the apparent arbitrary nature of some reported taboos; there is record of older men imposing taboos and restrictions at whim [24, 29, 54]. Some groups were prohibited from consuming specific foods at certain times, such as youths during initiation, women during pregnancy, lactation or menstruation, and those in certain kinship relationships during ceremonies and funerals [63, 112, 116, 140]. One common Law prohibited the consumption of the totemic animal or plant of a particular moiety; each moiety was responsible for the ritually-induced increase of their totemic species for the benefit of the rest of the group [27].

Nutritional Analysis of Traditional Foods

The composition of most traditional vegetable foods are typical of uncultivated plants world-wide, being high in fibre and relatively high in protein with a generally low energy density [41, 83, 128, 141–148]. Notable results include the much publicized green plum, *Terminalia ferdinandiana,* which has the highest concentration of ascorbic acid at 3 g/100 g of any plant known [149]. Seeds of Australian acacia species have been shown to be relatively high in linoleic and oleic acids [150]. The carbohydrate in most traditional plant foods is of low glycaemic index, producing lower glucose and insulin levels following oral ingestion than similar western foods and may be protective against diabetes [151, 152].

Liver used as traditional food has been found to contain between 18 and 27 mg of vitamin C per 100 g wet weight, comparable to many vegetables and fruits, and the ascorbic acid appeared to be present in a stable form in liver, suggesting, together with qualitative information about dietary preferences and food distribution patterns, that liver from small animals may have been a useful source of ascorbic acid in traditional times [153].

Although some animal foods such as witchetty grubs (*Cossidae* sp.) and green ants (*Oecophylla smaragdina*) have a relatively high fat content [154], most land animals are very lean, with traditional meat foods having a much lower carcass fat content and intramuscular lipid content than meat from domesticated animals, such as cattle and sheep [128]. Although lipid levels in the muscle of wild animals tend to be low irrespective of season, some animals have varying carcass fat depending on season. Most of this carcass fat is stored in discrete depots within the abdomen. These fat depots tend to be small and were traditionally shared by many people. Tropical seafood has been shown to contain both omega-6 (arachidonic acid) and omega-3 polyunsaturated acids (eicosapentaenoic and docosahexaenoic acids) [155]. Muscle lipid of land animals is mainly structural (phospholipid and cholesterol) and is relatively rich in highly polyunsaturated long-chain fatty acids of both the omega-3 and omega-6 families [128]. Marine animals do have a higher fat content; the lipid fraction of turtle (*Chelonia mydas*) fat is unusually high in lauric acid (C12:0) and both turtle and dugong (*Dugong dugon*) fat are unusually high in myristic acid (C14:0) [156]. Although the fat of these animals was particularly prized by coastal people, its distribution was strictly controlled by traditional Law, and relatively few marine animals would have been hunted successfully using traditional methods.

Therefore, on the basis of available evidence, the traditional diet was generally low in energy density but high in nutrient density, being high in protein, low in sugars, high in complex carbohydrate of low glycaemic index and high in micronutrients. Even though the traditional Aboriginal diet contained a high proportion of animal foods, it would have been low in total fat, extremely low in saturated fat and relatively high in polyunsaturated fatty acids including the long-chain highly polyunsaturated fatty acids of both the omega-3 and omega-6 families, and hence protective against cardiovascular disease and related conditions (see below).

Transitional Diet: Early Post-Contact

Social Setting

Post-contact dietary change of Aboriginal Australians was mainly influenced by non-Aboriginal political, economic and social policy. The process of general alienation of land and its devastation upon Aboriginal societies has been documented in detail [157]. Aboriginal groups from the more fertile and hospitable regions were driven from their land in the early years of settlement and Aboriginal society was generally obliterated in pastoral and agricultural areas [158]. The Aboriginal population was particularly susceptible to introduced infectious diseases including measles, influenza, syphilis, gonorrhoea, typhoid fever, whooping cough, diphtheria, leprosy and tuberculosis

[40], but trauma associated with resisting the European invasion is also believed to have contributed to the rapid decline of the population [158].

In more arid areas, Aboriginal groups were often prohibited from the best watering places, which soon became polluted by stock. Ecological pressure forced Aboriginal people to accept rations from railway sidings and telegraph stations, from pastoralists and miners, and from missions; one aspect of a reaction process which has been termed 'intelligent parasitism' [159].

In the first official phase of government intervention in Aboriginal affairs, a policy of protection and preservation was adopted from 1913 to 1960. This policy aimed to segregate Aborigines by the provision of trading and health facilities in remote regions and the development of Aboriginal reserves. However, introduced resources, particularly food, proved an irresistible attraction and eventually groups were centralized at cattle stations, Government settlements or missions [160].

At cattle stations, Aboriginal men were employed as stockmen and women as domestics; both were paid in rations. There is evidence that Europeans perceived rationing as a means for controlling the movement and presence of Aboriginal people [161, 162], while Aborigines *expected* distribution of rations from Europeans, due to the reciprocal nature of traditional food distribution practices [163, 164].

At many settlements and missions, communal dining rooms were established. Frequently children were housed in dormitories and separated from their parents, even at mealtimes, when it was hoped that children would learn 'appropriate' manners and values [125]. Hence Aboriginal people were deprived of all responsibility for their own diet, as for most other aspects of their lives [117, 157, 160, 161, 163, 164].

From the 1930s it was clear that the Aboriginal population was no longer dying out and policy became intermingled with assimilationist endeavours. The years of the Second World War provided opportunity for Aboriginal employment and increased contact with Europeans, particularly around the northern coast where air force bases were located [157]. After the war, trading posts were established in remote areas to encourage people to remain in their own lands [26]. Some failed due to shortage of staff and funds, but others developed into service centers and eventually settlements. These were intended to be transitional institutions, but many continue to this day.

With assimilation adopted as official government policy in 1961, Aboriginal people were further encouraged to centralize and became dependent on welfare handouts or allowances for employment which were set well below award wages [157].

In 1967, the national referendum granted Aborigines the right to be counted in census, the right to vote, the right to drink alcohol and the right to equal pay. The referendum effectively allowed the Federal government to legislate for all Aborigines, expediting 'monetization of rationing' and the granting of some social security entitlements [162]. With the introduction of a cash economy, standard charges were introduced for meals, settlement stores became more popular, and communal dining rooms eventually folded. It has been argued that monetization of rations contributed to poverty and consequent nutritional problems [162].

The First Introduced Foods

With decreased availability of and accessibility to traditional foods, Aboriginal people were increasingly forced to depend on European foods [165]. Early rations consisted of flour, sugar, tea [112, 129], and to a lesser extent meat (fresh, tinned or salted); these foods being those of 'pioneer Australia' [166]. The early popularity of such foods may be due to such factors as their relative durability, low bulk, transportability, inexpensiveness and the simple cooking and storage facilities required for their preparation.

The adoption of flour in particular marked the beginning of altered subsistence patterns [167]. Flour was an integral component of food rations, and a prestigious gift in early contact days [162]. It produced a damper similar to a traditional 'staple', but with far less labour; '... What for I want to walk about all day, ngulmandjmak (morning time) till gukak (dark time) when I got that kanditjawah (flour) right here in that drum' [168].

Transitional Diet

Flour, sugar and rice were the staple ration foods at settlements and missions, with supplementary and irregular quantities of fruit and vegetables from the local gardens [125]. Beef and lamb were available in pastoral areas; fish and marine products were harvested at the coastal settlements.

Sugar was eagerly sought, and was consumed in large quantities from early contact. During the 1960s, it was estimated that one group of central Australian people consumed 5 kg of sugar per person per week; the managers of the station store eventually imposed a ration of 2 kg per person per week [84]!

At most missions and settlements, rations were distributed 3 times daily prior to mealtimes. In early days, most people were encouraged to rely on traditional foods at the weekends, although rations were sometimes available to those who attended church services. At cattle stations, rations tended to be distributed less frequently, usually daily.

Administrative, transport and economic problems tended to affect the regular provision of complete rations at missions and cattle stations [169]. Hence early food supplies tended to be erratic, and rations were not necessarily adequate in either quality or quantity. Specific nutritional problems included inadequate supplies of energy, protein, iron, calcium, riboflavin, vitamin A and, particularly, ascorbic acid [170, 171]. Recourse to bush foods occurred at all communities whenever rationing proved inadequate.

During the 'assimilationist' years, communal feeding was established in an attempt to improve Aboriginal nutrition [172]. Compared with other Australian diets of the time, the diet provided included more flour, bread and meat and less fruit, vegetables and dairy products [173]. Many settlements and missions lacked the equipment, staff and regular transport required to provide a comprehensive, nutritious and hygienic communal feeding service [172]. Only certain groups, employees, school children, infants and mothers, tended to receive cooked meals; others received dry rations to prepare in camp [173]. Many Aborigines declined to be fed communally even when they had the option, preferring to spend 'training allowances' at the stores which were established as a development of ration depots during this time [112].

The extremely limited range of foods stocked in the first stores, and the fact that counter service limited direct access to products, may have contributed to the conservative choices made by Aboriginal customers [112, 174]. Popular foods were tinned meat, tinned fruit, biscuits, confectionery and jam as a supplement to the ubiquitous flour, tea, sugar and tobacco [162]. Perishable food was only available for a few days each week. Aboriginal people rarely consumed butter, margarine or green vegetables even when they were available [169]. Compared with total Australian food expenditure, less was spent on dairy products and eggs, and on fruit and vegetables, while more was spent on sugars, preserves and confectionary, bread and cereals, and meats [112]. More meat but less bread was available on cattle stations; in fringe camps around urban centres alcohol was a major component of the diet for some people [175].

Contemporary Aboriginal Diet and Meal Patterns

Social Setting
In 1972, land rights legislation and a policy of self-determination were introduced by the Australian government, facilitating the gradual return of local political power to Aboriginal people. Social security entitlements were extended and increased and award wages were maintained although few Aborigines were employed [176, 177]. By 1980, most Aborigines received social security entitlements, including unemployment benefits, and were economically dependent on the public sector. Aboriginal councils were established to administer settlements, while Aboriginal representative bodies, such as Land Councils

and Progress Associations, were also formed. Opportunity was also provided for community ownership and/or management of settlement retails stores [174]. 'Self-management' became the official policy in 1975.

These political changes coincided with decentralization called the outstation or homelands movement, whereby small family groups are supported to re-inhabit traditional lands in remote areas [178, 179]. Market foods are regularly transported to outstations and subsistence patterns are much altered from the past [172].

The food supply of all contemporary Aboriginal people is directly affected by the environment in which they live. Approximately two thirds of Aboriginal Australians now live in urban areas. Of the remaining population, about 15% reside in relatively large centralized communities in remote areas (those providing essential services in a locus), and 18.5% in rural towns or their surrounding 'fringe camps' or on cattle stations. About 5% dwell at outstations either permanently or temporarily throughout the year [180]. Unfortunately there is little published data on the contemporary diet and meal patterns of the majority of Aboriginal people who live in urban areas; most nutritional studies have focussed on remote and rural areas.

Persistence of Traditional Food Preferences
Market alternatives to the traditionally-preferred dietary items of meat and fat and sweet foods are now readily available. These include fresh, frozen and tinned meat, fatty cuts of beef and lamb, honey, treacle, golden syrup, jam, confectionery and refined sugar. All remain extremely popular.

Unlike some traditional food which may be taboo at certain times, European food is usually considered acceptable and 'They (people from a Queensland community) uncritically accepted European foods in all their forms as good for eating' [181]. The social function of traditional food has been seen to be more important than the fact that it tastes good and stops hunger; European food is now seen to fulfil the latter role [130].

Contemporary Role of Traditional Foods
Contemporary foraging patterns may be explained in terms of necessity, dietary preferences and cultural satisfaction [90, 102]. Because the adoption of flour in particular has removed the uncertainty of survival, it has enabled people to concentrate on the procurement of highly prized traditional foods where available [90].

In the short term, after establishment of 'new' settlements, there may be an increase in yields of traditional foods due to high initial availability and the use of western technology [172, 175]. Vehicles, boats, and hunting and fishing equipment such as axes, crowbars, guns, hooks, lines and lures may enable increased yields of some preferred indigenous foods such as perentie, magpie geese, turtle, dugong, kangaroo, emu and fish [168]. In some areas, introduced feral animals such as rabbits and buffalo are also popular [59, 168].

However, long-term evidence suggests that the range of traditional foods currently used is much reduced from the past. This is due to several factors including the effect of environmental degradation caused by stock and feral animals, the introduction of exotic plant species, the increasing incidence of hot, destructive bush fires due to poor land management practices, the restricted access to some areas of land, depletion of resources and population pressure around permanent settlements, high costs associated with the acquisition and maintenance of weapons, vehicles, and fuel, changing demographic patterns, and cultural loss from generation to generation [37, 182, 183]. Since the early 1970s, people in remote areas have relied on western foods from settlement stores for the major proportion of their diet [37, 54, 92, 112, 117, 125, 173–175].

Community Stores in Remote Centralized Communities

Early stores were established in small, unsuitable premises with inadequate facilities for the storage of bulk food supplies, particularly perishable items. With increased cash flow, store facilities have generally improved but still a very limited variety of food is offered relative to larger rural towns and urban centres. In particular, perishable items such as dairy foods, fruit and vegetables are frequently in short supply [174, 184]. These items carry the risk of high overheads which store managers may not be willing to bear.

Costs for handling and freight of goods to remote communities are unavoidably high, and few suitable local products are available for purchase [174]. Retail prices must also accommodate high accountancy costs, purchase and maintenance of capital items, wages and salaries and 'shrinkage' [174]. As a result, stock may be up to 66% more expensive than in capital cities [185].

Income and Budgeting: The Effect of the Cash Economy on Diet

Most income is derived from fortnightly unemployment benefits. The resultant two-weekly variation in dietary intake has been documented frequently, with a close relationship between dietary quality and 'pay day' [112, 175, 186, 187]. A typical pattern is the intake of a greater variety of foods and increased intake of fruit, vegetables and meat for 3 days after 'pay day', with bread or damper forming the major component of the diet during the 'off-pay' week. Some items, such as sweetened carbonated beverages, have no regular pattern.

With the exception of sugar, flour and tea, most foods are consumed within 24 h of purchase. Generally bread or damper and sweet tea are consumed at every meal. Vegetables or fruit may only be consumed 2–3 times per fortnight.

The relationship between diet and income is not necessarily straightforward; with increased income has also come increased demand for material goods and services, hence increased competition for the food dollar [181]. There is also evidence that distribution of income within the community is important; women tend to spend available income on market foods, while men tend to purchase other consumer goods [187].

Use of Drugs

In addition to direct effects on nutrient intake, the abuse of substances can direct substantial amounts of money away from the purchase of food. High rates of alcoholism [188], petrol sniffing [189], cigarette smoking [190] and the overuse of kava (a psychoactive drink, prepared from the root of *Piper methysticum* introduced from the South Pacific into some Northern Australian Aboriginal communities during the late 1970s, where it became a popular alternative to alcohol) [190, 191] have been reported in many areas.

Agriculture

Although vegetable gardens were cultivated at most settlements in early years, there are few functional examples of contemporary horticultural projects. Much discussion has focussed on the possibilities of agriculture as an economic or subsistence basis in Aboriginal communities and outstations [192]. However, most commentators do not address the difficulties confronting European agricultural incursions into tropical and arid regions of Australia [125, 193]. In addition, many authors have commented on the tension and stress caused by imposing an agricultural pattern on a hunting and gathering society [69, 175]. However, some family groups in rural areas have managed to cultivate gardens with the technical assistance of culturally sensitive support agencies and nurseries [69, 194].

Individual Dietary Intake

It is very difficult to measure individual Aboriginal diet because of a range of cultural, social and ethical factors [195, 196]. Various methods have been applied (table 1) but these have not been validated [186, 196–204]. In most of these studies the results were considered by the authors to be biased by underreporting or underrecording of usual dietary intakes. In particular, quantitative nutrient results tend to be inconsistent with other qualitative observations of food habits and available biological data.

Table 1. Assessment of individual dietary intake

Location	Subjects	n	Method	Major foods	Summary of nutrient intake	Comments	Reference
NSW rural town	children	29	24-hour recall	not reported	low: protein, iron, thiamine, riboflavin, ascorbic acid	abstract only available	Allen et al. [200] Heywood and Zed [203]
NSW rural town	2 families 4 adults 17 children	21	weighed intake over 6 days	bread damper golden syrup jam honey	low: energy, calcium, iron, ascorbic acid, thiamine, vitamin E	nonrandom sample ? dietary change during study period	Kamien et al. [203]
South Australian urban town	adults	98	diet history	bread jam tinned foods pasta icecream	energy: ♂ 0.8–1.4 MJ pcpd ♀ 0.6–0.8 MJ pcpd protein: ♂ 60–130 g pcpd ♀ 50–80 g pcpd CHO: ♂ 60–320 g pcpd ♀ 50–220 g pcpd	extremely high interindividual daily variability	Wise et al. [186]
Six Kimberley communities	children	129	at least 3 × 24-hour recall per child	meat flour sugar powdered milk	low intake: energy, fat low intake of most vitamins/ minerals, comparable carbohydrate intake as non-Aboriginal children	? inappropriate nutrient composition for meat refined CHO intake not reported	King et al. [198, 199]

Table 1 (Continued)

Location	Subjects	n	Method	Major foods	Summary of nutrient intake	Comments	Reference
NSW rural town	adults	38	24-hour recall	states similar to non-Aboriginals	low: energy, sugars and most other nutrients	biased sample evidence of under-recall	Sibthorpe [201]
South-west Australia rural town and 'fringe camp'	children	14	24-hour recall	bread flour	low: energy, vitamin C	most restricted diets in 'fringe camp'	Hithcock and Gracey [197]
Two Victorian rural towns and one urban health service	adults	522	short food habit question-naire	not applicable	not applicable	frequent consumption of fried and 'take-away' foods and salt dripping used for frying in rural areas	Guest and O'Dea [204]

pcpd = per capita per day.

Store Turnover

Most recent Aboriginal dietary studies have been conducted in remote areas, where it has been considered more logical and practical to measure intake of food and nutrients on a community rather than an individual basis [184].

Most centralized communities are serviced by a community store which is the only source of purchased food for several hundred kilometers [111, 174, 195, 205]. These stores now provide over 90–95% of dietary intake [184]. Under these circumstances the turnover of foodstuffs from isolated community stores has potential as a useful source of information about contemporary dietary intake. Different approaches to the collection of store food data have been used previously (table 2). However, these studies have generally collected data for short periods only, often not covering the financial and associated purchasing cycle involved, have not attempted to validate methods and have only been partially analysed [111, 174, 177, 181, 206–208].

A more systematic approach to the measurement of apparent per capita food and nutrient intake in remote Aboriginal communities has been described using the 'store turnover' method based on the analysis of community store food invoices [184, 196], which has been validated against biological indicators of nutritional status [209].

In all remote Aboriginal communities studied, the intake of energy, sugars and fat is excessive, while the intake of dietary fibre and several nutrients, including folic acid, is low (fig. 2). The diet lacks variety, with white sugar, flour, bread and meat providing in excess of 50% of total energy intake. Of the high fat intake, fatty meats contribute nearly 40% in northern coastal communities and over 60% in central desert communities. 60% of the high intake of sugars is derived from sugar per se in both regions; the mean intake of refined sugars is 258 g per person per day [184].

Compared with national Australian apparent consumption data, intakes of sugar, white flour and sweetened carbonated beverages are much higher in Aboriginal communities and intakes of wholemeal bread, fruit and vegetables are much lower [184] (table 3).

Traditionally-Orientated Outstations

Anthropologists and economists have concentrated on traditionally-orientated outstations. Their agenda generally has focused on traditional hunting and foraging activities, with quantitative assessment of the diet as one factor of an extensive analysis of economic and/or social aspects of contemporary lifestyle.

Even in these isolated outstations, purchased foods accounted for most of the energy intake, while bush foods provided the greatest proportion of

Table 2. Store-based dietary studies in remote, centralized communities

Location	Method	Major foods	Irregularly available foods	Summary of nutrient intake	Reference
Queensland community (i) 1970 (ii) 1972	noted individual purchases for unspecified number of days	fresh meat sugar (i) 202 g pcpd (ii) 245 g pcpd flour tinned meat	not reported	energy (i) 103% (ii) 70% protein (i) 103% (ii) 82% acceptable: thiamine low: calcium, ascorbic acid, iron, retinol, riboflavin	Taylor [181]
Western Australian community mid-1970s	noted 'a typical morning's sale'	flour 752 g pcpd sugar 360 g pcpd tinned meat tea jam	fresh fruit fresh meat	not analysed	Peterson [177]
South Australian community mid-1970s	noted purchasing patterns over 2 weeks	flour 325 g pcpd sugar 97 g pcpd tinned meat jam	not reported	not analysed	White [111]
Western Australian community mid-1970s	recorded purchases over 7 days	sugar flour meat	fresh fruit fresh vegetables	energy 16.8 MJ pcpd protein 104 g pcpd acceptable: iron low: calcium, retinol, ascorbic acid	Coles-Rutishauser [206]
Northern Territory community mid-1970s	noted purchases for 5 days after 'pay day'	sugar 130 g pcpd bread fresh meat flour	not reported	not analyzed	Kailis [208]
Four Northern Territory communities mid-1970s	interviews with store managers and records from order books	flour 120 g pcpd sugar 91 g pcpd meat bread	fresh fruit fresh vegetables	energy 114% RDA protein 267% RDA acceptable: calcium, ascorbic acid, thiamine low: iron, retinol, riboflavin	Young [174]

pcpd = per capita per day.

protein intake (table 4) [90, 168, 102]. All studies confirmed that processed plant foods, as purchased carbohydrate including sugar, provided most of the energy intake from store-purchased foods, but that animal foods, particularly those high in fat such as lizards, provided most of the energy from bush foods. In general, dietary patterns described are meat-orientated.

Table 3. Apparent consumption of selected foods (kg per capita per year) (after Lee et al. [184])

| Food | Aboriginal Communities | | Combined | Australia (ABS) |
	Central Desert Communities	Northern Coastal Communities		
Flour (white)	37.6	44.4	41.2	n/a
Bread (all)	34.1	30.5	32.3	45.5[1]
Beef	51.6	25.8	38.7	41.4[2]
Poultry	22.3	19.7	21.0	23.0
Lamb	22.8	3.3	13.1	16.9
Fish	0	4.8	2.4	4.0
Fruits	33.2	17.6	25.4	106.9
Vegetables	24.3	19.6	22.0	136.2
Sugar	54.1	50.3	52.2	8.2
Carbonated beverages	67.9	224.6	146	73.0
Fruit juice	48.3	12.8	30.6	n/a
Tinned meat	9.4	10.1	9.3	n/a
Pie/pastie	9.6	15.1	12.4	n/a
Snack foods[3]	1.8	2.7	2.3	n/a

Australia (ABS): Apparent Consumption of Foodstuffs and Nutrients (ABS, 1987 [340]).
n/a = Not available.
  [1] Includes flour used in bread-making.
  [2] Includes beef and veal.
  [3] Includes potato crisps, extruded snacks.

Contemporary Methods of Storing, Preparing, Cooking and Distributing Food

In remote communities, people tend to shop at the community store for the required foods every day, and sometimes twice a day prior to mealtimes. The foods are prepared immediately for consumption, and there is little wastage or 'leftovers'.

Many homes are without adequate refrigeration or domestic food storage [194]. People living a distance from the community stores, particularly in outstations, tend to purchase easily stored foods, such as flour and sugar. Much of this is stored in flour drums on the roofs of humpies, or in the fork of a tree to keep it from dogs and children [175].

Food is often prepared outside on an open fire. Even if gas or electric stoves are available, they are frequently not in good working order [194]. The availability of metal containers enables the boiling of meat and vegetables;

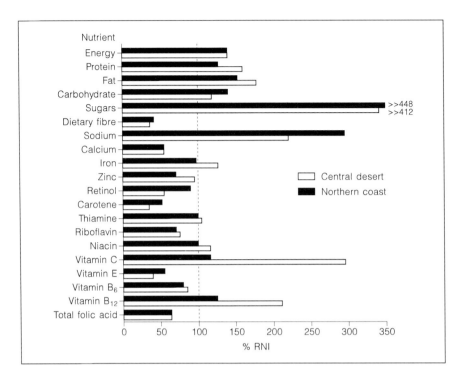

Fig. 2. The apparent per capita daily intake of nutrients in Aboriginal communities as a percentage of community-adjusted recommended nutrient intakes. After Lee et al. [184].

this is a more rapid cooking method than roasting, but one which also depletes the nutritional value of the diet due to leaching of nutrients into the cooking water [112]. Increasingly, meat and flour 'dampers' are fried in oil, dripping or margarine.

Communal feeding during the middle of this century meant that responsibility to share food resources declined and a breakdown in the well-defined traditional food distribution pattern was observed [172]. This tended to affect the more sensitive groups such as toddlers, pregnant and lactating mothers and the elderly [130, 172, 175].

Contemporary Meal Patterns in Remote Areas

Most people eat 2–3 meals per day. Breakfast may include oatmeal or a prepared cereal, such as 'Weetbix', with milk and sugar (up to 50 g), white bread or damper with butter or margarine and sometimes jam, and tea with milk and sugar (up to 40 g). In northern areas, 'flour porridge' of white flour,

---

Table 4. Daily per capita consumption of traditional and purchased foods in small, remote, decentralized, traditionally-orientated outstation communities[1]

Location	Central Australia	Arnhem Land Riverine	Arnhem Land Coastal
Reference	Devitt [90]	Altman [168]	Meehan [102]
Study year	1981–1982	1979–1980	1972–1973
Study period	3 × 1 month	10 × 1 month	3.6 × 1 month
Total number of days	109	n/a	n/a
Total intake per capita per day			
Weight, g	893	n/a	1,100
Energy, kJ	9,279	11,918	9,010
Protein, g	136	133	165
Total traditional foods per capita per day			
Weight, g (%)	342 (38.3)	n/a	803 (73.0)
Energy, kJ (%)	2,962 (31.9)	5,526 (46.2)	4,405 (48.9)
Protein, g (%)	100 (73.5)	107 (79.7)	135 (82.8)
Total purchased foods per capita per day			
Weight, g (%)	551 (61.7)	n/a	297 (27.0)
Energy, kJ (%)	6,317 (68.1)	6,392 (53.8)	4,605 (51.1)
Protein, g (%)	36 (26.5)	26 (20.3)	30 (18.2)
Reference requirements			
Energy, kJ (kCal)	8,965 (2,135)	10,486 (2,505)	8,581 (2,050)
Protein, g	56	65.5	n/a
Intake/requirement			
Energy, %	103	114	105
Protein, %	244	203	n/a
Intake of specific foods, g per capita per day *(% of total energy intake)*			
Sugar, g (%)	n/a (16.4)	313 (44)	n/a
Flour, g (%)	155 (n/a)	n/a (25)	n/a
Bread, g (%)	65 (n/a)	n/a (7)	n/a

[1] Data re-analysed on the basis of mean daily per capita intake over the total number of observation days.

n/a = Not available.

Table 5. Characteristics of hunter-gatherer and western lifestyle (after O'Dea [124])

	Hunter-gatherer lifestyle	Western lifestyle
Physical activity level	high	low
Principal characteristics of diet		
Energy density	low	high
Energy intake	usually adequate	excessive
Nutrient density	high	low
Nutrient composition of diet		
Protein	high	low-moderate
Animal	high	moderate
Vegetable	low-moderate	low
Carbohydrate	moderate (slowly digested)	high (rapidly digested)
Complex carbohydrate	moderate	moderate
Simple carbohydrate	usually low (honey)	high (sucrose)
Dietary fibre	high	low
Fat	low	high
Vegetable	low	low
Animal	low (polyunsaturated)	high (saturated)
Na:K ratio	low	high

sugar and water, and sometimes powdered milk, is a familiar breakfast food if little money is available.

A common meal for lunch and/or dinner is meat stew, with, or more frequently without vegetables, eaten with bread or damper, or sandwiches made from bread or damper. Tinned meat, or readily prepared prepackaged meals are also used for convenience. Take-away foods such as meat pies and rotisserie chicken are popular when available.

Sweetened carbonated beverages are consumed in large quantities, up to 2 litres per person per day in tropical or arid areas during the hottest part of the year. Snack foods, such as potato crisps, and confectionary, are consumed occasionally throughout the day.

Dairy foods, fruit and vegetables tend to be eaten irregularly in small quantities. In centralized communities, traditional foods, particularly animal foods, are very popular, but consumed relatively infrequently [210].

Major Components of Dietary Change

With the rapid change from a traditional to a sedentary lifestyle, there is a tendency for reduced physical activity, altered dietary consumption including increased energy intake, and concomitant weight gain. These changes have been qualitatively described [124] and are summarized in table 5.

The Nutritional Consequences of Traditional Diet and Meal Patterns

Early Assessment of Traditional Nutritional Adequacy

Past opinions about the adequacy of traditional nutrition have been contradictory; some early reports suggest that existence was a permanent struggle for survival [42, 211], while others believe that an 'inherited nutritive instinct' led to the evolution of a balanced diet [45, 117]. Contradictory nutritional assessments have been made frequently by the same author. For example, it was suggested that Aboriginal leanness was due to 'the scarcity of nourishing food and the amount of effort necessary to obtain a satisfing diet' [211] but also that 'through his (Aboriginals) keenly developed native instinct he had evolved a balanced diet' [212].

Sometimes observations reflected European values of the time, rather than nutrient value. For example, it was noted that 'In common with most races living under primitive conditions, the Aboriginal has no suitable dietary supplements to offer the weaning child until it is old enough to do full justice to the food of the tribe' [213]. This inaccurate observation has been repeated frequently [11], but probably reflects the view of non-Aboriginal observers that 'witchetty grubs' (*Cossidae* sp.) and tail meat from goannas (*Varanus* sp.), were not 'appropriate weaning food' [134, 214]. It has been noted that 'some medical writers appear to believe that because the level of nutrition differs from our own, it was inadequate, although they give no substantive reasons for this judgement' [32]. An example is the unqualified statement that Aboriginal Tasmanians appeared to suffer from a 'carbohydrate imbalance' [42].

More recent opinions have interpreted the long-term maintenance of the gene pool without supplement by migration [32], the wide variety and abundance of foods consumed and 'primitive methods of preparation' [45], as support for nutritional adequacy [123]. However it is now generally believed, that while the quality of the diet was usually good, that during poor seasons and drought, particularly in arid regions, environmental stress may have resulted in the deterioration of nutrition and health status [215].

Nutritional Status

All available evidence suggests that Aboriginal people were generally in good health prior to European settlement. Subjective impressions of early observers generally describe healthy people of athletic physique [27, 31, 43, 216–221]. Neither clinical evidence [38, 39, 41, 57, 171, 213, 216, 222–228], palaeopathological studies [229, 230], nor the study of traditional medicines [5, 98, 231–234] suggest widespread nutritional deficiencies. In particular there is no evidence of chronic diseases such as noninsulin-dependent diabetes and cardiovascular disease that are now widespread in contemporary Aboriginal communities (see below).

Body Mass

Early anthropometric studies generally described Aboriginal adults as shorter and lighter than contemporary Europeans. Low birth weights were documented in the central desert regions, but infants grew rapidly to the age of 4 months, when their weight was similar to European infants [235, 236]. However, all studies described a reduced velocity of weight gain after 4–6 months compared with white Australian children. It has been suggested that infants of low weight would advantage nomads, providing lighter burdens for women during the food quest [237].

Some observers have described severe loss of subcutaneous fat and muscle tone in some traditional women beyond early adult life, compared with relative maintenance of weight in older men [24, 171]. These observations have been supported by early anthropometric studies [238, 239] which indicate a greater coefficient of variation in the body mass index (BMI) of women between the age of 30 and 50 years than other Aboriginal age and sex groups [119] or contemporary European women [171]. The constant cycle of pregnancy and lactation ('reproductive strain' [171]), and greater variability in the care and status of older women, including discrimination in the allocation of food supplies as described above, have been suggested as explanations for the observed weight loss in older women [119]. In comparison, men were assured attentive care in older age due to their ritual dominance, and did not appear to suffer from nutritional deprivation.

The extreme leanness of traditional groups is indicated by the low BMIs ranging from 13.2 to 20 kg/m^2 described in comparison to European normal reference values of 20–25 kg/m^2 [41, 119, 238–241]. The apparent lack of obesity was considered so unusual that early writers ascribed differences between both races to hereditary factors, for example Aborigines must 'not physiologically store much fat' [45]. It is now believed that physical size of adults is determined more by a combination of adequate nutrition and freedom from infection in early life than by inheritance, while genetic factors affect relative dimensions and body build [239, 242]. Given this, the mean height increase of 5.5 cm for both men and women at a central Australian settlement over 30 years of acculturation, may be indicative of suboptimal energy intake under traditional conditions in this area during the early 1930s [243, 244].

Although these early anthropometric measurements suggest that some Aboriginal groups, in comparison with other populations, may have experienced lower energy intake relative to energy expenditure, it is not possible to comment on the nutritional consequences of this without reference to biochemical evidence.

*Summary of Biological Measurements of Nutritional Status
of Recent Nomads*

The few biochemical studies of traditional Aboriginal groups generally describe acceptable serum protein levels. The serum protein levels of stressed groups, such as the aged and nursing mothers, did not differ from others. Nomadic people in the central desert area had albumin levels within the European reference range, but γ-globulin levels were much higher [245]. High γ-globulin levels were also described for other desert nomads; but albumin concentrations were lower in this group than for Europeans [41]. Neither evidence of abnormal hepatic protein synthesis nor infection was apparent in other Aboriginal groups with similarly high levels of γ-globulin [246]. The significance of high levels of γ-globulin described for other hunter-gatherer societies [247–249] is also unknown.

Although few blood pressure measures are available for Aboriginal groups who had experienced little or no contact with Caucasian lifestyle, those measured in settlements during the 1960s were generally low compared with European levels and blood pressures are presumed to have been lower in traditional Aboriginal people [84, 250–254]. As with other traditional societies, traditional Aboriginal men in northern Australia did not experience an increase in diastolic blood pressure with age [255, 256]. However, many Aboriginal women showed a marked increase in blood pressure beyond 50 years of age [238]. This could not be explained by the decreased BMI of older women, but may be related to hormonal changes at menopause [119].

Early studies of nomadic Aboriginal groups also indicated that serum cholesterol levels were low [257–259] and atherosclerosis was rare [260].

Generally, nomadic Aboriginal men had high haemoglobin concentrations [261–263]. Haemoglobin levels in Aboriginal women (mean 16.3 g%) were very high relative to European women (13.9 g%) and there was no significant change over the reproductive life of Aboriginal women as experienced by European women. It has been argued that the higher haemoglobin levels in Aboriginal women were due to either higher dietary protein and iron intake, or the scanty and infrequent menstruation reported in traditional times [252, 262].

Ascorbic acid levels were high and, despite dramatic fluctuations in the availability of the vegetable component of the traditional diet, no evidence of scurvy has been recorded for truly traditional Aboriginal groups [171, 125, 264]. Cyanocobalamin levels were also very high relative to Caucasian groups [41, 261, 265]. Serum folate levels of nomadic people tended to be higher than in Aborigines living at early settlements and missions [266, 267].

Metabolic Consequences of Dietary Change

As early as 5 years after contact it was noted that Aboriginal groups in remote northern areas experienced a decline in health status as their diet changed and they became detribalized [26]. Early changes associated with increasing acculturation included increasing sodium/potassium ratio in sweat and urine, increasing blood pressure and greater weight for height [84].

The overall standard of health of contemporary Aboriginal Australians is very poor. For almost all disease categories, particularly for nutrition-related conditions, rates for Aborigines are worse than for non-Aboriginal Australians. Death rates are up to 4 times higher, and life expectancy is up to 21 years lower [180].

Infant Malnutrition

The infant mortality rate, which had been approximately 100 per thousand in the early 1960s, declined during the 1970s and is now relatively stable. However, it still remains up to 2.8 times the non-Aboriginal rate [180]. Birth weights of Aboriginal babies are 150–350 g lighter than non-Aboriginal babies, with up to 17% of Aboriginal infants having a low birth weight ($<2,500$ g) [268, 285]. Growth retardation amongst Aboriginal infants after the age of 4–6 months has consistently been noted, and Aboriginal children remain generally underweight when compared with European children of the same age [268, 269]. Theories that genetic differences account for the differing growth pattern between Aboriginal and European children are not supported by studies which indicate similar growth in similar environments [270, 271] or the greater stature reported for nomadic children compared to those Aboriginal children living on reserves and settlements [239]. Poor growth rates have been shown to be associated with malnutrition and repeated acute and chronic infections [272–277].

The synergism of malnutrition and infection is well recognized [278]. Folic acid, pyridoxine, vitamin C, vitamin A, zinc, copper, selenium, and vitamin E have been implicated in impaired cell-mediated immunity (CMI) and T-cell-dependent antibody responses, and iron deficiency has been implicated in impaired lymphocyte stimulation responses to mitogens and decreased neutrophil bactericidal capacity [278]. Lowered immune response, in conjunction with inadequate nutrient intake and environmental sanitation, results in recurrent infection and infestation, which negatively affects nutritional intake and status, creating a vicious cycle of malnutrition and infection [278].

Low birth weight can result in impaired immune response; several studies have demonstrated impairment of CMI, immunoglobulin and antibody response, and neutrophil function in neonates who are small for gestational age

[279]. The depressed CMI of these neonates has been shown to persist for up to 5 years [280]. Most Aboriginal infants experience their first episode of infection, particularly chronic respiratory infection and/or suppurative otitis media, during the first 6 months of life when breast milk would appear to contribute to adequate nutritional intake [281]. Although early cessation of breast-feeding has been described amongst urban Aboriginal women [282, 283], prolonged breast-feeding of infants to the age of aproximately 2 years has been more frequently noted in remote communities [135]. Evidence that lactoferrin concentration of breast milk is suppressed in undernourished Aboriginal mothers supports the need to ensure adequate maternal nutrition [284]. Birth weights have been shown to increase proportionally with energy intake during pregnancy, with maternal height and with maternal head circumference, indicating that early growth failure of Aboriginal female children and poor nutritional status of women of child-bearing age, may affect the birth weight of their future children [285, 286].

Clinical evidence of multiple vitamin deficiencies in 600 growth-retarded children were diagnosed in one Queensland community in the late 1960s [272]. Since then, various studies have suggested specific nutrients may be major contributing factors to poor health in Aboriginal children: zinc [287]; ascorbic acid [272, 288, 289]; vitamin D and iron [272], and more recently, following from international literature, vitamin A. It seems most unlikely, in the face of the complex factors contributing to poor dietary intake, infection and malnutrition, that administration of any single nutritional element or 'magic bullet' will have a positive and lasting effect on Aboriginal child health [269, 290, 291].

'Lifestyle' Diseases

The current leading cause of death for both Aboriginal males and females is diseases of the circulatory system, which occur up to 10 times more than in the rest of the population [180]. Previously, diseases of the respiratory system, specifically pneumonia and influenza, were the leading cause of death in Aborigines [292]. In general the recent reduction in communicable diseases has been offset by an increase in noncommunicable, or 'lifestyle' diseases, such as noninsulin-dependent diabetes (NIDDM), hypertension and cardiovascular diseases. These diseases tend to be consequent on rapid acculturation and associated decreased energy expenditure and overconsumption of energy-dense, nutrient-depleted foods.

In the absence of reliable comprehensive national data about individual diseases, community-based studies have been used to identify the prevalence of noncommunicable diseases. Methodological approaches to enable reliable comparison of results have not generally been considered. Sample sizes tend to be small and problems exist with the application of dissimilar sampling frames; differing, and frequently poor, response rates; standardization of measurements, and the application of different protocols and definitions.

Obesity and Body Fat Distribution

'Lifestyle' diseases amongst Aborigines tend to be associated with obesity, particularly with android (central) distribution of body fat. Both male and female Aboriginal adults tend to experience an increase in weight with increasing acculturation [244]. Although low BMI is common amongst young women [286], in older women a rapid onset of obesity, with a central distribution of subcutaneous fat, has been described. Body composition studies have also shown that for a given BMI, Aboriginal women have more body fat than Caucasian women [240, 293].

With increasing BMI, both male and female Aborigines tend to exhibit an android body profile (central distribution of fat), compared with the gynoid (peripheral) distribution of body fat most commonly seen in obese Caucasian women [240, 293]. Android distribution of body fat is associated with hypertriglyceridaemia, higher fasting glucose levels, hyperinsulinaemia, impaired glucose tolerance and hypertension in Caucasians, which increase an individual's susceptibility to 'lifestyle' diseases and the metabolic complications of obesity [294, 295]. The more android body fat distribution seen in Aboriginal women may help explain the similarly high prevalence of ischaemic heart disease and diabetes observed in Aboriginal men and women, in contrast to the male preponderance of these conditions in Caucasians [186, 205, 240, 296–298].

Cardiovascular Disease

Research into Aboriginal cardiovascular disease has concentrated on ischaemic heart disease, often describing prevalence of accepted risk factors and associated conditions, particularly NIDDM [186, 205, 209, 241, 297–302]. Of such studies, those measuring prevalence of cardiovascular risk factors in Aborigines compared to non-Aborigines, have most commonly shown less hypercholesterolaemia but more hypertriglyceridaemia in all age groups in both sexes, more obesity and hypertension particularly in younger men and women, and more cigarette smoking in all age groups. Studies in Aboriginal groups alone have most commonly shown lower serum cholesterol and triglyceride levels in women than men, lower serum triglycerides in both younger men and women, lower blood pressure in young women than young men, more smoking among younger people, and more obesity in older women than men. Serum triglyceride levels are increasingly elevated across nondiabetic, impaired glucose tolerance and diabetic groups. The early observation that cholesterol levels tend to rise with increasing 'westernization' of Aborigines, has been supported by the more recent studies.

Noninsulin-Dependent Diabetes Mellitus

The first case of NIDDM was described in an Aboriginal in 1923 [40]. Many studies have indicated high prevalence (8–19%) of diabetes amongst adults in Aboriginal communities [186, 205, 298, 302, 304–308], compared with a non-Aboriginal rate of 3.4% [309]. Prevalence of impaired glucose tolerance is also much higher in Aboriginal than non-Aboriginal Australians. A study identifying hyperinsulinaemia and impaired glucose tolerance in Aboriginal children between the age of 7 and 18 years, may indicate that the onset of this disease may be much earlier than previously recognized [310].

Both genetic predisposition and lifestyle 'triggers' have been implicated in the high prevalence of NIDDM and associated conditions. NIDDM prevalence tends to increase with the degree of westernization and related factors such as BMI [205, 240, 302], and decrease with increasing non-Aboriginal genetic admixture [311]. Prevalence is consistently higher in older adults. Even amongst lean, young Aboriginal people, mild impairment of glucose tolerance, hyperinsulinaemia and elevated total and very-low-density lipoprotein (VLDL), a group of metabolic characteristics consistent with underlying resistance to the glucose-lowering effects of insulin, have been observed [205, 301].

These observations are consistent with Neel's 'thrifty gene' hypotheses [312, 313]. Characteristics of a 'thrifty gene' may have been advantageous to lean hunter-gatherers whose lifestyle incorporated regular physical activity, a low fat diet, and a variable food supply on a day-to-day and seasonal basis, but led to increased susceptibility to NIDDM with an urbanized lifestyle and continuously available diet of high energy density [314, 315].

Resistance to the glucose-lowering effects of insulin, with normal or near normal sensitivity of mechanisms involved in fat deposition, has been postulated as a possible metabolic basis for the 'thrifty gene' [301]. It has been suggested that, in the traditional lifestyle with a high level of physical activity and variation in food availability and accessibility on both a seasonal and daily basis, both efficient hepatic gluconeogenesis not sensitive to suppression by insulin, and active hepatic lipogenesis, may have favoured survival by maximizing the response to insulin-sensitive processes involved in carbohydrate and lipid metabolism. In this way, conversion of large intakes of dietary protein during 'feasts' was promoted, and the efficient conversion of excess kilojoules to triglyceride as a long-term energy store in adipose tissue to cover periods of relative 'famine' was ensured [240, 301]. As the insulin secretory response to protein-rich meals is much less than to carbohydrate in Aboriginal people [315], the relatively low carbohydrate intake of the meat-orientated traditional

Aboriginal diet, combined with the slow digestion of complex carbohydrate in many plants used traditionally as foods [151], would have minimized post-prandial insulin response.

The contemporary lifestyle experienced by many 'westernized' Aboriginal people, which incorporates low physical activity and an energy-dense diet rich in rapidly absorbed carbohydrate and fat, is thought to produce hyperglycaemia and stimulate a high postprandial insulin response [316]. This produces increased glucose turnover in insulin-sensitive tissues and exacerbates selective insulin resistance, favouring those nonglucose regulatory metabolic pathways where insulin is functioning normally or near normally, that is, hepatic triglyceride and VLDL synthesis and accumulation of fat in adipose tissue [301, 315, 317]. The consumption of long chain saturated fatty acids present in the western diet have been shown to directly stimulate hepatic gluconeogenesis [318] and raise the circulating levels of free fatty acids which reduce glucose utilization in peripheral tissues and produce insulin resistance. While physical inactivity and high intakes of refined carbohydrate and saturated fat are maintained, insulin resistance, hyperinsulinaemia and glucose intolerance become more pronounced leading to obesity, NIDDM and hypertriglyceridaemia [301, 315].

Blood Pressure

A relatively high community prevalence of hypertension has been described in many contemporary Aboriginal communities, frequently in association with other 'lifestyle' diseases [186, 205, 299, 300, 304]. Obesity tends to be associated with hypertension, and may be of causal significance.

Anaemia and Haemoglobin Status

Compared with early data for nomadic Aborigines, there has been an increase in both incidence and prevalence of anaemia [267, 319]. Hookworm infestation may be implicated predominantly [320], although some studies have not shown significant differences in haemoglobin levels between those infected with various hookworm loads [264]. Dietary iron deficiency is doubtful in the face of the very high intakes of meat observed in remote areas, but may be more likely amongst children, particularly in urban areas. The impact of widespread dietary folate deficiency on anaemia requires further study in Aboriginal communities.

Dental Disease

Dental decay has increased in Aboriginal people since contact [208, 321–323]. Children and adolescents are particularly affected [45, 323]. There is general agreement that adoption of European diet, particularly more frequent and greater exposure to sugar and other high carbohydrate foods, is a major contributing factor to this increase. However, the varying fluoride level of artesian water in remote areas may complicate the relationship between dietary change and dental health [322, 323].

Vitamin and Mineral Status

Vitamin status has been measured infrequently in Aboriginal subjects and there is a general paucity of longitudinal data available. Studies have been conducted in a variety of Aboriginal groups and environments; people of Aboriginal descent in rural townships [290, 324], subgroups of full-descent populations, particularly children [272, 325], and groups living in remote areas [153, 191, 209, 266, 267, 303]. Samples have generally been small; in some studies subjects have often been selected from 'stress' groups of the community (that is, infants and pregnant and lactating mothers), perhaps in an attempt to describe the worst possible scenario [272, 290, 325]. Various methods of assays and functional tests have been applied in different studies, particularly as 'the state of the art' of analysis has changed over time. Different 'normal' ranges have also been applied. Therefore, quantitative comparison of published results and prevalence rates of deficiency states may be misleading.

Multiple biochemical vitamin deficiencies have frequently been described in the same subject and suggest the generally poor nutritional status of such individuals, rather than a specific micronutrient problem.

Relative to normal Caucasian levels, very low serum folates (1.7 ± 0.2 to 2.5 ± 0.2 µg/l) have generally been reported in acculturated groups of Aborigines, and have been observed in the majority of subjects [209, 266, 267, 290, 303, 324–326]. Very low red blood cell folates of 81.6 ± 3.0 µg/l have also been described amongst adults in a remote centralized community [209]. Low folate status is believed to be implicated in the high prevalence of neural tube defects described in Aboriginal infants [327].

Low plasma ascorbic acid levels have been reported in high-risk Aboriginal groups [264, 272, 290, 324] and very low levels of 4.1 ± 0.3 mg/l have been described in a remote community [209]. Ascorbic acid and folate results are statistically correlated, consistent with the very low contemporary dietary intakes of fruit and vegetables [209, 290].

In contrast, very high levels of serum cobalamin relative to the Caucasian reference range have been described for both traditional and acculturated Aboriginal groups [41, 261, 265, 267, 303, 320]. In the past, the high levels of the vitamin were attributed to increased levels of vitamin B_{12} binding protein which may be secondary to both acute and chronic infections [261]. Liver damage associated with alcoholism has also been associated with high vitamin

B_{12} levels [328]. However, in one small study, vitamin B_{12} concentrations were unrelated to previous alcohol intake [153], and liver damage would not explain the consistently high levels in traditionally-orientated groups with no access to alcohol. In one longitudinal community-based study, nutrient intake of vitamin B_{12} was positively correlated with observed fluctuations in individual changes in serum cobalamin concentration, suggesting that there is a dietary component to this common observation, and that the high serum cobalamin levels may reflect very high meat intakes [209].

Poor thiamine status has been described for most age and sex groups in a 'part Aboriginal' community, but was particularly marked for women of child-bearing age [290, 324]. Fortification of flour resulted in improvements in the thiamine status of this community [329]. Surprisingly large ranges of both red blood cell and serum thiamine concentrations, including some very high values, have been described in remote Aboriginal communities [209, 303]. These may be related to seasonally high intake of traditional foods rich in thiamine, such as the green turtle (*C. mydas*) [329]. Relative to the 'normal' European reference range, low levels of vitamin B_6 have been described in high-risk groups at four Aboriginal communities [209, 267, 324], but acceptable levels have been described more frequently [209]. Relatively low riboflavin status has been noted in one Aboriginal study [324].

Plasma retinol levels are generally acceptable in Aboriginal adults and children [153, 209, 324, 325]. However, very low plasma β-carotene levels (≤ 8 mg/100 ml) have been described frequently [209, 290, 324, 325] and are presumed to reflect low dietary intake of fruit and vegetables in Aboriginal communities.

Relative to 'normal' Caucasian concentrations, low levels of plasma vitamin E have been described in some Aboriginal groups [153, 209, 290, 324]. However, these results may not have been important as the Aboriginal diets tended to be low in polyunsaturated fatty acids; a ratio of serum α-tocopherol to total lipid ratio < 0.8 mg/g is considered acceptable for adults [330] and has been consistently described in Aboriginal subjects.

Several studies in Aboriginal communities have measured low zinc levels in hair [331–333] and studies focussing on the Kimberley area had suggested that zinc deficiency may contribute to growth retardation and undernutrition in Aboriginal children [287, 320, 331, 334]. However, a placebo-controlled double-blind trial of zinc supplements in the same region showed an increase in the concentration of plasma zinc in 200 children over 10 months, but no response in growth [335]. The relationship between the concentration of zinc in hair and zinc status remains controversial; similarly, plasma zinc concentration, which has also been found to be low in Aboriginal children [325], may not accurately reflect zinc status [336–338].

Metabolic Measurements of a Traditionally-Orientated Outstation Group

In an attempt to provide data for a community living as closely as possible to traditional lifestyle, metabolic parameters have been described for a small outstation community in north east Arnhem Land [241]. Fasting glucose and cholesterol levels were low relative to urbanized Aborigines and Caucasians. However, a high frequency of abnormal glucose tolerance, and associated hypertriglyceridaemia and hyperinsulinaemia, was described despite the leanness of the population (mean BMI 17 kg/m^2). Results were consistent with the concept of underlying insulin resistance. In contrast to the more acculturated groups described above, there was no evidence of suboptimal vitamin or mineral status, including folate, in this group [241]. Although this group uses western technology and derives a large proportion of nutrient intake from purchased carbohydrate, intake of both traditional plant and animal foods, and energy expenditure, was unusually high.

Dietary Intervention Based on Traditional Diet

Reversion to Traditional Diet and Lifestyle

An important study indicated that the main metabolic abnormalities of diabetes mellitus can be greatly improved, and also potentially prevented, by reversion to a traditional hunter-gatherer lifestyle even for an experimental period as short as 7 weeks [339]. During this study a small group of 14 Aboriginal diabetics travelled to ancestral coastal and inland territories where they existed entirely on traditional foods. Metabolic changes included decrease in fasting glucose, improved postprandial glucose clearance, improved insulin response, and reduction of fasting plasma triglyceride level. Additional improvements included a significant decrease in blood pressure, and increases in serum folate, vitamin B$_{12}$ and vitamin E [153]. O'Dea [339] has emphasized the implications of these findings to public health, and stressed the importance of physical activity, low energy dense diet and weight control in the management and prevention of diabetes in Aboriginal people.

Community-Based Intervention

A recent study has indicated that other improvements in risk factors for non-communicable disease can be brought about by Aboriginal people in a community setting when the hunter-gatherer lifestyle is adapted to a settled existence [209]. Dietary intervention strategies focussed on the consumption of purchased foods which were most like traditional foods, that is, low in energy density and high in nutrient density. Following 12 months' intervention, significant dietary changes included decreased intake of sugar and saturated

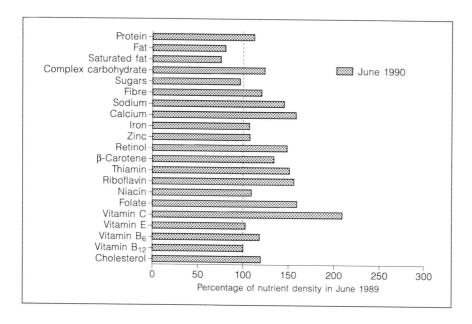

Fig. 3. Change in nutrient density over a 12-month dietary intervention in a remote, centralized Aboriginal community. After Lee et al. [209].

fat and increases in micronutrient density (fig. 3). These dietary improvements accompanied corresponding improvements in biochemical indices in the 68 adults in the community, including decrease in mean serum cholesterol (from 5.9 ± 0.2 to 5.2 ± 0.2 mmol/l), marked increases in red cell folate (from 82 ± 3 to 191 ± 9 µg/l), increases in serum folate, vitamin B_6 and plasma ascorbic acid, a decrease in mean systolic and diastolic blood pressure, normalization of BMI, and a normalization of haematologic indices [209].

Conclusion

It is clear that transition from traditional diet and meal patterns to 'westernized' food habits has heralded major nutritional problems for Aboriginal Australians. Much of this change is due to complex political, economic and social factors. Contemporary Aborigines are not generally in a position to, and may not wish to resume traditional hunter-gatherer lifestyle. However, Aboriginal people are demonstrating that the beneficial qualities of hunter-gatherer diet and meal patterns can be incorporated with increased physical activity into contemporary 'western' lifestyle. The resultant improvements in nutritional status and in some risk factors for noncommunicable disorders have important implications for public heatlh.

References

1   Mulvaney DJ: The Prehistory of Australia. Harmondsworth, Penguin, 1975, p 58.
2   Blainey G: Triumph of the Nomads: A History of Ancient Australia. South Melbourne, Macmillan, 1985, pp 15–24.
3   Flannery TFF: The Future Eaters: An Ecological History of the Australasian Lands and People. Chatswood, Reed Books, 1994.
4   Webb LJ: Eat, die, and learn: The botany of the Australian Aborigines. Aust Nat Hist 1973;17: 290–295.
5   Golson J: Australian Aboriginal food plants: Some ecological and cultural-historical implications; in Mulvaney DJ, Golson J (eds): Aboriginal Man and Environment in Australia. Canberra, Australian National University Press, 1971, pp 196–238.
6   Birdsell JB: Some environmental and cultural factors influencing the structuring of Australian Aboriginal populations. Am Nat 1953;87:171–207.
7   Lawrence R: Aboriginal habitat and economy: A historical perspective; in Mulvaney DJ, Golson J (eds): Aboriginal Man and Environment in Australia. Canberra, Australian National University Press, 1971, pp 249–261.
8   Maddock K: The Australian Aborigines: A Portrait of Their Society. London, Penguin, 1972.
9   Peterson N: The natural and cultural areas of Aboriginal Australia; in Peterson N (ed): Tribes and Boundaries in Australia. Canberra, Australian Institute of Aboriginal Studies, 1976, pp 50–71.
10 Jones R: Hunters in the Australian coastal savanna; in Harris D (ed): Human Ecology in Savanna Environments. New York, Academic Press, 1980, pp 107–147.
11 Tindale NB: Aboriginal Tribes of Australia. Canberra, Australian National University Press, 1974.
12 Rose FGG: The Traditional, Mode of Production of the Australian Aborigines. London, Angus & Robertson, 1987, p 53.
13 Smyth RB: The Aborigines of Victoria. Melbourne, Government Printer, 1878, vol 1+2.
14 Curr EM: The Australian Race. London, Trubner, 1886, vol 1+2.
15 Curr EM: The Australian Race. London, Trubner, 1886, vol 3+4.
16 Sturt C: Narrative of an Expedition into Central Australia during the Year 1844. New York, Greenwood Press, 1969, vol 1+2.
17 Eyre EJ: Journals of Expeditions of Discovery into Central Australia and Overland from Adelaide to King George's Sound, in the Years 1840–1841. London, T&W Boone, 1845.
18 Grey G: Journal of Two Expeditions of Discovery in North West and Western Australia. London, T&W Boone, 1841.
19 Leichhardt L: Journal of an Overland Expedition in Australia from Morton Bay to Port Essington 1844–1845. London, T&W Boone, 1847.
20 Lindsay D: Mr D. Lindsay's Explorations through Arnhem's Land. South Australian Parliamentary Papers No 239, 1884.
21 Lindsay D: Explorations in the Northern Territory of South Australia. Papers of the Proceedings of the Royal Society of Tasmania (South Australia Branch) 1890;2:1–16.
22 Giles E: Australia Twice Traversed. London, Sampson Low, Marston, Searle & Rivington Ltd, 1889.
23 Carnegie DW: Spinifex and Sand. London, C. Arthur Pearson, 1898.
24 Chaseling WS: Yulengor: Nomads of Arnhem Land. London, Epworth Press, 1957.
25 Long JPM: Arid region Aborigines: The Pintubi; in Mulvaney DJ, Golson J (eds): Aboriginal Man and Environment in Australia. Canberra, Australian National University Press, 1971, pp 262–270.
26 Kyle-Little S: Whispering Wind: Adventures in Arnhem Land. London, Hutchinson, 1957.

27   Spencer B, Gillen FJ: The Native Tribes of Central Australia. London, Macmillan, 1899.

28   Spencer B, Gillen FJ: The Northern Tribes of Central Australia. London, Macmillan, 1904.

29   Spencer WB: Native Tribes of the Northern Territory of Australia. London, Macmillan, 1914.

30   Spencer B: Wanderings in Wild Australia. London, Macmillan, 1928.

31   Tindale N: Natives of Groote Eylandt and of the West Coast of the Gulf of Carpentaria. Rec. South Aust Mus 1925;3:61–134.

32   Thompson DF: The seasonal factor in human culture: Illustrated from the life of a contemporary nomadic Group. Proc Prehist Soc 1939;5:209–221.

33   Thompson DF: Arnhem Land: Explorations amongst an unknown people. Part 1. Geogr J 1948; 112:146–164.

34   Thompson DF: Arnhem Land: Explorations amongst an unknown people. Part 2. Geogr J 1949; 113:1–8.

35   Thompson DF: Arnhem Land: Explorations amongst an unknown people. Part 3. Geogr J 1949; 114:53–67.

36   Thompson DF: The Bindibu expedition: Exploration among the desert Aborigines of Western Australia. Geogr J 1962;128:1–14, 143–157, 262–278.

37   Peterson N: The traditional pattern of subsistence to 1975; in Hetzel BS, Frith HJ (eds): Symposium on the Nutrition of Aborigines in Relation to the Ecosystem of Central Australia. Melbourne, CSIRO, 1978, pp 25–35.

38   Breinl A: Report on health and disease in the Northern Territory. Bull NT Aust 1912;1:32–55.

39   Holmes MJ: Health report for the year 1912. Bull NT Aust 1913;6.

40   Basedow H: Diseases of the Australian Aborigines. J Trop Med Hyg 1932;35:177–185.

41   Elphinstone JJ: The health of Australian Aborigines with no previous association with Europeans. Med J Aust 1971;ii:293–301.

42   Noetling F: The food of the Tasmanian Aborigines. Papers and Proceedings of the Royal Society of Tasmania, 1910, pp 279–305.

43   Basedow H: The Australian Aboriginal. Adelaide, Preece, 1925, pp 120–154.

44   Daley C: Food of the Australian Aborigines. Vic Nat 1932;48:23–31.

45   Campbell AH: Food, food values and food habits of the Australian Aborigines in relation to their dental conditions. Aust J Dent 1939;43:1–15, 45–55, 73–87, 141–156, 177–198.

46   Cleland JB, Johnston TH: Notes on native names and use of plants in the Musgrave Ranges. Oceania 1937;8:208–215.

47   Cleland JB, Johnston TH: Notes on native names and use of plants in the Musgrave Ranges. Oceania 1938;8:329–342.

48   Cleland JB: Our natives and the vegetation of Southern Australia. Mankind 1957;5:149–162.

49   Hyam GN: The vegetable foods of the Australian Aborigines. Vic Nat 1939;56:95–98, 115–119.

50   Hyam GN: The animal food of the Australian Aborigines. Vic Nat 1940;57:136–140.

51   Roth WE: Food, Its Search, Capture and Preparation. North Queensland Ethnography Bulletins, vol 3. Brisbane, Government Printer, 1901.

52   Malinowski B: The Family among the Australian Aborigines. London, University of London Press, 1913.

53   Rose FGG: The Traditional Mode of Production of the Australian Aborigines. London, Angus Robertson, 1987, p 4.

54   McArthur M: Food consumption and dietary levels of the Aborigines living on naturally occurring foods; in Mountford CP (ed): Records of the American-Australian Scientific Expedition to Arnhem Land, vol 2: Anthropology and Nutrition. Melbourne, Melbourne University Press, 1960, pp 90–136.

55   McCarthy FD, McArthur M: The food quest and the time factor in Aboriginal economic life; in Mountford CP (ed): Records of the American-Australian Scientific Expedition to Arnhem Land, vol 2: Anthropology and Nutrition. Melbourne, Melbourne University Press, 1960, pp 145–194.

56   Kirk RL: Aboriginal Man Adapting. Melbourne, Oxford University Press, 1983, pp 69–75.

57   Woodburn J: Hunters and gatherers today and reconstruction of the past; in Geller E (ed): Soviet and Western Anthropology. London, Duckworth, 1980, p 74.

58   Sahlins MD: Notes on the original affluent society; in Lee RB, Devore R (eds): Man the Hunter. Chicago, Aldine, 1968, pp 85–89.

59 Calaby JH: Man, fauna and climate in Aboriginal Australia; in Mulvaney DJ, Golson J (eds): Aboriginal Man and Environment in Australia. Canberra, Australian National University Press, 1971, pp 80–93.

60 Yengoyan AA: Structure, event and ecology in Aboriginal Australia; in Peterson N (ed): Tribes and Boundaries in Australia. Canberra, Australian Institute of Aboriginal Studies, 1976, pp 121–132.

61 Flood J: Archaeology of the Dreamtime. Sydney, Angus & Robertson, 1992.

62 Penny DH, Moriarty J: The Aboriginal economy – then and now; in Hetzel BS, Frith HJ (eds): Symposium on the Nutrition of Aborigines in Relation to the Ecosystem of Central Australia. Melbourne, CSIRO, 1978, pp 19–24.

63 Spencer B, Gillen FJ: The Native Tribes of Central Australia (facsimile edition). Adelaide, Anthropological Publications, 1969.

64 Mulvaney DJ: The Prehistory of Australia. Harmondsworth, Penguin, 1975, p 375.

65 Mulvaney DJ: The chain of connection: The material evidence; in Peterson N (ed): Tribes and Boundaries in Australia. Canberra, Australian Institute of Aboriginal Studies, 1976, pp 72–94.

66 Johnston TH, Cleland JB: The history of the Aboriginal narcotic, pituri. Oceania 1935;4:201–223.

67 Thompson DF: Economic Structure and the Ceremonial Exchange Cycle in Arnhem Land. Melbourne, Macmillan, 1949.

68 Jones R: Fire-stick farming. Aust Nat Hist 1969;16:224–228.

69 Latz PK, Griffin GF: Changes in Aboriginal land management in relation to fire and to food plants in central Australia; in Hetzel BS, Frith HJ (eds): Symposium on the Nutrition of Aborigines in Relation to the Ecosystem of Central Australia. Melbourne, CSIRO, 1978, pp 77–86.

70 Allen H: The Bagundji of the Darling Basin: Cereal gatherers in an uncertain environment. World Archaeol 1974;5:309–322.

71 Roth WE: Ethological Studies among the North-West-Central Queensland Aborigines. Brisbane, Government Printer, 1897.

72 Basedow, H: The Australian Aboriginal. Adelaide, Preece, 1925, p 129.

73 McCarthy FD: Habitat, economy and equipment of the Australian Aborigines. Aust J Sci 1957; 19:88–97.

74 Blainey G: Triumph of the Nomads: A History of Ancient Australia, rev. ed. South Melbourne, Macmillan, 1982, pp 194–197.

75 Mulvaney DJ: The Prehistory of Australia. Harmondsworth, Penguin, 1975, p 241.

76 Harvey A: Food preservation in Australian tribes. Mankind 1945;3:191–192.

77 Ashwin A: From South Australia to Port Darwin with sheep and horses in 1870–1871. Proceedings of the Royal Geological Society Australia, South Australia, 1932, p 32.

78 Tindale NB: Adaptive significance of the panara or grass seed culture of Australia; in Wright RVS (ed): Stone Tools as Cultural Markers. Canberra, Australian Institute of Aboriginal Studies, 1977.

79 O'Connell JF, Latz PK, Barnett P: Traditional and modern plant use among the Alyawara of Central Australia. Econ Bot 1983;37:80–109.

80 Finlayson HH: The red centre, Man and beast in the heart of Australia. Sydney, Angus & Robertson, 1935.

81 Gould RA: Yiwara: Forages of the Australian desert. New York, Scribner, 1973.

82 Thompson DF: Bindibu Country. Melbourne, Nelson, 1975.

83 Peterson N: Aboriginal use of Australian Solanaceae; in Hawkes J (ed): The Biology and Taxonomy of the Solanaceae. London, Academic Press, 1977.

84 Macfarlane WV: Aboriginal desert hunter-gatherers in transition; in Hetzel BS, Frith HJ (eds): Symposium on the Nutrition of Aborigines in Relation to the Ecosystem of Central Australia. Melbourne, CSIRO, 1978, pp 49–63.

85 Berndt CH: Digging sticks and spears, or, the two-sex model; in Gale F (ed): Woman's Role in Aboriginal Society. Canberra, Australian Institute of Aboriginal Studies, 1978.

86 Hamilton A: Dual social systems: Technology, labour and women's secret rites in the eastern Western Desert of Australia. Oceania 1980;1:4–19.

87 Bell D: Daughters of the Dreaming. Sydney, McPhee Gribble, Allen & Unwin, 1983.

88   Meehan B: Who feeds the multitudes? The contribution women make to the diet of Aborigines in Tropical Australia; in Women in Food Chains. Melbourne, Food Justice Centre of Friends of the Earth, 1980.

89   Altman JC: Hunter-gatherer subsistence production in Arnhem Land: The original affluence hypothesis re-examined. Mankind 1984;14:179–190.

90   Devitt J: Contemporary Aboriginal women and subsistence in remote, arid Australia, PhD thesis, Department of Anthropology and Sociology, University of Queensland, 1988.

91   Irvine FR: Wild and emergency foods of Australian and Tasmanian Aborigines. Oceania 1957;28: 113–142.

92   Silberbauer GB: Ecology of the Ernabella Aboriginal community. Anthropol Forum 1971;3:21–36.

93   Meggitt MJ: Notes on the vegetable foods of the Walbiri of Central Australia. Oceania 1956;28: 143–145.

94   Specht RL: An introduction to the ethnobotany of Arnhem Land; in Specht RL, Mountford CP (eds): Records of the American-Australian Scientific Expedition to Arnhem Land, vol 3: Botany and Plant Ecology. Melbourne, Melbourne University Press, 1958.

95   Worsley PM: The utilisation of natural food resources by an Australian Aboriginal tribe. Acta Ethnogr 1961;10:1–2, 158–189.

96   Gould RA: Subsistence behaviour among the Western Desert Aborigines of Australia. Oceania 1969;39:253–274.

97   Lawrence R: Aboriginal habitat and economy. Department of Geography, Canberra, Occasional Paper No 6, Australian National University, 1965.

98   Levitt D: Plants and People: Aboriginal Uses of Plants on Groote Eylandt. Canberra, Australian Institute of Aboriginal Studies, 1981.

99   Cribb AB, Cribb JW: Wild Food in Australia. Sydney, Collins, 1976.

100 Sweeney G: Food supplies of a desert tribe. Oceania 1947;17:289–299.

101 Peterson N: Camp site location among Australian hunter-gatherers: Archaeological and ethnographic evidence for a key determinant. Archaeol Phys. Anthropol Oceania 1973;8:173–193.

102 Meehan B: Shell Bed to Shell Midden. Canberra, Australian Institute of Aboriginal Studies, 1982, pp 144–151.

103 Rose FGG: The Traditional Mode of Production of the Australian Aborigines. London, Angus & Robertson, 1987, p 56.

104 Gould RA: Living Archaeology. Cambridge, Cambridge University Press, 1980.

105 Jones R, Bowler J: Struggle for the savanna: Northern Australia in ecological and prehistoric perspective; in Jones R (ed): Northern Australia: Options and Implications. Canberra, Research School of Pacific Studies, Australian National University, 1980, pp 3–33.

106 Tindale N: The Pitjandjara; in Bicchieri MG (ed): Hunters and Gatherers Today. New York, Holt, Rinehart & Winston, 1972.

107 Lockwood D: The Lizard Eaters. Melbourne, Cassell, 1964.

108 Tindale N: On some Australian Cossidae including the moth of the witjuti (witchetty) grub. Trans. R Soc South Aust 1953;76:56–65.

109 Chewings C: Back in the Stone Age. Sydney, Angus & Robertson, 1936, p 4.

110 Lamilami L: Lamilami Speaks. Sydney, Ure Smith, 1974.

111 White IM: Pitfalls to avoid: The Australian experience; in Elliot K, Whelan J (eds): Health and Disease in Tribal Societies. Amsterdam, Elsevier, 1977, pp 269–292.

112 Middleton M, Francis S: Yuendemu and Its Children – Life and Health on an Aboriginal Settlement. Canberra, DAA, 1977.

113 Waddy J: Classification of food from a Groote Eylandt Aboriginal point of view; in Manderson L (ed): Shared Wealth and Symbol: Food Culture and Society in South-East Asia and the South Pacific. Cambridge, Cambridge University Press, 1986.

114 Cleland JB, Johnston TH: The ecology of the Aborigines of central Australia: Botanical notes. Trans R Soc South Aust 1933;57:113–124.

115 Marbutt JA: The Australian arid zone as a prehistoric environment; in Mulvaney DJ, Golson J (eds): Aboriginal Man and Environment in Australia. Canberra, Australian National University Press, 1971, pp 66–79.

116 Berndt RM, Berndt CH: Man, Land and Myth in North Australia – The Gunwinggu People. Sydney, Ure Smith, 1970.

117 McArthur M: Introduction to the report of the nutrition unit; in Mountford CP (ed): Records of the American-Australian Scientific Expedition to Arnhem Land, vol 2: Anthropology and Nutrition. Melbourne, Melbourne University Press, 1960, pp 1–13.

118 Rae CJ, Lamprell VJ, Lion RJ, et al: The role of bush foods in contemporary Aboriginal diets. Proc Nutr Soc Aust 1982;7:45–49.

119 White NG: Sex differences in Australian Aboriginal subsistence: Possible implications for the biology of hunter-gatherers; in Newcombe F, Ghesquierre J, Martin R (eds): Human Sexual Dimorphism. London, Taylor & Francis, 1985, pp 323–361.

120 Specht RL: The climate, geology, soils and plant ecology of the northern portion of Arnhem Land; in Specht RL, Mountford CP (eds): Records of the American-Australian Scientific Expedition to Arnhem Land, vol 3: Botany and Plant Ecology. Melbourne, Melbourne University Press, 1958, pp 333–414.

121 Scarlett NH: Riitja and Gathul: The role of monsoon and mangrove forests in Yualngu traditional economy. Canberra, Australian Institute of Aboriginal Studies, 1976.

122 Basedow H: Notes on the natives of Bathurst Island, North Australia. J R Anthropol Inst 1913; 43:291–323.

123 Wadsworth G: The Diet and Health of Isolated Populations. Boca Raton. CRC Press, 1984.

124 O'Dea K: Traditional diet and food preferences of Australian Aboriginal hunter-gatherers. Phil Trans R Soc Lond 1991;334:233–241.

125 McArthur M: Food consumption and dietary levels of the Aborigines at the settlements; in Mountford CP (ed): Records of the American-Australian Scientific Expedition to Arnhem Land, vol 2: Anthropology and Nutrition. Melbourne, Melbourne University Press, 1960.

126 Basedow H: The Australian Aboriginal. Adelaide, Preece, 1925, p 108.

127 Gould RA: Notes on hunting, butchering and sharing of game among the Nganatjara and their neighbours in the Western Australian Desert. Kroeber Anthropol Soc Pap 1967;36:41–66.

128 Naughton JM, O'Dea K, Sinclair AJ: Animal foods in traditional Australian Aboriginal diets: Polyunsaturated and low in fat. Lipids 1986;11:684–690.

129 Wilson WE: The food consumption of Australian Aborigines: Natural versus civilised diets. Aust Med J 1954;ii:599–605.

130 Stacy SJG: Nutritional integration of the Aborigine. Food Nutr Notes Rev 1975;32:163–168.

131 Meehan B: Shell bed to shell midden. Canberra, Australian Institute of Aboriginal Studies, 1982, pp 137–138.

132 Bourne GH: Foods of the Australian Aboriginal. Proc Nutr Soc Aust 1953;12:58–61.

133 Hamilton A: Nature and Nurture. Canberra, Australian Institute of Aboriginal Studies, 1981.

134 Cowlishaw GK: The determinants of fertility among Australian Aborigines. Mankind 1981;13:37–55.

135 Hamilton A: Child health and child care in a desert community; in Reid J (ed): Body, Land and Spirit: Health and Healing in Aboriginal Society. St Lucia, University of Queensland Press, 1982, pp 49–71.

136 Blainey G: Triumph of the Nomads: A History of Ancient Australia, rev ed. South Melbourne, Sun Books/Macmillan, 1982, p 135.

137 Meehan B: Shell bed to shell midden. Canberra, Australian Institute of Aboriginal Studies, 1982, p 26.

138 Campbell TD, Lewis AJ: The Aborigines of South Australia: Dental observations recorded at Ooldea. Aust J Dent 1926;30:371–376.

139 Rose FGG: The Traditional Mode of Production of the Australian Aborigines. London, Angus & Robertson, 1987, p 51.

140 Ackerman K: Altered food taboos: Effects on the geriatric population of south-west Kimberley. Oceania 1975;46:122–125.

141 Dadswell IW: The chemical composition of some plants used by Australian Aborigines as food. Aust J Exp Biol Med Sci 1934;12:13–18.

142 Fysh CF, Hodges KJ, Siggins LY: Analysis of naturally occurring foodstuffs of Arnhem Land; in Mountford CP (ed): Records of the American-Australian Scientific Expedition to Arnhem Land, vol 2: Anthropology and Nutrition. Melbourne, Melbourne University Press, 1960, pp 136–138.

143 Morrison FR, Penfold A de R: Individual essential oils of the plant families; in Guenther E (ed): The Essential Oils. New York, Van Nostrand, 1952, vol 5, pp 187–192.

144 Williams LR, Casali J, Horne V: Evaluation of some Australian Plant species for potential as hydrocarbon-producing crops. Chem Aust 1981;48:344–345.

145 Jones RJ, Hegarty MP: Screening pasture plants for possible toxic effects on livestock; in Wheeler JL, Mochrie RD (eds): Forage Evaluation: Concepts and Techniques. Melbourne, CSIRO, 1981, pp 237–241.

146 Rivett DE, Tucker DJ, Jones GP: The chemical composition of seeds from some Australian plants. Aust J Agric Res 1983;34:427–432.

147 Brand JC, Cherikoff V, Lee A, et al: Nutrients in important bushfoods. Proc Nutr Soc Aust 1982; 7:50–54.

148 Brand Miller J, James KW, Maggiore PMA: Tables of Composition of Australian Aboriginal Foods. Canberra, Aboriginal Studies Press, 1993.

149 Brand JC, Cherikoff V, Lee A, et al: An outstanding food source of vitamin C. Lancet 1982;ii: 873–875.

150 Brown AJ, Cherikoff V, Roberts DCK: Fatty acid composition of seeds from the Australian Acacia species. Lipids 1987;22:490–494.

151 Thorburn AW, Brand JC, Truswell AS: Slowly digested and absorbed carbohydrate in traditional bushfoods: A protective factor against diabetes? Am J Clin Nutr 1987;45:98–106.

152 Thorburn AW, Brand JC, O'Dea K, et al: Plasma glucose and insulin responses to starchy foods in Australian Aborigines: A population now at high risk of diabetes. Am J Clin Nutr 1987;46: 282–285.

153 O'Dea K, Naughton AJ, Rabuco L, et al: Lifestyle change and nutritional status in Kimberley Aborigines. Aust Aborig Stud 1987;1:46–51.

154 Cherikoff V, Brand JC, Truswell AS: The nutritional composition of Australian Aboriginal bush-foods. 2: Animal foods. Food Technol Aust 1985;37:208–211.

155 O'Dea K, Sinclair AJ: Increased proportion of arachidonic acid in plasma lipids after two weeks on a diet of tropical seafood. Am J Clin Nutr 1982;36:868–872.

156 Lee AJ: Survival tucker: Aboriginal dietary intake and a successful community-based nutrition intervention project, PhD thesis, University of Sydney, 1992, p 341.

157 Rowley CD: The Destruction of Aboriginal Society, Aborigines in Australian Society. Canberra, Australian National University Press, 1970, vol 4.

158 Reynolds H: The Other Side of the Frontier: Aboriginal Resistance to the European Invasion of Australia. Melbourne, Penguin, 1982.

159 Elkin AP: Reaction and interaction: A food-gathering people and European settlements in Australia. Am Anthropol 1951;53:164–186.

160 Long JPM: Aboriginal settlements: A survey of institutional communities in Eastern Australia. Aborigines in Australian Society. Canberra, Australian National University Press, 1970, vol 3.

161 Brady M: Leaving the spinifex: The impact of rations, missions and the atomic tests on the southern Pitjantjatjara. Rec South Aust 1986;20:35–45.

162 Rowse T: White flour, white power: From rations to citizenship, PhD thesis, University of Sydney, 1988.

163 Hamilton A: Blacks and whites: The relationship of change. Arena 1972;30:34–48.

164 Berndt RM, Berndt CH: Acculturation and native policy. Oceania 1942;13:52–70.

165 Gould RA: Progress to oblivion, Ecologist 1972;2:17–22.

166 Walker RB, Roberts DCK: Colonial food habits; in Truswell AS, Wahlqvist ML (eds): Food Habits in Australia: Proceedings of the First Deakin/Sydney Universities Symposium on Australian Nutrition, Victoria 1988, pp 40–59.

167 Ross FGG: The Traditional Mode of Production of the Australian Aborigines. London, Angus & Robertson, 1987, p 31.

168 Altman JC: Hunter-gatherers today: An Aboriginal economy in north Australia. Canberra, Australian Institute of Aboriginal Studies, 1987.

169 Cordon M: Observations on food habits of Europeans and Aborigines in the Northern Territory. Food Nutr Notes Rev 1962;19:3–8.

170   Cleland JB: Scurvy. Med J Aust 1929;ii:867.
171   Billington BP: The health and nutrition status of the Aborigines; in Mountford CP (ed): Records of the American-Australian Scientific Expedition to Arnhem Land, vol 2: Anthropology and Nutrition. Melbourne, Melbourne University Press, 1960, pp 27–54.
172   Sinclair H: Factors affecting Aboriginal nutrition. Med J Aust (Special Suppl) 1977;i:1–4.
173   Wilson WE: A dietary survey of Aborigines in the Northern Territory. Aust Med J 1953;i: 536–537.
174   Young E: Outback stores: Retail services in north Australian Aboriginal communities. Darwin, Australian National University NARU, 1984.
175   Cutter T: Nutrition and food habits of the central Australian Aboriginal; in Hetzel BS, Frith HJ (eds): Symposium on the Nutrition of Aborigines in Relation to the Ecosystem of Central Australia. Melbourne, CSIRO, 1978, pp 63–72.
176   Stanley D: Aboriginal communities on cattle stations in the Northern Territory of Australia. Australian Economic Papers, 1976.
177   Peterson N: Aboriginal involvement with the Australian economy in the central reserve during the winter of 1970; in Berndt RM (ed): Aborigines and Change: Australia in the '70s. Canberra, Australian Institute of Aboriginal Studies, 1979, pp 136–147.
178   Coombs HC: Decentralisation trends among Aboriginal communities. Search 1974;5:135–143.
179   Coombs HC: Kulinma: Listening to Aboriginal Australians. Canberra, Australian National University Press, 1978.
180   Thomson N: A review of Aboriginal health status; in Reid J, Trompf P (eds): The Health of Aboriginal Australia. Sydney, Harcourt Brace Jovanovich, 1991, pp 37–79.
181   Taylor JC: Diet, health and economy: Some consequences of planned social change in an Aboriginal community; in Berndt RM (ed): Aborigines and Change: Australia in the '70s. Canberra, Australian Institute of Aboriginal Studies, 1979.
182   Cane S, Stanley O: Land Use and Resources in Desert Homelands. Canberra, NARU, Australian National University, 1985.
183   Gibson M: Peoples of the North, Anthropology and Tradition: A Contemporary Aboriginal Viewpoint; in Proceedings of the Menzies Symposium, Nutrition and Health in the Tropics.57th ANZAAS Congress, Townsville, Darwin, MSHR, 1987.
184   Lee AJ, O'Dea K, Mathews J: Apparent dietary intake in remote Aboriginal communities. Aust J Publ Health 1994;18:190–196.
185   Sullivan H, Gracey M, Hevron V: Food costs and nutrition in remote areas of Northern Australia. Med J Aust 1987;147:334–337.
186   Wise PH, Edwards FM, Thomas DW, et al: Hyperglycaemia in the urbanised Aboriginal – The Davenport survey. Med J Aust 1970;ii:1001–1006.
187   Rowse T, Scrimgeour D, Knight S, et al: Food purchasing in an Aboriginal community. 1. Survey results. Aust J Public Health 1994;18:63–66.
188   Brady M: Drug and alcohol use among Aboriginal people; in Reid J, Trompf P (eds): The Health of Aboriginal Australia. Sydney, Harcourt Brace Jovanovich, 1991, pp 173–217.
189   Brady M, Morice R: Defiance or despair? Petrol sniffing in an Aboriginal Community; in Reid J (ed): Body, Land and Spirit: Health and Healing in Aboriginal Society. St Lucia, University of Queensland Press, 1982, pp 72–88.
190   Watson C, Flemming J, Alexander K: A Survey of Drug Use Pattern in Northern Territory Aboriginal Communities, 1986–1987. Darwin, NTDHCS, 1988.
191   Mathews JD, Riley MD, Fejo L, et al: Effects of the heavy usage of kava on physical health: Summary of pilot survey in an Aboriginal community. Med J Aust 1988;148:548–555.
192   Hetzel BS, Frith HJ (eds): Symposium on the Nutrition of Aborigines in Relation to the Ecosystem of Central Australia. Melbourne, CSIRO, 1978.
193   MacKenzie CJC: European incursions and failures in northern Australia; in Jones R (ed): Northern Australia: Options and Implications. Canberra, Research School of Pacific Studies, Australian National University, 1980, pp 43–72.
194   Report of Uwankara Palyanyku Kanyintjaku: An environmental and public health review within the Anangu Pitjantjatjara lands, Adelaide, Nganampa Health Council Inc, 1987.

195 Coles-Rutishauser IHE: Food intake studies in Australian Aborigines: Some Methodological considerations; in Proc 13th International Congress of Nutrition. London, Libbey, 1985, pp 706–710.

196 Lee AJ, Smith A, Bryce S, et al: Measuring dietary intake in remote Australian Aboriginal communities. Ecol Food Nutr, in press.

197 Hitchcock NE, Gracey M: Dietary patterns in a rural Aboriginal community in South-West Australia. Med J Aust (Special Suppl) 1975;ii:12–16.

198 King RA, Smith RM, Spargo RM: Dietary patterns of Aboriginal children in the Kimberley. Proc Nutr Soc Aust 1985;10:173.

199 King RA, Smith RM, Wilkinson GN, et al: Nutrient intake of Aboriginal children in the Kimberley. Proc Nutr Soc Aust 1988;13:164.

200 Allen JR, Heywood PF, Mensch MG, et al: Dietary methods used in an ascorbic acid supplementation trial in Australian Aboriginal and Caucasian school children. Food Nutr Notes Rev 1977;34:12–17.

201 Sibthorpe B: All our people are dyin': Food and health in a rural Aboriginal community, PhD thesis, Canberra, Australian National University, 1989.

202 Kamien M, Woodhill JM, Nobile S, et al: Nutrition in the Australian Aborigine: A dietary study of two Aboriginal families. Food Technol Aust 1975;27:93–103.

203 Heywood PF, Zed CA: Dietary and anthropometric assessment of the nutritional status of Aboriginal and white children in Walgett, NSW. Proc Nutr Soc Aust 1977;2:21–27.

204 Guest CS, O'Dea K: Food habits in Aborigines and persons of European descent of southeastern Australia. Aust J Public Health 1993;4:321–324.

205 Bastian P: Coronary heart disease in tribal Aborigines – The West Kimberley Survey. Aust N Z J Med 1975;9:284–292.

206 Coles-Rutishauser IHE: Growing up in Western Australia: If you are Aboriginal. Proc Nutr Soc Aust 1979;4:27–32.

207 Sladden TJ: Cardiovascular disease risk factors in an Aboriginal community, MSc thesis, University of Sydney, 1987.

208 Kailis DG: Groote Eylandt Studies. 3. The influence of diet on the prevalence of dental caries in Aboriginal children at Groote Eylandt, NT Australia, 1973. Proc Nutr Soc Aust 1979;4: 118.

209 Lee AJ, Bailey APV, Yarmirr D, et al: Survival tucker: Improved diet and health indicators in an Aboriginal community. Aust J Public Health 1994;18:277–285.

210 Lee AJ: Survival tucker: Aboriginal dietary intake and a successful community-based nutrition intervention project, PhD thesis, University of Sydney, 1992, pp 184–187.

211 Bleakley W: Aborigines of Australia. Brisbane, Jacaranda Press, 1961, p 6.

212 Bleakley W: Aborigines of Australia. Brisbane, Jacaranda Press, 1961, p 17.

213 Davidson WS: Health and nutrition of Warburton Range natives of Central Australia. Med J Aust 1957;ii:21–22.

214 Thomson N: Aboriginal nutrition: The need for a cultural and historical perspective. Proc Nutr Soc Aust 1982;7:20–29.

215 O'Dea K: The hunter-gatherer lifestyle of Australian Aborigines: Implications for health; in McLean AJ, Wahlqvist ML (eds): Nutrition, Pharmacology and Toxicology. London, Libbey, 1988, pp 26–36.

216 Cleland JB: Disease amongst the Australian Aborigines. J Trop Med Hyg 1928;31:53–59, 65–70, 141–145, 157–160, 173–177, 196–198, 202–206, 216–220, 232–235, 262–266, 281–282, 290–294, 307–313, 326–330.

217 MacPherson J: Medicine amongst the Australian Aborigines. Br Med J 1903;ii:96.

218 White SA: Aborigines of the Everard Range. Trans R Soc South Aust 1915;39:725–731.

219 Basedow H: Anthropological notes made on the South Australian government north-west prospecting expedition, 1903. Trans R Soc South Aust 1904;28:12–51.

220 Stanner WEH: The Daly River Tribes: A report of fieldwork in North Australia. Oceania 1933;3: 377–405.

221 Vanderwal R: The Aboriginal photographs of Baldwin Spencer. South Yarra, Curry O'Neil, 1982.

222 Basedow H: Notes on the natives of Bathurst Island, North Australia. J R Anthropol Inst 1913; 43:291–323.

223 Breinl A, Holmes MJ: Medical report on the data collected during a journey through some districts of the Northern Territory. Bull NT Aust 1915:15.

224 Hackett CJ: Boomerang leg and yaws in Australian Aborigines. Trans R Soc Trop Med Hyg 1936; 30:137–150.

225 Black EC, Cleland JB: Pathological lesions in Australian Aborigines, Central Australia (Granites), and the Flinders Ranges. J Trop Med Hyg 1938;41:69–83.

226 Mann I: Report on the ophthalmic findings in the Warburton Range natives of Central Australia. Med J Aust 1957;ii:610–612.

227 Packer AD: The health of the Australian native. Oceania 1961;32:60–70.

228 Abbie AA: The health of the Australian Aborigines. Organorama 1966;3:13–16.

229 Sandison AT: Notes on skeletal changes in pre-European contact Australian Aborigines. J Hum Evol 1980;9:45–47.

230 Prokopec M: Demographical and morphological aspects of the Roonka population. Archaeol Phys Anthropol Oceania 1979;14:11–26.

231 Webb LJ: The use of plant medicines and poisons by Australian Aborigines. Mankind 1969;7: 137–146.

232 Devanesen D, Henshall TS: A study of plant medicines in Central Australia. Trans Menzies Found 1982;4:161–166.

233 Scarlett, N, White N, Reid J: Bush medicines: The pharmacopoeia of the Yolngu of Arnhem Land; in Reid J (ed): Body, Land and Spirit: Health and Healing in Aboriginal Society. St Lucia, University of Queensland Press, 1982, pp 154–191.

234 Aboriginal Communities of the Northern Territory of Australia: Traditional Bush Medicines: An Aboriginal Pharmacopoeia. Darwin, Greenhouse, 1988.

235 Abbie AA: Physical standards of nomadic Aboriginal children. Med J Aust 1974;i:470–471.

236 Parsons PA: Growth in a sample of Australian Aborigines from one to twenty-three months of age. Growth 1965;29:207.

237 Hamilton A: Socio-Cultural Factors in Health among the Pitjantjatjara: A Preliminary Report. Sydney, Department of Anthropology, Macquarie University, 1971.

238 Abbie AA: Studies in Physical Anthropology. Canberra, Australian Institute of Aboriginal Studies, 1968, vol 1.

239 Abbie AA: Studies in Physical Anthropology. Canberra, Australia Institute of Aboriginal Studies, 1968, vol 2.

240 O'Dea K: Body fat distribution and health outcome in Australian Aborigines. Proc Nutr Soc Aust 1987;12:56–75.

241 O'Dea K, White NG, Sinclair AJ: An investigation of nutrition-related risk factors in an isolated Aboriginal community in Northern Australia: Advantages of a traditionally orientated lifestyle. Med J Aust 1988;148:177–180.

242 Coles-Rutishause IHE: Body mass and body composition in Australian Aboriginal women; in Proceedings of the Menzies Symposium, Nutrition and Health in the Tropics. 57th ANZAAS Congress, Townsville, Darwin, MSHR, 1987, pp 226–232.

243 Barrett MJ, Brown T: Increase in average height of Australian Aborigines. Med J Aust 1971;ii: 1169–1172.

244 Brown T, Barrett MJ: Increase in average weight of Australian Aborigines. Med J Aust 1973;ii: 25–27.

245 Curnow DH: The serum proteins of Aborigines in the Warburton Ranges area. Med J Aust 1957; ii:608–609.

246 Wilkinson GK, Day AJ, Peters JA, et al: Serum proteins of some Central and South Australian aborigines. Med J Aust 1958;ii:158–160.

247 Neel JV, Sal Zano FM, Junqueira PC, et al: Studies on the Xavante Indians of the Brazillian Mato Grosso. Am J Hum Genet 1964;16:52–140.

248 Truswell AS, Hansen JDL: Serum lipids in bushmen. Lancet 1968;ii:684.

249 Brading I: The serum protein pattern in some Pacific natives. Med J Aust 1958;12:49–52.

250 Nye LJJ: Blood pressure of the Australian Aboriginal, with a consideration of possible aetiological factors in hyperpiesia and its relation to civilisation. Med J Aust 1937;ii:1000–1001.

Lee

251 Casley-Smith JR: Blood pressures in Australian Aborigines. Med J Aust 1959;i:627–633.

252 Abbie AA: Physical changes in Australian Aborigines consequent upon European contact. Occeania 1960;31:140–144.

253 Abbie AA, Schroder J: Blood pressures in Arnhem Land Aborigines. Med J Aust 1960;ii: 493–496.

254 Van Dongen R, Davigongs V, Abbie AA: Aboriginal blood pressures at Beswick, south-west Arnhem Land, and correlation with physical dimensions. Med J Aust 1962;ii:286–289.

255 Lowenstein FW: Blood pressure in relation to age and sex in the tropics and subtropics. Lancet 1961;ii:389–392.

256 Prior IAM, Stanhope JM, Grimley JE, et al: The Tokelau Island migrant study. Int J Epidemiol 1974;3:225–232.

257 Schwartz CJ, Casley-Smith JR: Serum cholesterol levels in atherosclerotic subjects and in the Australian Aborigines. Med J Aust 1958;ii:84–86.

258 Charnock JS, Casley-Smith J, Schwartz CJ: Serum magnesium-cholesterol relationships in the central Australian Aborigine and in Europeans with and without ischaemic heart disease. Aust J Exp Biol Med Sci 1959;37:509–516.

259 Schwartz CJ, Day AJ, Peters JA, et al: Serum cholesterol and phospholipid levels of Australian Aborigines. Aust J Exp Biol Med Sci 1957;35:449–456.

260 Schwartz CJ, Casley-Smith JR: Atherosclerosis and the serum mucoprotein levels of the Australian Aborigine. Aust J Exp Biol Med Sci 1958;36:117–120.

261 Davis RE, Pitney WR: Some haematological observations on Aborigines in the Warburton Ranges area. Med J Aust 1957;ii:605–608.

262 Casley-Smith JR: The haematology of the central Australian Aborigines. 1. Aust J Exp Biol Med Sci 1958;36:23–38.

263 Casley-Smith JR: The haematology of the central Australian Aborigines. 2. Aust J Exp Biol Med Sci 1959;37:481–488.

264 Hodges KJ: Report of the biochemical assessments of nutritional status; in Mountford CP (ed): Records of the American-Australian Scientific Expedition to Arnhem Land, vol 2: Anthropology and Nutrition. Melbourne, Melbourne University Press, 1960, pp 72–89.

265 Pitney WR: Serum vitamin B_{12} concentrations in the Western Australian Aborigines. Aust J Exp Biol Med Sci 1962;40:73–80.

266 Davis RE, Kelly A, Byrne G: Serum folate levels in the Australian Aboriginal. Med J Aust 1965; ii:21–22.

267 Davis RE, Smith BK, Curnow DH: Pyridoxal, folate and vitamin B_{12} concentrations in Western Australian Aborigines. Aust J Exp Biol Med Sci 1975;53:93–105.

268 Propert DN, Edmonds R, Parsons PA: Birth weights and growth rates up to one year for full-blood and mixed-blood Australian Aboriginal children. Asut Paediatr J 1968;4:134–143.

269 Gracey M: The nutrition of Australian Aborigines; in Walhqvist ML, Truswell AS (eds): Recent Advances in Clinical Nutrition. London, Libbey, 1986, pp 57–68.

270 Maxwell GM, Elliot RB: Nutritional state of Australian Aboriginal children. Am J Clin Nutr 1969; 22:716–724.

271 Cockington RA: Growth of Australian Aboriginal children related to social circumstances. Aust N Z J Med 1980;10:322–325.

272 Jose DG, Welch JS: Growth retardation, anaemia and infection, with malabsorption and infection of the bowel – The syndrome of protein-calorie malnutrition in Australian Aboriginal children. Med J Aust 1970;i:349–356.

273 Edwards LD: Malnutrition and disease in pre-school Aboriginal children in the Walgett area of NSW. Med J Aust 1970;ii:1007–1012.

274 Gracey M: Undernutrition in the midst of plenty: Nutritional problems of young Australian Aborigines. Aust Paediatr J 1976;12:180–182.

275 Gracey M, Bourke V, Robinson J: Patterns of intestinal infection in Australian Aboriginal children. Med J Aust 1980;ii:375–380.

276 Moodie PM: Mortality and morbility in Australian Aboriginal children. Aust Paediatr J 1969;1: 180–185.

277 Harris MF, Nolan B, Davidson A: Early childhood pneumonia in Aborigines of Bourke, New South Wales. Med J Aust 1984;i:705–707.

278 Gershwin ME, Beech RS, Hurley IS: Nutrition and Immunity. San Diego, Academic Press, 1985.

279 Chandra RK: Nutrition, immunity and infection: Present knowledge and future directions. Lancet 1983;ii:688–691.

280 Neumann CG: Maternal nutrition and neonatal immunoglobulins; in Jellife DB, Jellife EFB (eds): Advances in International Maternal and Child Health. Oxford, Oxford University Press, 1980, vol 2.

281 Scrimgeor D: Growth Failure in Aboriginal Children. London, Tropical Child Health Unit/Institute of Child Health, 1983.

282 Phillips PE, Dibley MJ: A longitudinal study of feeding patterns of Aboriginal infants living in Perth. Proc Nutr Soc Aust 1983;8:130–133.

283 Coyne T, Dowling M: Infant feeding practices among Aboriginals in rural NSW. Proc Nutr Soc Aust 1978;3:91.

284 Houghton MR, Gracey M, Burke V, et al: Breast milk lactoferrin levels in relation to maternal nutritional status. J Paediatr Gastrointest Nutr 1985;4:230–233.

285 Rae CJ: Maternal nutritional status among Aborigines in the Northern Territory: Impact on birth weight, MPH thesis, University of Sydney, 1989.

286 Gracey M, Spargo RM, Bottrell C, et al: Maternal and childhood nutrition among Aborigines of the Kimberley region. Med J Aust 1984;141:506–508.

287 Cheek DB, Spargo RM, Holt AB: Evidence for zinc deficiency in Aboriginal settlements in North Western Australia. Med J Aust (Special Suppl) 1981;i:4–5.

288 Kalokerinos A: Some aspects of Aboriginal infant mortality. Med J Aust 1969;i:185.

289 Kelokerinos A: Every second child. Melbourne, Nelson, 1974.

290 Nobile S: Blood vitamin levels in Aboriginal children and their mothers in Western NSW. Med J Aust 1974;i:601–607.

291 Gracey M, Spargo RM: The state of health of Aborigines in the Kimberley region. Med J Aust 1987;146:200–204.

292 Moodie PM: Aboriginal Health. Canberra, Australian National University Press, 1973.

293 Rutishauser IHE, McKay H: Anthropometric status and body composition in Aboriginal women of the Kimberley region. Med J Aust (Special Suppl) 1986;144:8–10.

294 Krotkiewski M, Bjorntorp S per A, Sjostrom L, et al: Impact of obesity in metabolism in men and women: Importance of regional adipose tissue distribution. J Clin Invest 1983;72:1150–1162.

295 Haffner SM, Stern MP, Hazuda HP, et al: The role of behavioural variables and fat patterning in explaining ethnic differences in serum lipids and lipoproteins. Am J Epidemiol 1986;123: 831–839.

296 Zimmet PZ, King HOM, Bjorntorp S per A: Obesity, hypertension, carbohydrate disorder and the risk of chronic diseases. Med J Aust 1986;145:256–262.

297 Stanton KG, McCann V, Knuiman M, et al: Diabetes in part-Aborigines of Western Australia. Diabetologia 1985;28:16–21.

298 O'Dea K, Lion RJ, Lee AJ, et al: Diabetes, hyperinsulinemia and hyperlipidaemia in a small Aboriginal community in Northern Australia. Diabetes Care 1990;13:830–834.

299 Simons L, Whish P, Marr B, et al: Coronary risk factors in a rural community which includes Aborigines: Inverell Heart Disease Prevention Program. Aust N Z J Med 1981;11:386–390.

300 Edwards FM, Wise PH, Thomas DW, et al: Blood pressure and electrocardiographic findings in the South Australian Aborigines. Aust N Z J Med 1976;6:197–205.

301 O'Dea K, Trianedes K, Hopper JL, et al: Impaired glucose tolerance, hyperinsulinaemia, and hypertriglyceridaemia in Australian Aborigines from the desert. Diabetes Care 1988;11:23–29.

302 Wise PH, Edwards FM, Craig RJ, et al: Diabetes and associated variables in the South Australian Aboriginal. Aust N Z J Med 1976;6:191–196.

303 Gault A: Health Survey, Urapuntja Health Service. Alice Springs, Institute of Aboriginal Development, 1990.

304 Duffy P, Morris H, Neilson G: Diabetes mellitus in the Torres Strait region. Med J Aust (Special Suppl) 1981;i:8–11.

305 Finlay-Jones RA, McCormish MJ: Prevalence of diabetes mellitus in Aboriginal lepers: The Derby Survey. Med J Aust 1972;ii:135–137.

306 Cameron WI, Moffitt PS, Williams DDR: Diabetes mellitus in Australian Aborigines of Bourke, New South Wales. Diabetic Res Clin Pract 1986;2:307–314.

307 Williams DRR, Moffitt PS, Fisher JS, et al: Diabetes and glucose tolerance in New South Wales coastal Aborigines: Possible effects of non-Aboriginal genetic admixture. Diabetologia 1987;30:72–77.

308 McGrath M, Collins V, Zimmet P, et al: Lifestyle disorders in Australian Aborigines. Melbourne, International Diabetes Institute, 1991.

309 Glatthaar C, Welbourn TA, Stenhouse NS, et al: Diabetes and impaired glucose tolerance – A prevalence estimate based on the Busselton 1981 survey. Med J Aust 1985;143:436–440.

310 White K, Gracey M, Schumacher L, et al: Hyperinsulinaemia and impaired glucose tolerance in young Australian Aborigines. Lancet 1990;335:735.

311 Guest CS, O'Dea K: Diabetes in Aborigines and other Australian populations. Aust J Public Health 1992;16:340–349.

312 Neel JV: Diabetes mellitus, a thrifty genotype rendered detrimental by progress? Am J Hum Genet 1962;14:353–358.

313 Neel JV: The thrifty genotype revisited; in Kobberling J, Tattersall R (eds): The Genetics of Diabetes Mellitus. London, Academic Press, 1982, pp 283–293.

314 Reaven GH, Bernstein R, Davis B, et al: Nonketotic diabetes mellitus: Insulin deficiency or insulin resistance? Am J Med 1976;60:80–88.

315 O'Dea K, Spargo R: Metabolic adaptation to a low carbohydrate-high protein ('traditional') diet in Australian Aborigines. Diabetologia 1982;23:494–498.

316 Collier G, McClean A, O'Dea K: Effect of co-ingestion of fat on the metabolic responses to slow and rapidly absorbed carbohydrates. Diabetologia 1984;26:50–54.

317 O'Dea K, Spargo RM, Ackerman K: The effect of transition from traditional to urban life-style on the insulin secretory response in Australian Aborigines. Diabetes Care 1980;3:31–37.

318 Blumenthal SA: Stimulation of gluconeogenesis by palmitic acid in rat hepatocytes: Evidence that this effect can be dissociated from the provision of reducing equivalents. Metabolism 1983;32:971–976.

319 Holt AB, Spargo RM, Iveson JB, et al: Serum and plasma zinc, copper and iron concentrations in Aboriginal communities of North Western Australia. Am J Clin Nutr 1980;33:119–132.

320 Crotty JM: Anaemia and nutritional disease in Northern Territory native children. Med J Aust 1958;ii:322–325.

321 Barrett MJ, Williamson JJ: Oral health of Australian Aborigines: Survey methods and prevalence of dental caries. Aust Dent J 1972;17:37–50.

322 Schamschula RG, Cooper MH, Agus HM, et al: Oral health of children using surface and artesian water supplies. Community Dent Oral Epidemiol 1981;9:27–31.

323 Brown T: Denotal decay in Aborigines; in Hetzel B, et al (eds): Better Health for Aborigines? St Lucia, University of Queensland Press, 1974.

324 Kamien M, Nobile S, Cameron P, et al: Vitamin and nutritional status of a part-Aboriginal community. Aust N Z J Med 1974;4:126–137.

325 Cheek DB, McIntosh GH, O'Brian V, et al: Malnutrition in Aboriginal children at Yalata, South Australia. Eur J Clin Nutr 1989;43:161–168.

326 Watson DS, Tozer RA: Anaemia in Yirrkala. Med J Aust (Special Suppl) 1986;144:513–515.

327 Bower C, Forbes R, Seward M, et al: Congenital malformations in Aborigines and non-Aborigines in Western Australia, 1980–1987. Med J Aust 1989;151:245–248.

328 Jones PN, Mills EH: Serum vitamin B_{12} concentrations in liver disease. J Lab Clin Med 1955;46:927–931.

329 Lee AJ: Survival tucker: Aboriginal dietary intake and a successful community-based nutrition intervention project, PhD thesis, University of Sydney, 1992, pp 307.

330 Kamien M, Woodhill JM, Nobile S, et al: Nutrition in the Australian Aborigines – Effects of the fortification of white flour. Aust. N Z J Med 1975;5:123–133.

331 Roberts DCK: Vitamin E; in Truswell AS, Dreosti IE, English RM, et al (eds): Recommended Nutrient Intakes, Australian Papers. Sydney, Australian Professional Publications, 1990, pp 159–176.

332 Eastwell HD: Low zinc levels in Aborigines. Med J Aust 1991;ii:201.
333 Smith RM, Spargo RM, Cheek DB: Zinc status and the growth of Aboriginal children in the North-West of Australia. Proc Nutr Soc Aust 1982;7:37–44.
334 Reilly C, Harrison F: Nutritional implications of levels of zinc, copper, iron and lead in hair of British and Australian children. Proc Nutr Soc Aust 1983;8:209.
335 Cheek DB, Spargo RM, Holt AB: Hair zinc and copper and retarded growth in Aboriginal children of North Western Australia. Aust Paediatr J 1982;18:139–140.
336 Smith RM, King RA, Spargo RM, et al: Growth-retarded Aboriginal children with low plasma zinc levels do not show a growth response to supplementary zinc. Lancet 1985;i:923–924.
337 Klevey LM, Bistrian BR, Fleming CR, et al: Hair analysis in clinical and experimental medicine. Am J Clin Nutr 1987;46:233–236.
338 Solomons NW; Zinc and copper in human nutrition; in Karcioglu ZA, Sarper RM (eds): Zinc and Copper in Medicine. Springfield, Thomas, 1980, pp 224–275.
339 O'Dea K: Marked improvement in carbohydrate and lipid metabolism in diabetic Australian Aborigines after temporary reversion to traditional lifestyle. Diabetes 1984;33:596–603.
340 Australian Bureau of Statistics: Apparent Consumption of Food and Nutrients, Australia, 1985–86. Canberra, AGPS, 1987.

Dr. Amanda Lee, Menzies School of Health Research
PO Box 41096 Casuarina, NT 0811 (Australia)

Simopoulos, AP (ed): Metabolic Consequences of Changing Dietary Patterns.
World Rev Nutr Diet. Basel, Karger, 1996, vol 79, pp 53–69

....

Food Variety of Adult Melbourne Chinese: A Case Study of a Population in Transition

Bridget H.-H. Hsu-Hage, Mark L. Wahlqvist

Monash University, Department of Medicine – Monash Medical Centre,
Clayton, Melbourne, Vic., Australia

Contents

Introduction

Food variety, together with *adequacy, energy control* and *moderation* are considered important aspects of a preferred diet both in occidental and oriental societies. Nutrients essential for human life are not all found in one food (with the exception of human breast milk in the first months of life) but amongst many. This has led to dietary guidelines which have been adopted by several countries, to include a variety of foods in the diet [1–3]. Several studies have investigated the relationships between food variety, or dietary diversity, and either nutrient adequacy in the diet [4–6], intake quality [7], or more recently health outcomes [8–10]. Many researchers attribute poor nutritional status to the lack of food variety in the diet, noticeably amongst vulnerable groups, such as the aged, children and women, those who are chronically ill, socio-economic disadvantaged, migrants or minority ethnic groups, and athletes [11–30]. Few, however, have examined the determinants of food intake variety in population groups [16].

The purposes of this study were to investigate socio-economic determinants of food variety, and to consider food variety in relation to food intake patterns and nutrient intake, to nutritional status assessed by anthropometry and to the cardiovascular risk factors, blood pressure, plasma lipids, and fasting blood glucose, in a representative sample of adult Chinese, living in Melbourne, Australia. Methods for assessing food intake and its variety [31–33], and measurements for anthropometry, blood pressure, plasma lipids, and fasting blood glucose in this Chinese population have been reported elsewhere [34].

Adult Melbourne Chinese

The majority of Melbourne Chinese are a relatively recent immigrant group to Australia (table 1). More than 95% of Melbourne Chinese were born overseas, who have arrived in Australia at different times from different countries, and speak different dialects at home [35, 36]. Adult Melbourne Chinese represent a population in transition, whose traditional values about food and health are under challenge and undergoing modification for survival in a new environment. At the same time, some of the variety of food intake which characterizes the majority European Australian population was made possible by the Chinese who immigrated to Australia in the mid-19th century at the time of the 'gold rush' and thereafter [37]. Diversity in dialects amongst Melbourne Chinese allows one approach to a consideration of the socio-cultural determinants of dietary change. In a socio-cultural model, determinants of eating habits include traditional food culture, food availability and accessibility, food preparation skills and facilities and the household economy [38, 39]. In a world of new foods, migrant populations are particularly sensitive to these determinants [40, 41] in addition to various extraneous factors in food selection. These include language skill, health motives, nutrition awareness, food sensitivity (perceived or real) and sensory preferences [42, 43].

Socio-Economic Factors

Age, education and income of Melbourne Chinese are important socio-demographic determinants of food variety. Older age groups, the less educated,

Table 1. Socio-demographic characteristics of the study population, by gender

	Men (n = 269)	Women (n = 276)
Age, years		
25–34	23.4	34.4
35–44	34.9	33.0
45–54	23.0	15.2
55–64	10.3	9.4
65+	8.2	8.0
Mean ± SD	44.6 ± 12.4	42.4 ± 12.6
Length of stay in Australia[a], years		
Mean ± SD	12.1 ± 9.0	8.8 ± 5.8
Country of birth		
Australia	4.1	3.3
PR China	24.2	23.6
Hong Kong	11.2	13.4
Malaysia/Singapore	27.1	22.1
Vietnam	24.2	26.8
Others	9.3	10.9
Education level, years		
0–6	12.3	28.7
7–9	22.3	17.8
10–12	20.1	27.9
13+	45.4	25.7
Occupational status		
Professional/administrative	28.6	24.3
Clerical/sales	24.2	18.9
Tradesman/services	43.9	33.0
Domestic duties	3.3	23.9
Gross household income[b], AUD pa		
<12,000	8.6	14.0
12,000–21,999	20.7	24.5
22,000–39,999	35.7	35.9
≥40,000*	35.0	25.6

[a] Overseas born only, 258 for men and 267 for women.

[b] 266 for men and 273 for women.

and low income families had a lower food variety compared to the young, the educated, and/or high-income families. Those in the manual labour or service workforce or those who stay at home also had a lower food variety than professionals or administrative occupation groups. As the educated Melbourne Chinese were younger, mostly professional or in the administrative occupation group, and had a higher income, these findings were consistent with its population profile. Those born in China, generally known to be older, less educated and more adherent to country of ancestry or traditional eating habits, reported a lower food variety than those born in Australia, independently of age (table 2). This was consistent with the positive relationships of food variety with age, education level, and food acculturation index (table 3). The positive relationship between food variety and length of stay in Australia, independently of age, suggested that increased food variety can be achieved with increased exposure to the world of new foods. The process may be accelerated by education level or English language skills (the latter not measured in this study).

The ways by which the nutritional status of immigrants may be compromised has also been reported by Pelto [17], who attributed undernutrition in children of recent immigrants to the 'new environment'. It has been reported that nutritional status is comparable between children of ethnic minorities and nonminority children of similar economic status in England, Australia, and the USA [17]. In a study of food habits and nutritional status of agricultural migrant workers in Southern Brazil, the traditional diet of these workers was considered inadequate both in quality and quantity [25]. The traditional rice and bean-based diet amongst these agricultural migrant workers was shown to be of limited variety; the use of fresh fruits and vegetables, while locally available and in abundance, was infrequent.

In a recent report, Kinsey [11] examined correlates of families' socioeconomic status and food expenditure and consumption in the USA and found that income was a key determinant of food purchase and consumption patterns. Age and ethnic backgrounds, on the other hand, contribute to dietary diversity. Women's participation in the work force has led to increased consumption of foods away from home, with a tendency for variety to decrease. The extent of dietary diversity in the black and white adult Americans has been investigated by Kant et al. [16]. These investigators reported that American blacks consumed less food variety. As income and level of education increase, the food variety in the diet increases. From the changing food intake pattern viewpoint, Popkin et al. [44] reported major changes in American women's diet between 1977 and 1985; in particular, increased dietary diversity associated with a decreased intake within most food groups. Educated women were more likely to make changes. During the same period, Krondl et al. [23] conducted a study of food selection amongst elderly Americans and found that many maintained food dietary variety; women showed a greater use of a wider range of food items, in particular, vegetables and fruits. Ethnic differences in food intake variety has been reported amongst culturally diverse low-income families. The same study however failed to show a relationship between food variety and nutrient intake quality [19]. This probably was due to the fact that, for

Table 2. Prevalence of low food variety in subgroups of adult Melbourne Chinese

Parameters	Low food variety		Unadjusted		Age-adjusted	
	n	%	OR	p value	OR	p value
Age group, years						
25–34[1]	37	23.4	1.0		NA	
35–44	33	17.8	0.7	0.0000		
45–54	26	25.0	1.1	NS		
55–64	24	44.4	2.6	0.0263		
≥65	25	56.8	4.3	0.0001		
Length of stay in Australia, years						
<10[1]	83	28.1		NS	NA	
≥10	62	24.8	0.8			
Country of birth						
Australia[1]	2	10.0	1.0		1.0	
PR China	55	42.3	6.6	0.0000	1.9	0.0046
Hong Kong	16	23.9	2.8	NS	1.2	NS
Malaysia/Singapore	24	17.9	2.0	NS	0.8	NS
Vietnam	34	24.5	2.9	NS	1.3	NS
Others	15	25.5	3.1	NS	1.2	NS
Education level, years						
0–6	55	49.1	7.1	0.0000	2.2	0.0000
7–9	40	36.7	4.9	0.0122	1.6	0.0075
10–12	27	20.6	1.9	0.0472	0.7	NS
13+[1]	23	11.9	1.0		1.0	
Occupational status						
Professional/administrative[1]	16	11.1	1.0		1.0	
Clerical/sales	29	24.8	2.6	NS	0.9	NS
Tradesmen/services	68	32.5	3.9	0.0322	1.6	0.0041
Domestic duties	32	42.7	6.0	0.0001	1.3	0.0123
Household income, AUD pa						
<12,000	27	44.3	7.8	0.0004	1.6	0.0327
12,000–21,999	49	40.2	6.6	0.0006	1.9	0.0004
22,000–39,999	51	26.4	3.5	NS	1.1	NS
≥40,000[1]	15	9.2	1.0		1.0	

Low food variety is where the diet consisted of <40% of the maximum achievable variety.
OR = Odds ratio.
[1] Comparison group for odds ratio calculation.

Table 3. Correlation between food variety and selected socio-demographic character-istics

	Unadjusted			Age-adjusted[1]	
	n	r	p	r	p
Age, years	545	−0.24	0.0001	NA	
Length of stay in Australia, years	525	0.11	0.0093	0.17	0.0001
Education level	545	0.43	0.0001	0.38	0.0001
Food acculturation[2]	545	0.14	0.0014	0.10	0.0242

[1] Overseas-born only (n = 516); Education level: 1 = 0–6 years, 2 = 7–9 years, 3 = 10–12 years, 4 = 13+ years.
[2] A food acculturation index was calculated based upon number of Chinese and non-Chinese type foods consumed in the 12-month period prior to the survey. The classification of Chinese and non-Chinese type foods is as defined by Hage [53].

the several nutrients examined, their sources were not sufficiently varied to ensure a spread of difference in nutrient intake quality (unlike the data from Melbourne Chinese shown in tables 6 and 7 below). Children of immigrants to Lima City, Peru, in a low-income peripheral settlement, were reported to have a relatively high prevalence of malnutrition, attributable to a lack of dietary diversity and the low-energy value of the weaning foods. Income available to mothers and spent on food were major determinants of dietary diversity in the homes of these Peruvian migrants [22].

Food Intake Patterns at the Cultural Cross-Roads

A noticeable difference, observed in Melbourne Chinese, between those with a low and a high food variety is the discrepancy in total amount of food consumed (table 4). Apart from the intake of rice, those with a low food variety in the diet invariably consumed less meat, dairy, other vegetables, fruits, beverages and all other foods than did those with a high food variety. The intake of rice was associated positively with the intake of traditional Chinese foods, such as pork, poultry, fish, leafy green, cruciferous vegetables, legumes, dried vegetables, tea and soup [33]. The intake of these traditional Chinese foods, with the exception of pork, was not found to be significantly higher in those with a low food variety in the diet; pork intake was significantly lower. One possible explanation is that, in Melbourne, pork is less available than red meat, a novel food for traditional Chinese. There is a lack of difference in the

Table 4. Comparison of mean daily food intake in those with a low or a high food variety score

Food items, g/day	Low food variety (n = 145) mean ± SD	High food variety (n = 400) mean ± SD	p value
Rice	487 ± 322	428 ± 256	0.027
Wheat	100 ± 76	115 ± 118	
Cereals – total	588 ± 328	544 ± 276	
Pork	39 ± 44	51 ± 42	0.0040
Poultry	26 ± 23	26 ± 22	
Red meat	28 ± 32	35 ± 29	0.0089
Fish	20 ± 18	19 ± 16	
Other seafood	15 ± 17	21 ± 18	0.0007
Eggs	16 ± 16	20 ± 21	0.025
Meats – total	144 ± 96	172 ± 89	0.0013
Dairy	78 ± 116	116 ± 168	0.0026
Leafy green	22 ± 24	21 ± 22	
Cruciferous vegetables	16 ± 15	16 ± 12	
Legumes	27 ± 38	30 ± 34	
Dried vegetables	4 ± 7	4 ± 5	
Other vegetables	109 ± 90	128 ± 81	0.018
Vegetables – total	178 ± 128	199 ± 108	
Fresh fruits	214 ± 154	249 ± 195	0.027
Fruit juice	21 ± 60	45 ± 81	0.0002
Other fruits	3 ± 10	14 ± 29	<0.0001
Fruits – total	237 ± 176	308 ± 225	0.0007
Tea	305 ± 388	279 ± 267	
Coffee	161 ± 222	258 ± 357	0.0002
Nonalcoholic beverages	74 ± 121	136 ± 177	<0.0001
Alcoholic beverages	29 ± 100	44 ± 138	
Beverages – total	569 ± 503	717 ± 534	0.0037
Nuts and seeds	5 ± 19	9 ± 87	
Sweets	19 ± 27	30 ± 32	<0.0001
Soups	91 ± 74	80 ± 73	
Snacks	36 ± 38	51 ± 41	<0.0001
All other foods	151 ± 86	171 ± 129	0.042
Water	1,764 ± 669	1,939 ± 665	0.0069
Total food consumed	2,321 ± 799	2,647 ± 852	<0.0001

Low food variety is where the diet consisted of <40% of the maximum achievable variety; high food variety is where it was ≥40%.

intake of vegetables and of traditional Chinese foods between those with a low and a high food variety; most of the differences were found in new foods, such as red meat, dairy food, fruit juice, other fruits, coffee, nonalcoholic beverages, sweets and snacks. There is no previous study to confirm our findings that increase in the intake of a particular food group may contribute to an increased dietary diversity. It, however, can be postulated from the study of this Chinese population that increase in food consumption is a key to secure dietary diversity. Furthermore, results derived from this Chinese population suggested that introduction of new foods is a way of increasing food variety amongst migrant groups.

Nutrient Intake

The most impressive finding was the generally low essential nutrient intakes in those with a low food variety; the only insignificant findings between the two groups were alcohol intake, percentage of energy from protein and alcohol (table 5). It should be noted that alcohol contributed less than 1% of total energy intake for Melbourne Chinese. Taking together energy requirements and recommended nutrient intake as a recommended nutrient density (RND = recommended nutrient intake/recommended energy intake), the nutritional value of the diet can be evaluated as a nutrient density score (NDS = estimated nutrient density/recommended nutrient density) [45]. Protein intake nutrient density is not significantly different between the two groups nor were those NDS for iron, zinc, retinol equivalents, thiamin, niacin equivalents, and vitamin C (table 6). This indicates that both energy intake and food variety are important for a nutritionally adequate diet, and confirms food intake analyses (table 4) as discussed in the previous section.

In those whose diet consisted of less than 40% of the maximum achievable variety (over a 12-month period), 92.4% had at least one nutrient fall below two thirds of the Australian Recommended Daily Intakes (RDIs) compared to 75.8% who had all nutrients equal to or above two thirds of RDIs (table 7). Those with a low food intake variety were at a 2-fold risk for having an essential nutrient intake level fall below two thirds of the recommended intake (for protein, calcium, phosphorous, magnesium, iron, zinc, retinol equivalents, thiamin, riboflavin, or vitamin C).

Nutrient intake quality was generally low in those with a low food variety. The intake quality for calcium, magnesium, zinc, retinol equivalents, and riboflavin in those with a low food intake variety was compromised. There was a significantly high prevalence of poor NDS for phosphorous, magnesium,

Table 5. Comparison of mean daily nutrient intake in those with a low or a high food variety score

Nutrients	Low food variety (n = 145) mean ± SD		High food variety (n = 400) mean ± SD		p value
Total energy, kJ/day	7,201	± 2,725	8,193	± 3,406	0.0005
Protein – total, g/day	71	± 33	80	± 32	0.0016
Carbohydrates – total, g/day	259	± 105	283	± 117	0.030
Fat – total, g/day	49	± 21	60	± 43	<0.0001
Alcohol, g/day	2.20	± 7.2	2.61	± 7.1	
Protein, % energy	15.9	± 3.0	16.1	± 2.4	
Carbohydrates, % energy	54.6	± 8.1	53.1	± 7.0	0.049
Fat, % energy	24.7	± 6.2	26.0	± 6.0	0.029
Alcohol, % energy	0.76	± 2.5	0.85	± 2.2	
Dietary fibre, g/day	17	± 6.4	20	± 10	0.0002
Dietary cholesterol, mg/day	205	± 128	253	± 142	0.0004
Potassium, μg/day	49	± 19	63	± 26	<0.0001
Calcium, mg/day	389	± 209	492	± 262	<0.0001
Phosphorous, mg/day	910	± 405	1,081	± 475	<0.0001
Magnesium, mg/day	224	± 79	269	± 125	<0.0001
Iron, mg/day	10	± 4.2	12	± 4.3	<0.0001
Zinc, mg/day	8.7	± 4.4	9.9	± 4.1	0.0027
Retinol equivalents, μg/day	513	± 474	690	± 495	0.0002
Thiamin, mg/day	0.85	± 0.43	1.02	± 0.46	<0.0001
Riboflavin, mg/day	0.89	± 0.45	1.16	± 0.57	<0.0001
Niacin equivalents, mg/day	26	± 11	30	± 11	0.0002
Vitamin C, mg/day	101	± 65	128	± 77	<0.0001

Low food variety is where the diet consisted of <40% of the maximum achievable variety; high food variety is where it was ≥40%.

retinol equivalents, thiamin, and riboflavin. The risk ranged from 1.5- to 2-fold of those who had a high food intake variety.

Two important aspects of dietary diversity are nutritional adequacy and dietary quality; both rely on essential nutrients as a yardstick and use the RDIs [4, 6, 7]. The use of RND as a point of reference for the assessment of dietary quality in this study, which takes into account energy requirements and RDIs, has been previously reported. Randall et al. [5] found that nutrient intake in young American adults (18–34 years old) was directly related to both number of foods consumed and total energy intake, as well as to nutrient density scores. For energy-providing nutrients, such as fat, differences in nutri-

Table 6. Comparison of mean NDS in those with a low or a high food variety score for selective nutrients

Nutrients	Low food variety (n = 145)	High food variety (n = 400)	p value
	mean ± SD	mean ± SD	
Protein – total	1.72 ± 0.38	1.76 ± 0.29	
Calcium	0.59 ± 0.30	0.66 ± 0.28	0.0077
Phosphorous	1.10 ± 0.25	1.18 ± 0.23	0.0012
Magnesium	0.94 ± 0.21	1.01 ± 0.19	0.0002
Iron	1.60 ± 0.59	1.58 ± 0.62	
Zinc	0.87 ± 0.25	0.90 ± 0.21	
Retinol equivalents	0.86 ± 0.82	1.00 ± 0.61	
Thiamin	1.16 ± 0.37	1.21 ± 0.36	
Riboflavin	0.81 ± 0.35	0.91 ± 0.36	0.0042
Nacin equivalents	2.10 ± 0.49	2.14 ± 0.45	
Vitamin C	3.73 ± 2.40	4.13 ± 2.24	

Low food variety is where the diet consisted of <40% of the maximum achievable variety; high food variety is where it was ≥40%.

ent intake adequacy are largely accounted for by differences in total energy intake alone. The intake of essential nutrients, such as cholesterol, calcium, and retinol equivalents, however, is best differentiated by nutrient density.

Similar to most studies, we found that increased food intake variety is the key to adequacy in essential nutrient intakes and, to a lesser extent, an improved nutrient intake quality in this transitional population of ethnic Chinese. It can be noted that the average daily intake for calcium, zinc, retinol equivalents, and riboflavin in adult Melbourne Chinese falls well below that recommended for Australian populations (table 6). For these nutrients, efforts in public health nutrition education should be ones that encourage increases in various nutrient-specific food sources as well as increased intakes of those foods which are nutrient dense (table 8) [5]. This may include efforts to retain in the diet some traditional foods, such as, in the case of Chinese, tofu, leafy greens and pulses which have been identified as major sources of calcium in southern Chinese [46]. At the same time, traditional, vegetarian or designer diets may be intrinsically biased towards deficiency or excess of essential nutrients [11, 22, 25, 28, 47–50]. The introduction of new foods or variety may overcome this problem. Food-Based Dietary Guidelines (FBDG), now being recommended after the WHO Cyprus workshop of 1995, address these issues [Wahlqvist, pers. commun.].

Table 7. Odds ratio for those whose intakes fall below two thirds of the RDIs in those with a low food variety score

Nutrients	2/3 RDIs	n	%	OR	95% CL	p value
Total energy	<1.5 BMR	39	26.9			
	≥1.5 BMR	84	21.0	1.38	0.89, 2.15	
Protein[1]	<55 g/day	33	22.8			
	≥55 g/day	42	10.5	2.51	1.54, 4.11	<0.0001
Calcium[2]	<800 mg/day	116	80.0			
	≥800 mg/day	268	67.0	1.97	1.25, 3.10	0.003
Phosphorous	<1,000 mg/day	39	26.9			
	≥1,000 mg/day	46	11.5	2.83	1.78, 4.51	<0.0001
Magnesium[3]	<320 mg/day	53	36.6			
	≥320 mg/day	78	19.5	2.38	1.57, 3.59	<0.0001
Iron[4]	<7 mg/day	35	24.1			
	≥7 mg/day	38	9.5	3.03	1.86, 4.95	<0.0001
Zinc	<12 mg/day	75	51.7			
	≥12 mg/day	146	36.5	1.86	1.27, 2.73	0.001
Retinol equivalents	<750 µg/day	95	65.5			
	≥750 µg/day	168	42.0	2.62	1.78, 3.87	<0.0001
Thiamin[5]	<1.1 mg/day	40	27.6			
	≥1.1 mg/day	58	14.5	2.25	1.43, 3.53	<0.0001
Riboflavin[6]	<1.7 mg/day	98	67.6			
	≥1.7 mg/day	172	43.0	2.76	1.87, 4.10	<0.0001
Vitamin C[7]	<40 mg/day	3	2.1			
	≥40 mg/day	7	1.8	1.19	0.30, 4.65	
Adequacy	at least one nutrient falls <2/3 RDIs	134	92.4			
	all nutrients ≥ 2/3 RDIs	303	75.8	3.90	2.10, 7.24	<0.0001

Low food variety is where the diet consisted of <40% of the maximum achievable variety; high food variety is where it was ≥40%. BMR = Basal metabolic rate (estimated using the Scholfield equation [54]). [1] 45 g/day for women; [2] 1,000 mg/day for women aged 55 years and over; [3] 270 mg/day for women; [4] 12 mg/day for women <55 years of age and 5 mg/day for women aged ≥55 years; [5] 0.8 mg/day for women <55 years of age and 0.7 mg/day for women aged ≥55 years; [6] 1.2 mg/day for women <55 years of age and 1.0 mg/day for women aged ≥55 years; [7] 30 mg/day for women.

Nutritional Status

Mean systolic blood pressure, fasting glucose, abdominal circumference, waist-to-hip ratio, total body fat, and percentage body fat amongst those with a low food intake variety were significantly higher than their counterparts with

Table 8. Odds ratio for nutrient intake quality (by NDS) fall below that recommended for intake (as RND) in those with a low food variety score

Nutrients	n	%	OR	95% CL	p value
Calcium					
NDS <1	130	89.7			
NDS ≥1	364	91.0	0.86	0.45, 1.62	
Phosphorous					
NDS <1	52	35.9			
NDS ≥1	89	22.3	1.95	1.30, 2.94	0.001
Magnesium					
NDS <1	91	62.8			
NDS ≥1	210	52.5	1.53	1.03, 2.25	0.033
Iron					
NDS <1	35	24.1			
NDS ≥1	84	21.0	1.20	0.76, 1.88	
Zinc					
NDS <1	115	79.3			
NDS ≥1	288	72.0	1.49	0.95, 2.35	
Retinol equivalents					
NDS <1	109	75.2			
NDS ≥1	248	62.0	1.86	1.21, 2.84	0.004
Thiamin					
NDS <1	52	35.9			
NDS ≥1	106	26.5	1.55	1.04, 2.32	0.033
Riboflavin					
NDS <1	113	77.9			
NDS ≥1	269	67.3	1.72	1.11, 2.68	0.016
Vitamin C					
NDS <1	8	5.5			
NDS ≥1	11	2.8	2.07	0.83, 5.15	
Quality					
At least one NDS falls <1	143	98.6			
All NDS ≥1	389	97.3	2.02	0.46, 8.98	

Low food variety is where the diet consisted of <40% of the maximum achievable variety.

a high food variety (table 9). Food intake variety, expressed as a continuum, also correlated significantly to systolic blood pressure, fasting glucose, stature (positive), waist-to-hip circumference, total body fat, fat free mass (positive), and percentage body fat (table 10). However, after adjusting for age, food variety related only to systolic blood pressure and stature.

Table 9. Comparison of selected health outcomes in those with a low or a high food variety score

Parameters	Low food variety (n = 145)		High food variety (n = 400)		p value
	mean ± SD		mean ± SD		
SBP, mm Hg	121.9	± 25.5	113.5	± 17.8	0.0003
DBP, mm Hg	70.5	± 12.1	70.2	± 10.4	
Total cholesterol, mmol/l	5.48	± 1.18	5.40	± 1.10	
Triglycerides, mmol/l	1.46	± 0.97	1.38	± 0.92	
HDL cholesterol, mmol/l	1.41	± 0.38	1.44	± 0.38	
LDL cholesterol, mmol/l	3.41	± 1.10	3.33	± 0.98	
Fasting glucose, mmol/l	4.83	± 2.04	4.35	± 1.09	0.0083
Body weight, kg	58.12	± 9.67	58.22	± 10.35	
Stature, cm	160.8	± 7.72	162.0	± 8.21	
BMI, kg/m^2	22.43	± 2.95	22.11	± 3.15	
Abdominal circumference, mm	838	± 88	817	± 96	0.0274
Hip circumference, mm	918	± 60	918	± 60	
Waist-to-hip ratio	0.91	± 0.0680	0.89	± 0.067	0.0005
Total body fat, kg	16.3	± 5.89	15.0	± 6.01	0.0324
Fat free mass, kg	41.9	± 8.84	43.2	± 9.10	
Body fat, %	28.0	± 9.24	25.8	± 9.13	0.0101

Low food variety is where the diet consisted of <40% of the maximum achievable variety; high food variety is where it was ≥40%.

The underlying hypothesis for increased food variety is that there are related health benefits. Studies of children show improvement in human growth during the vulnerable years of life. Novotny [20] found that increased dietary diversity, along with parental factors, accounted for a significant variation of growth as measured by weight-for-age and height-for-age, and indirectly influenced weight-for-height in a group of preschool children under 5 years of age in Gualanceo, Ecuador. For children living in extreme nutritionally-deprived environments, it was found that food availability, and hence dietary diversity, accounted for differences in type of malnutrition and its impact on the relative retardation of growth [21]. The effect of dietary diversity on growth has also been demonstrated in preschoolers in the affluent society whose diets may be limited in type of animal food through the choice of their parents. Children of vegetarian parents are smaller, lighter and leaner by reference to the standard growth charts (Harvard or Tanner-Whitehouse). The observation

Table 10. Correlation between food variety and selected health outcomes

Health outcomes	Unadjusted			Age-adjusted	
	n	r	p	r	p
SBP, mm Hg	545	−0.22	0.0001	−0.09	0.0326
DBP, mm Hg	545	−0.03		0.06	
Total cholesterol, mmol/l	543	−0.08		−0.01	
Triglycerides, mmol/l	543	−0.07		−0.02	
HDL cholesterol, mmol/l	543	0.05		0.02	
LDL cholesterol, mmol/l	543	−0.07		−0.01	
Fasting glucose, mmol/l	543	−0.09	0.0472	−0.03	
Body weight, kg	545	0.04		0.05	
Stature, cm	545	0.13	0.0033	0.09	0.0461
BMI, kg/m²	545	−0.05		−0.01	
Abdominal circumference, mm	538	−0.08		0.00	
Hip circumference, mm	538	0.00		0.01	
Waist-to-hip ratio	538	−0.12	0.0054	−0.01	
Total body fat, kg	544	−0.10	0.0214	−0.03	
Fat free mass, kg	544	0.11	0.0094	0.07	
Body fat, %	544	−0.13	0.0027	−0.05	

[1] Overseas-born only (n = 516).

that a diet with limited variety or animal foods is associated with risk for slow growth in children, however, does not imply an association between increased food variety and human obesity [48]. Results from the study of Melbourne Chinese are consistent with current literature; this indicates that, in spite of a higher intake of most foods and total energy (and energy-providing nutrients) amongst the Melbourne Chinese with a high food intake variety, the anthropological assessments and health outcomes are somewhat favourable.

Other aspects of health outcome include disease risk factors. By using NDSs, Randall et al. [5] found that at least in an affluent society the intake of fat, sodium/potassium, and total energy were profoundly influenced by dietary diversity. Assuming that key nutritional factors associated with the elevation of blood pressure include sodium/potassium and body fatness, the association between food variety and systolic blood pressure in this study of Melbourne Chinese is an observation that warrants further investigation. More recently, the effect of food variety on human health has shifted its attention to specific disease outcomes, such as macrovascular disease and disease mortality. Wahlqvist et al. [8] found that food variety explained 13–19% of the variation in arterial wall indices in a comparative study of apparently healthy and individuals with type II diabetes. Using fasting blood glucose as a risk indicator, we have confirmed in this study of apparently healthy adult Melbourne Chinese, the potential benefit of a high food variety for blood glucose and, therefore, possibly the prevention of diabetes and its complication [51, 52]. The advocacy for food variety in human health is better appreciated when disease mortality is considered. Kant et al. [9, 10] in two consecutive studies of American populations showed an increased risk of CVD, cancer and all-cause mortality associated with diets lacking of several major food groups.

Conclusions

In today's world of rapid transition, nutritionists are faced with the problem of undernutrition on the one hand, and overnutrition on the other. The profound effects of food variety on human nutritional problems are a continuum and operate at the individual as well as population level. In this paper, we illustrate that: (1) determinants of food variety are complex and include social, cultural, economic, political, and environmental factors; (2) consumption of greater amounts of specific food and a variety of foods, which should take place in physically active individuals, holds the key to adequate intake of essential nutrients conducive to growth and health, and (3) nutrient intake quality can only be achieved when adequacy of intake is safeguarded.

References

1   Milio N: Toward healthy longevity. Lessons in food and nutrition policy development from Finland and Norway. Scand J Soc Med 1991;19:209–217.
2   Fukuba H: Food policy for health in Japan. Nutr Health 1992;8:177–190.
3   Palmer S: The implications of dietary recommendations for dietary patterns and health. In Vivo 1989;3:135–141.
4   Krebs-Smith SM, Clark LD: Validation of a nutrient adequacy score for use with women and children. J Am Diet Assoc 1989;89:775–783.
5   Randall E, Nichaman MZ, Contant CF Jr: Diet diversity and nutrient intake. J Am Diet Assoc 1985;85:830–836.
6   Guthrie HA, Scheer JC: Validity of a dietary score for assessing nutrient adequacy. J Am Diet Assoc 1981;78:240–245.
7   Krebs-Smith SM, Smiciklas-Wright H, Guthrie HA, et al: The effects of variety in food choices on dietary quality. J Am Diet Assoc 1987;87:897–903.
8   Wahlqvist ML, Lo CS, Myers KA: Food variety is associated with less macrovascular disease in those with type II diabetes and their healthy controls. J Am Coll Nutr 1989;8:515–523.

9 Kant AK, Schatzkin A, Harris TB, et al: Dietary diversity and subsequent mortality in the First National Health and Nutrition Examination Survey Epidemiologic Follow-Up Study. Am J Clin Nutr 1993;57:434–440.

10 Kant AK, Schatzkin A, Ziegler RG: Dietary diversity and subsequent cause-specific mortality in the NHANES I Epidemiologic Follow-Up Study. J Am Coll Nutr 1995;14:233–238.

11 Kinsey JD: Food and families' socioeconomic status. J Nutr 1994;124:1878S–1885S.

12 McNabb SJ, Welch K, Laumark S, et al: Population-based nutritional risk survey of pensioners in Yerevan, Armenia (see comments). Am J Prev Med 1994;10:65–70.

13 Earland J, Freeman P: Community nutrition survey in an urban settlement in Papua New Guinea. P N G Med J 1993;36:10–15.

14 Volkert D: (Nutritional needs of the aged) Anforderungen an die Ernährung alter Menschen. Zentralbl Hyg Umweltmed 1993;194:80–88.

15 Pardoe EM: Development of a multistage diet for dysphagia. J Am Diet Assoc 1993;93:568–571.

16 Kant AK, Block G, Schatzkin A, et al: Dietary diversity in the US population, NHANES II, 1976–1980. J Am Diet Assoc 1991;91:1526–1531.

17 Pelto GH: Ethnic minorities, migration and risk of undernutrition in children. Acta Paediatr Scand Suppl 1991;374:51–57.

18 Al-Shoshan AA: Some sociodemographic factors influencing the nutritional awareness of the Saudi teens and adults: Preliminary observations. J R Soc Health 1990;110:213–216.

19 Suitor CW, Gardner JD, Feldstein ML: Characteristics of diet among a culturally diverse group of low-income pregnant women. J Am Diet Assoc 1990;90:543–549.

20 Novotny R: Preschool child feeding, health and nutritional status in Gualaceo, Ecuador. Arch Latinoam Nutr 1987;37:417–443.

21 Coulter JB, Omer MI, Suliman GI, et al: Protein-energy malnutrition in northern Sudan: Prevalence, socio-economic factors and family background. Ann Trop Paediatr 1988;8:96–102.

22 Herold P, Sanjur D: Homes for the migrants: The pueblos jovenes of Lima – A study of socioeconomic determinants of child malnutrition. Arch Latinoam Nutr 1986;36:599–624.

23 Krondl M, Lau D, Yurkiw MA, et al: Food use and perceived food meanings of the elderly. J Am Diet Assoc 1982;80:523–529.

24 Hulse JH: Food science and nutrition: The gulf between rich and poor. Science 1982;216:1291–1294.

25 Desai ID, Garcia Tavares ML, Dutra de Oliveira BS, et al: Food habits and nutritional status of agricultural migrant workers in Southern Brazil. Am J Clin Nutr 1980;33:702–714.

26 Grivetti LE: Nutritional success in a semi-arid land: Examination of Tswana agro-pastoralists of the eastern Kalahari, Botswana. Am J Clin Nutr 1978;31:1204–1220.

27 Bowering J, Lowenberg RL, Morrison MA, et al: Influence of a nutrition education program (EFNEP) on infant nutrition in East Harlem. J Am Diet Assoc 1978;72:392–397.

28 Grandjean AC: Nutrition for swimmers. Clin Sports Med 1986;5:65–76.

29 Grandjean AC: Vitamins, diet, and the athlete. Clin Sports Med 1983;2:105–114.

30 Wahlqvist ML, Hsu-Hage BH-H, Kouris-Blazos A, et al: The IUNS cross-cultural study of "Food habits in later life". An overview of key findings. Asia Pacific J Clin Nutr 1995;4:233–243.

31 Hsu-Hage BH-H, Wahlqvist ML: A food frequency questionnaire for use in Chinese populations and its validation. Asia Pacific J Clin Nutr 1992;1:211–223.

32 Hodgson JM, Hsu-Hage BH-H, Wahlqvist ML: Food variety as a quantitative descriptor of food intake. Ecol Food Nutr 1993;32:137–148.

33 Hsu-Hage BH-H, Ibiebele KI, Wahlqvist ML: Food intakes of adult Melbourne Chinese. Aust J Public Health 1995;19:623–628.

34 Hsu-Hage BH-H, Wahlqvist ML: Cardiovascular risk in adult Melbourne Chinese. Aust J Public Health 1993;17:306–313.

35 Have BH-H, Oliver RG, Powles JW, et al: Telephone directory listings of presumptive Chinese surnames: An appropriate sampling frame for a dispersed population with characteristic surnames. Epidemiology 1990;1:405–408.

36 Hsu-Hage BH-H, Wahlqvist ML: The authors' response to letter to the Editor – Telephone directory listings of presumptive Chinese surnames. Epidemiology 1993;4:87.

37   Wahlqvist ML: History of nutrition in Australia; in Wahlqvist ML (ed): Food and Nutrition in Australia. Melbourne, Nelson, 1988, pp 12–21.

38   Sagkubs M: Culture and Practical Reason. Chicago, University of Chicago Press, 1976.

39   Axelson ML: The impact of culture on food-related behavior. Annu Rev Nutr 1986;6:345–363.

40   Powles J, Ktenas D, Sutherland C, et al: Food habits in southern European migrants: A case of migrants from the Greek Island of Levkada; in Truswell AS, Wahlqvist ML (eds): Food Habits in Australia. Melbourne, Gordon, 1988.

41   Chong R, Holowaty M, Krondl M, et al: The effect of culturally determined satiety meaning on food practices. J Can Diet Assoc 1976;37:245–249.

42   Krondl M, Coleman P: Social and biocultural determinants of food selection. Prog Food Nutr Sci 1986;10:179–203.

43   Anderson GH, Krasnegor NA, Miller GD, et al: Diet and Behavior. Multidisciplinary Approaches. Berlin, Springer, 1990.

44   Popkin BM, Haines PS, Reidy KC: Food consumption trends of US women: Patterns and determinants between 1977 and 1985. Am J Clin Nutr 1989;49:1307–1319.

45   Australian Department of Community Services and Health: National Dietary Survey of Adults, 1983, No 2: Nutrient Intakes. Canberra, Australian Government Publishing Service, 1987.

46   Hsu-Hage BH-H, Wahlqvist ML: Culturally specific sources of food component: Lesson from studies amongst Chinese (abstract). 7th Asian Congress of Nutrition, Beijing, Oct 7–11, 1995.

47   Doolan N, Appavoo D, Kuhnlein HV: Benefit-risk considerations of traditional food use by the Sahtu (Hare) Dene/Metis of Fort Good Hope, N W T Arctic Med Res 1991 (suppl):747–751.

48   Dwyer JT, Palombo R, Valadian I, et al: Preschoolers on alternate life-style diets. Associations between size and dietary indexes with diets limited in types of animal foods. J Am Diet Assoc 1978; 72:264–270.

49   Brown PT, Bergan JG: The dietary status of 'new' vegetarians. J Am Diet Assoc 1975;67:455–459.

50   Stare FJ: Fortification of foods in industrial and developing countries. Bibl Nutr Dieta. Basel, Karger, 1979, vol 28, pp 201–205.

51   Satinsky AL: A key to preventing diabetic retinopathy: The link between nutrition and blood sugar. J Ophthalmic Nurs Technol 1994;13:263–266.

52   Quinn S: Diabetes and diet. We are still learning. Med Clin North Am 1993;77:773–782.

53   Hage BH-H: Food habits and cardiovascular health in adult Melbourne Chinese, PhD thesis, Monash University, Department of Medicine, 1992.

54   Schofield MN: Predicting basal metabolic rate, new standards and review of previous work. Hum Nutr 1985;39C:5–41.

Prof. Mark L. Wahlqvist, Monash University, Department of Medicine, Block E Level 5, 246 Clayton Road, Clayton, Melbourne, Vic. 3168 (Australia)

Simopoulos, AP (ed): Metabolic Consequences of Changing Dietary Patterns.
World Rev Nutr Diet. Basel, Karger, 1996, vol 79, pp 70–108

....

Traditional Diets and Meal Patterns in South Africa

Demetre Labadarios[a,1]*, Alexander R.P. Walker*[b,2]*, Renée Blaauw*[a]*,
Betty F. Walker*[b,2]*

[a] Department of Human Nutrition, Faculty of Medicine, University of Stellenbosch
    and Tygerberg Hospital, Tygerberg, and
[b] Human Biochemistry Research Unit, Department of Tropical Diseases, School of
    Pathology of the University of the Witwatersrand, and the South African Institute
    for Medical Research, Johannesburg, South Africa

Contents

[1] Financial assistance from the South African Medical Research Council is acknowledged.
[2] For research funding, gratitude is expressed to the South African Medical Research
Council, South African Sugar Association, National Cancer Association and Anglo-American De Beers Chairmans Fund.

Introduction

South Africa is considered by many as an excellent example of coexisting first and third world nutritional experiences and problems. It has a rich heritage of indigenous foods, of the dietary experience of the hunter-gatherers, Bushmen, Khoisan or San, of rural Africans in different regions, and of urban dwellers. The intention of this review is to describe resources of food, meal patterns, their nutritional adequacy, and health/ill-health sequelae, past and current. While the primary focus is on the African population (approximately 30 million), mention will also be made of the experience of the white population (5 million), the 'Coloured' (Euro-African-Malay) population (3 million), and of the Indians (1 million), who arose from immigration around a century ago. While information is extensive on some of the aspects mentioned, on other aspects, unfortunately, it is relatively meagre.

Geography of South Africa

Of the earth's six continents, Africa holds a prominent position. It separates the Indian and Atlantic Oceans. Its land mass extends into the Northern and Southern hemispheres, and there is a very wide range of climate and therefore of vegetation. The Continent includes six very large areas, namely, Sahara, Egypt, West and East Africa, Central and Southern Africa. The latter is composed of six countries, namely, Namibia, Botswana, Mozambique, Zambia, Zimbabwe, and South Africa (fig. 1). South Africa enjoys a subtropical climate. A small proportion of the land in the north lies within the Tropic of Capricorn. The country has an area one fifth of that of the United States, and 3 times that of the United Kingdom.

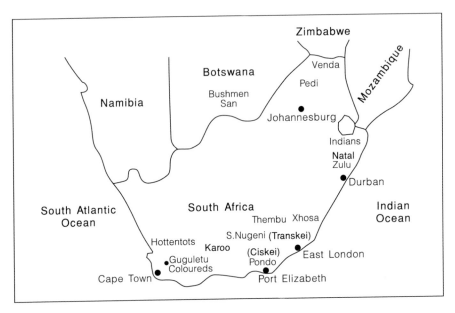

Fig. 1. Map of South Africa showing relative location of different races.

African Populations

Historically, traces of earliest man were found along the enormous rift of the Great Lakes in Central Africa. Later descendants were identified by Dr. S. Leaky and by Prof. Raymond Dart. The populations included three main ethnic groups who once lived and roamed over the Continent. There were the Negroid people, who were black skinned, and who left traces of their origin in the Congo basin. There were brown skinned Hamites stemming from the East, and who lived mainly in the North. The third group, the copper skinned Bushmen, Khoisan or San, can be traced throughout the Continent; their descendants are now very limited, both in regions and in numbers [1].

Contact between Negroes and Hamites resulted in a new ethnic group, the Negroid African. These people gradually moved southwards across the Limpopo River, and occupied the luxuriant Eastern regions and the central plateau of South Africa. Towards the end of the 18th century, they began to settle in organized groups and then became divided into smaller units, each of which had their own cultural patterns and languages. Clan members were united through age groups, and each member had an importance in that particular age category. These groupings lasted throughout life.

In South Africa, the present African population, as distinct from the San, resulted from migrations from Central Africa in the 17th–19th centuries. In

Table 1. Indigenous foods of Africans in southern Africa

Cereals	*Sorghum vulgare* ('kaffir corn'), millet, maize
Legumes	Jugo beans, mung beans, cowpeas, also groundnuts
Vegetables	'kaffir melon', water melon, gourd, pumpkin
Wild plants	Pigweed, purslane, lamb's-quarters, Black Jack
Wild fruits	Sour plum, wild plum, monkey apple, Kei apple, prickly pear
Insects	Caterpillars, beetles, ants, locusts
Other foods	Honey, wild birds, small game
Beverages	Milk, mostly sour, light beer, strong (intoxicating) beer, and other potent traditional and modern beers

the far past the people were hunter-gatherers. They depended on indigenous foods and small game, as do the small groups of present-day San or Bushmen in northwestern Botswana. However, within the last 150 years or so the way of life of rural Africans changed to one of pastoralism and dependency subsistence, with the rearing of cattle. It was women who tilled the land, sowed the seed, husbanded the plants, and eventually harvested and threshed the crop. The men were responsible for the cattle. Erratic rainfall, low soil fertility, no fertilizer and no crop rotation, led to low harvests [1].

In more recent times, major changes have taken place, for many rural Africans now work on white-owned farms, or they migrate to towns and cities seeking employment. Access to villages has greatly improved. Changes in village life usually include the store, the clinic, the school, improved water supply and transport to towns.

South African Populations

In South Africa, the main subdivisions of Africans are Zulu in KwaZulu/Natal, Xhosa in Eastern Province, Tswana in the Centre and North West, and Sotho, Shangaans, Pedi and Venda in the North and East of the country (fig. 1).

Indigenous Foods

In Africa, commonly consumed indigenous foods (table 1) used to be the sole source of nourishment for all populations, especially of the hunter-gatherer type [1–3]. But with the immigration of western populations, particularly to southern Africa, the African diet has changed with the gradual introduction

Table 2. Common foodstuffs of the San (Bushmen)

Plants	Mongongo, fruit and nut, Morethlwa berry, sour plum, tsama melon, fruit of baobab tree, morula fruit and nut, tsi bean
Animals	Kudu, wildebeeste, gemsbok, steenbok, duiker, wart hog, ant bear, porcupine, spring hare, common hare

of processed foods, e.g. refined cereal products and sugar, and of new vegetables and fruits. Of indigenous foods, much the same as that of other populations in Africa, cereals and legumes contribute most of the carbohydrate and protein moieties as well as fat. Many plant foods are rich sources of minerals, especially calcium and iron, and of vitamins, especially vitamins A, B complex and C.

Regarding indigenous preparations, dishes were prepared from mealies (maize), green or dried, and samp, which is coarsely ground maize. Porridges (gruels) were made from mealie meal, millet, sorghum, and mealie rice, and fermented milk. Cereals were also made into dumplings. Simple dishes were made from stewed unripe sorghum or mealie ears, whole grain stews, and cooked cereal with sour milk. Cereals were also cooked with various mixed vegetables. Dried vegetable leaves (morogo), and mushrooms were consumed in season. Numerous dishes included beans and groundnuts. Meat included wild birds, rodents and insects. Beverages included milk, mostly sour, light beer, strong (intoxicating) beer, and other potent traditional and modern beers.

Rural Africans

Hunter-Gatherers, Bushmen, Khoisan, San

Hunting and gathering were the only methods of obtaining food until about 10,000 years ago. Understandably, many of the highly developed and densely populated countries in the world were once thinly inhabited by hunter-gatherers.

At present, in numbers, the San probably do not exceed 10,000, although the precise figure is uncertain. Among these people, there was considerable variety in the foodstuffs consumed [4]. For example, it was noted that those in the Dobe region in Botswana ate 85 species of plants and 54 species of animals, although only 9 of the plant species were eaten in large amounts, and only 17 of the animal species were consistently hunted [5] (table 2).

Some animals were taboo to certain members of the community, for example premenstrual girls, and some animals were taboo to all classes, for example the vervet monkey, a close relative to man. Few species of plants were taboo in contrast to the animal sources. The San knew where food was to be found at each season of the year and they arranged their schedule of activities to take maximum advantage of the resources. Plant foods were abundant, local and predictable, whereas meat was of secondary importance. Nine species of plants provided three quarters of their diet. The mongongo nut available the whole year round was the most important and provided about half of their total. Every territory had enough food to sustain at least some of its members throughout the year, but such arrangements were flexible enough to permit people to collect and eat freely in territories other than their own. There were no recorded instances of one camp going hungry, while there was still food available at other camps [5, 6].

The !Kung San appeared to spend less than half of their days in subsistence and they appeared to enjoy more leisure time than members of many agricultural and industrial societies. These observations were made during the dry season when neighbouring farmers experienced stock losses and crop failures.

As to the nature of the foodstuffs gathered, it differed regionally. Among the most common of foods was the fruit of the mongongo tree, a good source of carbohydrate [6]. The tsi bean, a tuber weighing up to 10 kg, with seeds; the tsa plant, with its root swellings; both are good sources of fat and protein. The all-purpose tsama melon was important throughout low rainfall areas like the Kalahari Desert, on account of its high water content.

On an average day, food collection habits were as follows: the women would gather wild leaves, fruits, roots, bulbs, and water. The latter was often found in small quantities in forks of trees, and, as mentioned, the wild melon pulp contained very large amounts of water. It was preserved in ostrich eggs, and used only in dire necessity. Rodents, snakes, tortoise and grubs were also found by the women [7]. The men hunted usually small animals.

The food gathered was shared among the other members of a group. This occurred especially when a large animal was killed. When it occurred, after eating, the people would spend the night in dancing; the sharing of food had very strong effects on the social organization within the group. Plant foods were not shared to the same extent.

Health Study Made in 1976

The diet, meal patterns and nutritional status of the San, at Dobe, Botswana, have been studied [8]. Their foodstuffs were those as already described. Examinations were carried out on 100 adults and 60 children. They confirmed that the people were generally short. The men averaged 160.9 cm; however, some of the younger men were quite tall, measuring up to 175 cm. Most were very thin. Among adults, there appeared to be a mild degree of undernutrition. However, there was very little evidence of malnutrition, even in the children. Among girls, their relatively late age at onset of menarche, about $15\frac{1}{2}$ years, could be attributed in measure to their low body fat content. Clinical examination and biochemical investigations (blood and urine) indicated a good state of protein nutrition, and of vitamin and mineral status. There were only a few exceptions, principally, in persons who had been ill or who had been injured.

As to disorders/diseases, there was very little evidence of dental caries. Obesity was absent. Blood pressure did not rise with age, as is usual with primitively living rural African populations; none had hypertension. Serum cholesterol concentration was very low, averaging around 120 mg/dl (3.1 mmol/l). Triglycerides also were low averaging 100 mg/dl (1.12 mmol/l). These low levels were attributed to a combination of a diet relatively low in energy intake, moderate in fat intake and high in polyunsaturated fats, to the absence of obesity, and, of course, to the liberal amount of physical exercise. Mongongo nuts, their major source of vegetable fat, are rich in polyunsaturated fat. There was no evidence of coronary heart disease, and, as is characteristic of rural African populations, there was only an occasional case of rheumatic heart disease.

It was concluded that there was no evidence that the hunter-gatherers were unhealthy because of their diet [8, 9]. Indeed, the authors reported that in several respects the San were considered to be more healthy than people in western countries. Provided they did not die from infections or from injuries, the hunter-gatherers at Dobe could live to a good old age. In brief, the diet consumed was associated with little nutritional deficiency and no evidence of nutritional excess.

Health Study Made in 1987

A repeat health and nutrition survey was carried out in the Dobe region on the same population [9]; included in the sample were a number of the individuals who had been examined 20 years previously [9]. It proved possible to trace 49 of the latter. Some had been children at the time of the last examination, but 39 had been adults at that time. An additional 100 San subjects, 29 of whom were children, were also examined.

As to dietary patterns, it was reported that the diet remained similar to that consumed formerly.

All the children appeared healthy and had not changed significantly regarding their mean height-and-weight-for-age. There were fewer children below the 5th percentile of US NCHS reference standards; the proportion was 5%, in 1987, compared to 15% in 1976. This observation thus indicates a positive secular trend in height and weight, which has been associated with a measure of change from a hunting and gathering lifestyle, to that of pastoralism. The change described suggests that the shorter height of San may be nutritionally rather than genetically determined. There was little evidence of acute malnutrition or of starvation.

Regarding adults, the mean heights of men and women differed significantly from such noted in 1976. Mean weight and body mass index (BMI) had increased, for men, from 47.9 to 48.9 kg, and from 18.2 to 19.1, respectively, and for women from 40.8 to 42.6 kg, and from 17.8 to 19.0, respectively. There was no rise in average blood pressure levels. Mean serum cholesterol levels in adults compared with the value in the previous survey, had risen by 6.5%. This presumably was due in part to the introduction of milk into the diet. Mean haemoglobin levels of children rose from 12.9 to 14.1 g/dl, and of men from 14.7 to 15.6 g/dl, respectively. Peripheral blood films, made on 125 of the children and adults, were negative for malaria, trypanosomiasis and filaria. Swabs regarding sexually transmitted diseases, gonorrhoea, chlamydia, and trichomonas, were negative.

While both children and adults were lean, they appeared to be in good health with no evidence of specific nutritional disease. The skin, hair and mucous membranes showed no abnormality, and there was no clinical evidence of anaemia. The teeth were worn, often down to the gums, but there was very little evidence of caries. The level of physical activity was high, especially in women who had to gather food, and examination of the cardiovascular and central nervous systems revealed no abnormality.

Namibian San

The nutrition and health status of 51 adult San, in northeast Namibia, was also investigated in 1989 [10]. This community of people had been forced to abandon their traditional hunter-gatherer lifestyle, and had merged with pastoral-urbanized Hereros of Bantu origin. Their diet was very unbalanced and consisted very largely of refined white maize meal; it was the only food consistently eaten. Because of the arid nature of the region, the maize meal had to be purchased. Mixed with water, it was cooked in cast iron pots over wood fires. The porridge was usually flavoured with some sugar, salt, or, occasionally, with fat derived from milk or cooked beef, which had been bartered from Herero herdsmen. Meals, such as these were usually eaten in communal gatherings between 2 and 3 times a day.

During the period of 3-day diet recall, only 3 San had eaten meat; the remainder generally obtained small quantities towards the end of the month when they had some money. Unlike Hereros, 50% of San denied ever having drunk fresh milk, and 30% occasionally obtained sour milk. During the recall period only 20% had a milk product in their diet. None had eaten vegetables, and 45% claimed never to have eaten fruit. During the rainy season, November to March, wild leafy vegetables were used to flavour porridge; otherwise only onions, cabbage and bananas were purchased by some at the end of the month. No traditional foods had been collected from the land, and hunting was not considered for the provision of food. Locally brewed cereal-based beer was very popular with the men. When it was available, it generally replaced part of the already inadequate diet. Excessive consumption occurred particularly at weekends; 50% of men interviewed on Monday had consumed between 2 and 4 litres/day with little food, and many still had signs of intoxication at the time of the interview. The beer consumption by women was considerably less.

The observations made showed that the nutrition and health of the San who have abandoned their traditional way of life, and were desperately poor, had deteriorated. Not one overweight San was seen. No female was obese, indeed, if anything, women were thinner than men. Oral hygiene was uniformly poor. Most of the old people were either partially or totally edentulous, any remaining teeth being loose. Gingivitis was also common. While clinical manifestations of nutritional deficiencies were difficult to identify, the skin and mucosal changes seen were possibly related to combined deficiencies of protein and vitamins A and C, whereas anaemia was associated with folate deficiency. Low plasma albumin concentrations were considered to be an index indicative of chronic disease.

Cape Town San

A similar study conducted by one of us in 1993 [11] in another small, displaced San community living in Ceres (250 km north of Cape Town) has shown that their diet was similarly unbalanced and was characterized by a very low daily energy intake ($<5,500$ kJ; $<1,300$ kcal), an almost complete lack of fruit and vegetables and a high consumption of refined carbohydrates. Biochemically, they all had an inadequate protein intake and multiple vitamin deficiencies. Oral hygiene was very poor, dental caries were common as was tuberculosis, asthma among the children, and chronic bronchitis.

Comment

Clearly, a high measure of everyday good health is compatible with the diet and manner of existence described of the San who still subsist as in the past. However, the plight of the modern San in Namibia and Cape Town is grave and their future bleak. This population, in the changed circumstances, is not likely to survive as an independent ethnic group, and almost inevitably will become absorbed into local African/Western communities, with further deterioration in health.

Pedi Africans

These people, who form part of the Sotho-speaking people, occupy various rural regions in Northern Transvaal (fig. 1). General information was published on the past food habits, for a group of Pedi living in the Pietersburg district [12]. Two meals were eaten daily; breakfast was about 11 a.m., and the second meal at sunset. Each meal included a cereal food, a relish, and vegetables. Home-pounded cereal products were preferred, 'kaffir corn', millet, or sweet reed. Frequently, jugo and mung beans, introduced from India, were eaten, with peanuts. The relish included fresh vegetable leaves (morogo), sometimes mixed with pumpkin seeds, and morula nuts and water melon. At times, beetles and mopani worms were included. Home-made beer was taken intermittently throughout the day by the men. Meat was seldom available. Beverages consumed consisted virtually of sour milk and cereal. Morula beer is very potent and apt to make one 'cause bodily harm to others' when one is under its influence.

In 1959, a comprehensive investigation of the Pedi people was made [13]. It was found that the women were the chief tillers of the ground, but because they were prohibited from dealing with cattle, the men perforce had to plough the land. Once it was cleared of trees and stones, its cultivation lay in the hands of the women. Fertilizer was not used, nor was cattle manure spread on the land, because women were barred from the cattle kraal.

The chief crops were *Sorghum vulgare,* i.e. 'kaffir corn', millet, maize, cow pea, sweet reed, Njugo beans, mung beans, gourds, water melon, and pumpkin. Rainfall was uncertain, so that the land had to be tilled and weeded regularly in order to harvest a crop. Numerous wild plants and fruits were eaten, and some were dried for winter use. Domestic animals included cattle, sheep, goats, donkeys, dogs, and cats. Edible insects such as caterpillars, mopani worms, beetles, locusts, ants, and termites were gathered. The food described protected these people from deficiency diseases such as kwashiorkor and pellagra. When maize was increasingly introduced, being deficient in niacin and tryptophan, these diseases began to become common.

Dwellings were not built near water, for they would be too vulnerable to any enemy. Large clay pots were used to fetch water; this was the duty of the women and girls. Sometimes the water source would be some distance away, and it would be shared by the animals. About 15 litres were needed for a household per day. As for cooking, gourd shells and a three-legged iron 'kaffir pot', were used.

Traditionally, there was profound paternal respect. One manifestation was for the head of the house to have delicacies reserved for him, even by the herd boys after a day's hunting. Well-cooked food was an accepted norm. Women and children ate after the men had finished. Food was prepared primarily for the man. Since women and children ate what was left over, it will be apparent that in times of scarcity, they suffered thereby. The Pedi people were reported as kind and sociable, and given to warm hospitality. A sheep or goat would be slaughtered to welcome a relative. Food was shared; even children were taught to share everything; it was considered a bad deed to be selfish.

As to meal times, there were 2 meals a day, at noon and at night. Sitting on the ground, the food was served cold and eaten using their fingers; hot foods were considered bad for the teeth. The main food at both meals was porridge. There were three kinds, sorghum ('kaffir corn'), millet, and maize; the latter was preferred. A relish of vegetables or fish was prepared as a side dish. When eating, a ball of maize meal the size of an hen's egg was rolled and then dipped into the relish. There was no seasoning with the porridge, but generous amounts of salt were added to the relish. Porridge was also prepared with 'kaffir beans', and Njugo beans. A large portion was considered sufficient for the day. Porridges were also made from 'kaffir melon'; thin porridge was ladled into a bowl and served hot, perhaps once daily and was greatly enjoyed.

Among children the most common disease was gastroenteritis. Among adults, diseases included helminthiasis, pneumonia, scabies, ringworm, tropical ulcers, tuberculosis, and venereal diseases.

Recent Changes in Pattern of Foodstuffs
Starting in 1920–1930, there were major changes. Sorghum was replaced by maize meal. Men went to towns and cities for work. New, but not necessarily better, feeding habits were acquired, often resulting in a lower consumption of minerals and vitamins. The modern diet of Pedi farm workers was described [13] in 1959:

Beverages: Fermented gruel was still commonly consumed. Observations indicated that the local African was rapidly becoming a tea drinker, and despite its high ruling price, there was a keen and general demand for it. Also becoming popular were mineral waters, including Coca-Cola. A very popular snack was a bottle of lemonade and a raisin bun, or half loaf of white bread.

Cereals: The survey revealed that cereal meal porridge, together with meat, constituted virtually the entire diet of the local African farm worker. This was largely due to the fact that both mealie meal and meat were supplied as free rations. It was submitted, however, that, even if supplies had to be bought, mealie meal would still form the basis of their diet. As indicated previously, the African has developed a preference for refined white mealie meal.

Bread: The survey revealed that bread had become a common foodstuff. As with mealie meal, preference was given to the white refined article. There was also a regular, although not big, demand for the cheaper brands of biscuits.

Meat: This food figured prominently in the local diet, for, as mentioned, African employees had started to receive a ration of meat, free, 4 times per week. Additional supplies would be bought at the store. Although canned meat (bully beef) was accepted readily, the demand was limited because of the cheapness of fresh meat.

Fish: Although the Pedi tradition forbade fish as food, there was a tendency then to accept it as such, especially the article canned in tomato sauce.

Eggs: Despite the fact that the majority owned fowls, eggs were seldom eaten. The reason for this was that an egg was regarded as a potential fowl, which was of far greater consequence.

Milk and milk products: These were little consumed, due to shortage of supplies. Condensed milk, which was used exclusively in tea and coffee, was bought regularly. As to butter and cheese consumption, as in the traditional diet, the amounts eaten were low. The consumption of sugar was still low.

Vegetables: Those cultivated and indigenous included, tomatoes, cabbages, onions, potatoes, and especially sweet potatoes; which were rapidly gaining favour in the local African diet. What was to be deplored, however, was the tendency to ignore the very valuable and abundant supplies of indigenous spinaches (morogo).

The tradition of 2 meals per day was still usual. Thus of 2,420 meal-days surveyed, in 1,078 (i.e. 44.5%) there was no food consumed before noon, and 1,405 (i.e. 58%) had no food after the evening meal.

This survey, therefore, indicated a disconcerting decline in the serving of traditional foods dishes. Thus, whilst baker's bread was used on 533 occasions, the traditional *dinkgwa* (cereal meal 'breads') was served only 19 times. Similarly, tea was served 1,125 times, and the traditional *metôgô* (non-intoxicating beverages) only 759 times. In the traditional dietary of the Pedi, morogo was a more popular staple food than meat. Yet, the survey indicated that meat was served 3,458 times and morogo 757 times. This was largely because meat was supplied to the households, whereas spinach had to be collected from the veld. In this regard, the continued consumption of insect dishes was explained by the fact that cured mopani worms were available at the co-operative store in the village. Remarkably, the relaxation in traditional feeding among the local Africans has been attributed to the indolence of the women, who now accepted the food provided as sufficient for their family's needs. Furthermore, there has been an unfortunate and completely unjustified tendency to discredit indigenous foods.

As to dietary balance, the survey revealed that, although there was a slight tendency to eat more than two different foods simultaneously, the traditional two-dish meal still prevailed, namely, a bulky carbohydrate-rich porridge, supplemented with a protein-containing relish. Of the possible 4,840 noon and evening meals, 3,197 (i.e. 66%) consisted of only porridge and meat, and in the case of one group studied, these foods constituted 93.8% of their regular meals.

Table 3. Recommended minimum daily ration scale for farm labourers

	Males	Females
Skim milk powder, g, or	40	40
Skim milk, ml	400	400
Meat, fish, eggs, cheese, g	65	65
Dry beans, peas, nuts, g	55	55
Fresh vegetables, including potatoes, sweet potatoes, amadumbes (tubers), g	335	335
Margarine, g	25	20
Oil, ml	10	10
Brown or whole-wheat bread, g	210	180
Cereal products, mainly maize, g	530	370
Sugar, g	40	30
Coffee and tea, g	7	7
Salt, g	15	15
Condiments, etc. per week, g	40	40
Energy value, kJ	13,000	10,500
kcal	3,200	2,500

In 1969, another study [14] on the dietary habits of Pedi children revealed that at breakfast the majority had porridge, morogo, and bread, and a third had tea. A few had eggs or meat. A fifth had nothing. For supper, the majority ate porridge and morogo. A tenth had meat, very few had milk or an egg. Other foods eaten included potatoes, and soup. Very occasional foods included sweets and cool drinks.

In 1970, the Department of Health [15] defined the provision of supplementary food to workers on farms (table 3). The energy value calculated for males was 13,000 kJ (3,200 kcal), and for females, 10,500 kJ (2,500 kcal). Fresh vegetables could be replaced in part, by the same weight of fresh fruit and/ or by dehydrated vegetables, at the rate that 5 g dehydrated vegetables = 70 g fresh vegetables. Bread could be replaced by other cereal products; 100 g bread = 70 g cereal products. It was stated that preference, as far as possible, should be given to unrefined cereal products. The ration for cereal products includes the mean for *mahewu* and other such drinks.

Venda Africans

In 1971, a detailed study of Venda Africans, who live in Northern Transvaal, was made [16]. Most of the land of these people lies in the Tropic of Capricorn, and it enjoys a climate warmer than much of the rest of the

Transvaal (fig. 1); hence there are tropical fruits and vegetation. At the time of the investigation, home-pounded maize was the staple food, indeed, only 2% of the people studied consumed bread. Consumption of meat, and also of milk, was irregular. Vegetable consumption was high, although that of fruit was very low; actually, the men considered fruit to be suitable only for women and children. The consumption of indigenous foods was not mentioned. People ate 2 meals a day, the first at noon and the main meal at sunset. Energy consumption, also protein consumption, mostly of plant origin, was considered satisfactory. Animal fat intake was low. Sugar consumption too was very low. Vitamin C was derived almost entirely from vegetables.

In 1993, a study in a rural area of Venda was made [17] at Tshikundama-lema, a tribal area near Sibasa, capital of the region. In the area studied the climate was hot and dry. The land was mainly bushveld with a variety of trees, sandy soil and few natural resources. There were still no tarred roads, railway, post offices, telephones, electricity, regular sanitation nor running water. The terrain is mountainous and communication remains difficult. Cultivation is wholly for food consumption, and not for income. As in other African societies, the women do most of the agricultural work. They fetch water daily from the river, besides carrying out their family and household duties.

This investigation took place during October, after the long dry winter and before locally grown vegetables and veld spinaches and fruits became available. Thus, it was at a time of the year when the smallest variety of foods was consumed. The study included 61 subjects, 20 men and 41 women. Their average ages were 36.6 ± 10.0 and 33.0 ± 6.9 years, respectively. The authors reported that the diet consumed was fairly monotonous. The meal times, and their patterns, remained much the same as those described earlier [16]. A porridge of maize meal and *morogo* (green leafy vegetable) was eaten more than once daily, sometimes alternately with other traditional maize dishes. It was cooked with beans, peanuts or pumpkin. Peanuts, which were locally grown, were well liked and eaten often. Tea was the usual beverage. Brown bread was available sometimes, and was taken daily by some, without the addition of margarine or other fat. Dried mopani worms were considered a great delicacy by half the population and were taken once a week or so. Locusts, abundant in the spring, were eaten by 38% of the subjects studied. Some fruits, available at that time, were eaten 4 or 5 times a week, a remarkable change from the past. Most people drank *maphapfe,* which is home brewed beer, and *mabundu,* which is a thin fermented maize porridge; these were taken throughout the day, starting at breakfast time. Fish was seldom eaten, once or twice a month. Rice was eaten on Sundays. Meat, chicken, beef or goat, like eggs, were eaten 2 or 3 times a week. Wild plants or 'spinaches' (*imifino*), were important articles of their diet.

In terms of dietary intake, carbohydrate intake was high; in only 6 of the 61 subjects studied, did carbohydrates supply less than 70% of the total daily energy intake. The intake of dietary fibre was not as high as expected, an average of 21 g daily. Sugar in tea was usual. The diet was low in fat, supplying an average of 21% energy, with a high polyunsaturated/saturated fatty acid ratio (P/S), which was contributed mainly by the consumption of peanuts, some fat in meat, and occasionally sunflower oil. Calcium and iron intake was higher than usual, on account of a high intake of spinaches (*imifino*). This wild leafy plant contains 264 mg calcium and 6.1 mg iron per 100 g fresh weight. A more than adequate intake of vitamin A was attributable to the *morogo* (a wild spinach), which provides 966 retinol equivalents of vitamin A per 100 g uncooked weight. In comparison with recommended dietary allowances (RDAs) [18], mean intakes of vitamin D, B_6, and folic acid were low in both men and women. Vitamin C levels were also low due to the season. In brief, the diet described was considered to be reasonably well balanced. The intake of micronutrients, were likely to be much higher during the summer months when more vegetables and fruits were available.

The BMI of men and women averaged 22.5 ± 3.1 and 25.4 ± 4.2, respectively. Average systolic blood pressure for men and women was 125.8 ± 18.7 and 110.0 ± 7.8 mm Hg, respectively, and diastolic pressure 74.7 ± 10.2 and 66.8 ± 6.9 mm Hg, respectively. Percentages with hypertension (WHO criteria) [19] were 15 and 0 for men and women, respectively. Haemoglobin values averaged 12.3 and 10.8 g/dl for men and women, and serum cholesterol level 4.7 ± 1.1 and 4.4 ± 1.3 mmol/l, respectively.

Smoking practice was moderate in men, but absent in women, who, however, were fond of snuff. Helminthic infections were not tested for, although they are likely to be low in the highveld, in comparison to the situations in the lowveld, e.g., in areas in Eastern Transvaal and KwaZulu/Natal, where schistosomiasis and hookworm infestations are near endemic [20].

Xhosa Africans

The regions of the previous so-called homelands of the Transkei and the Ciskei are situated in the south-east of South Africa (fig. 1). The population is South Nguni people, the Pondo, Thembu, and Xhosa. The climate is temperate, Mediteranean, and there is adequate rainfall. The land consists mainly of rural grasslands. The produce includes tomatoes, pineapples, vegetables, citrus fruit, dairy farming, and goat rearing. There are Boer goats for meat, and Angoras for mohair.

Dietary surveys made in 1967 and 1972 [21] found that maize was eaten daily, 'kaffir corn' was only used by 31% of people and not on a daily basis. It was, however, used by a high percentage of people for beer-brewing. Meat (goats, sheep, small animals, birds, chicken) was not eaten more than once a month. As cattle represent wealth, they were rarely killed. Fresh milk was rarely used. In some areas, pregnant women were forbidden to drink milk and beer and to eat meat and eggs. Women ate edible wild plants (*imifino*) picked in the veld, but this habit was not shared by the men.

A typical diet consisted of coffee and tea, sour porridge in the mid-morning, samp and beans or pumpkin, mixed with mealie meal or *imifino* in the afternoon and thick crumbly mealie meal porridge with sour milk in the evening [21].

Further dietary surveys were done between 1981 and 1987 [22–25]. The first survey [22], made in the ex-Transkei, was undertaken on 212 children aged at 2–4 years, 328 aged 6–9 years and 140 school pupils older than 16 years of age. Maize was the staple foodstuff. The methods of preparation differed from district to district. Various legumes were popular. The main vegetable was pumpkin, which grew among the mealies, and which has good keeping qualities. Wild plant leaves and weeds (*imifino*) were popular. Most households owned a few cattle, sometimes goats and sheep. The number of cattle possessed gave prestige to the household. Unproductive animals were not slaughtered, neither was improvement in milk production ever considered. Only small amounts of milk and meat were included in the daily diet.

There were the usual 2 meals a day, the evening one being the main one. It was considered that the majority of people had adequate energy and protein intake. Vitamin A was supplied by yellow maize and pumpkin. The only occasional, but at times, excessive consumption of meat, resulted in consider-able variability in vitamin A intake, derived chiefly from the cherished liver, which became available when an animal died or was killed for a festive occasion. Animal protein made up a total of 20% protein. There was a very low intake of calcium. It was considered that there were long-standing deficiencies of nicotinic acid, riboflavin and ascorbic acid.

The dietary survey in 1984 [23] was undertaken at the request of the ex-Ciskeian authorities. The groups studied included 67 children aged 6–23 months, 148 at 2–3 years, at 7–8 years, 118 schoolchildren, and 44 lactating mothers. Of the total daily energy intake, cereals provided 67–76%, sugar 6–9%, and fruit 1% (table 4). Energy intake for all of the groups studied approximated to the RDAs [18]. Protein contributed 11% to the total daily energy in the 3 older age groups and was derived mainly from cereals.

Of the school-going children, 28% lay under the 5th centile of US NCHS reference standards [26]. Of the younger children, 1.1% were wasted and stunted. This situation was similar to that of other groups of rural children who have been studied elsewhere in the country. The diet of lactating mothers was considered to be inadequate, in that the intakes of most nutrients were

Table 4. 24-Hour recall of food intake and diet history of rural Africans in the Ciskei

Cereals	Maize, wheat and sorghum
Other plant foodstuffs	Cake, biscuit, commerical soups, thickened gravy, sorghum beer
Milk	Fresh, sour, evaporated and powdered cow's milk, goat's milk, sheep's milk, with some cheese and custard
Other	Meat and fish of all kinds (fresh and tinned), eggs and Pro-Nutro
Legumes	Dried beans, dry peas and soya beans
Vegetables	Potatoes, sweet potatoes and green mealies
Other foods	Tomato and onion gravy and home-made soups, and many types of fresh and canned fruits
Fat	Margarine, plant fat, lard, oil
Sugar	Added to most carbohydrate-rich foods, mainly as simple sugars, e.g. cold drinks, jam, sweets and jelly; honey and condensed milk were also consumed

General meal of rural Africans

Breakfast	Soft maize porridge, with or without milk
Midday and evening	Maize, samp and beans, crumbly or stiff maize meal porridge, and occasionally vegetables including potato, with sour milk, soup or meat.
	Bread, mainly home-made maize meal, sometimes formed the entire meal, or was eaten with or between meals

well below the RDAs. Notwithstanding, breastfeeding was usual, and practiced for long periods.

The third survey in 1985 [24] determined the nutritional status of 1,725 Zulu adults in KwaZulu. Thirty-nine percent of the males were undernourished and 17% of the females were obese. The staple diet consisted of maize meal, eaten 2–3 times per day. Bread was consumed once a day and rice 1–2 times per month. Meat and meat products were used 2–3 times per month and a large seasonal variation was found in vegetable intake. Eighty-seven percent of the diet was from carbohydrate (mostly refined) with a low contribution to daily energy by protein (7%) and fat (6%). Fibre intake was < 10 g/day and 20% of respondents complained of constipation.

The fourth survey in 1987 [25] studied the diet in 578 rural households in three districts of the ex-Transkei. It was found that about one third of families had below-minimum energy intake, and the majority consumed a diet deficient in protein, minerals and vitamins. Between 50 and 60% of the respondents did not consume meat, fish, milk or eggs. Vegetables were added to only 23% of meals and legumes to 32% of meals. An interesting observation in one of the districts was that 'some respondents were found to be selling vegetables to buy bread and maize'!

Comment on Rural Africans

It will be apparent that the rural dwellers of the past had two major health/disease problems. The first problem lay in securing enough food to eat. If there was enough of it and it was varied, as was usually the case, then the diet was certainly compatible with sustained good health. The second problem concerned the very young, among whom high losses were apt to occur at weaning time, from infections as well as from inadequate or incorrect feeding practices.

In later years, however, when there were increased purchases of food, and much less reliance on home-grown or gathered foodstuffs, the change in diet was accompanied by deterioration in health. This has been particularly well manifested by the experience of the San in Namibia and in Cape Town. But in all of the rural groups on whom there is information, there have been rises in admissions to rural hospitals, respecting increases in hypertension-related diseases and in diabetes.

Urban Africans

Cape Town
Nutrition/Health Study in 1974

Early, published information on the subject is very limited. In 1974, a survey was published [27] on 80 families of Africans who lived in Guguletu (fig. 1), a large African township near Cape Town. Five groups of people were questioned regarding their eating patterns. Group A were well-off, and included university lecturers, shopkeepers, taxi drivers, and nurses. Group B were garage attendants, road workers, hospital porters and caretakers. Group C were poor families with a low income, and included old age pensioners, and fathers who were unemployed or were away from home. Group D included 20 families who had moved recently from a coastal town. Group E was composed of 20 men who lived in bachelor quarters, where 2 or 3 occupied a single room.

Most of the staple foods were purchased for cash at a supermarket near the railway station. There was a great disparity between prices in the supermarket and those in the local trading stores, being sometimes as much as a third or more higher in the latter. Obviously, this situation was disadvantageous for the poorer segment who could not afford transport, or who were too old to walk a distance and carry the provisions.

Primus stoves were the usual mode of heating and cooking. A few households possessed a stove which was also used for heating; only a few had electricity; there was one that had gas. The three-legged iron pots were employed for festive occasions. Aluminium saucepans were the usual cooking vessels. Heavy cast iron pots or cauldrons in a variety of sizes were used for baking bread, and for roasting meat or chicken. Storage facilities depended on income; only a few households had a refrigerator. A basin of cold water was used to keep milk cool, and a tin box under the bed was used as a store for dry goods. Metal-lined bins were used for keeping samp and maize meal dry and vermin-free.

General Dietary Practices

As to the daily eating pattern, a hurried cup of tea at about 5 a.m. constituted breakfast for most of the adults before setting off to work. For breakfast, children had maize meal porridge or bread. Snacks of bread or leftovers were eaten at home at any time of the day. At work, men took a pause from work from 9 to 10 a.m. for tea and bread, with polony, or a tin of pilchards. Sometimes they roasted some meat over a fire if they were working on the roads or were involved in construction works.

The principal meal of the day was in the evening. In general, coarse (samp) or refined maize meal was the main constituent. Some meat or a relish from vegetables might be served, with or without beans. Soups were made from split peas or lentils, during the winter; such, provided a good meal. Peanuts were immensely popular with all children and adults. On Sunday, many households had a western type of breakfast, or had porridge or cold cereal, which was followed by bacon and eggs and sausage. Sunday lunch was a full meal which consisted of meat, rice and potatoes. Only at weekends did the majority of households have vegetables such as squash, pumpkin, cabbage, tinned peas, or beans in tomato sauce, or had pudding, which consisted of jelly with custard, or tinned fruit, peaches or guavas. Trifle was a special treat. Soft drinks usually accompanied lunch on Sunday.

Bread was a favoured food, because of its availability at all times. Other popular foods were quickly prepared food such as Minit meal and Minit samp. As a drink, tea was tending to replace *maheu,* a non-alcoholic maize gruel, as it was prepared quickly, whereas the gruel took 12 h before being ready for consumption. Sugar was used a great deal, 5 lb (2.25 kg) were bought weekly (this implies a consumption of 50 g or so daily for each person).

Rice and potatoes were becoming more popular; these were eaten on Sundays in well-off households. Fresh fish was difficult to obtain, but fish and chips were increasing considerably in popularity. Fruit was sold by hawkers, particularly outside schools at 'break' times. Beer, brewed by local shebeens, was popular, since the municipal sorghum beer was disliked. Shebeens were a regular feature in township life. Many Africans were noted as showing an increasing fondness for fat, and a tendency to use oil for cooking. Fat was often added to samp and beans, when there was no meat. Of relevance, urban

Africans had no access to various seeds or insects (e.g. locusts); these have a high fat content and are very popular in the rural areas.

Children were fed by a schoolfeeding scheme. The food consisted of bread and soup, or of milk on alternate days, during lunch breaks. Elderly women would sell chicken legs, hard boiled eggs and fat cakes (vetkoek), also mineral drinks at break. Young children were specially favoured by all, and tremendous care was lavished on babies by African mothers who, at weaning time, would often purchase proprietary baby-food preparations.

Typical Diet of a Poor Family

Tea was served with fresh milk and sugar at 5 a.m. Women and children usually ate an early morning meal when the men had gone to work. Bread was baked or steamed at home, and maize meal eaten, prepared with the addition of sugar. During the day, tea, bread and any left-overs from the previous evening were consumed. As mentioned, children had the benefit of schoolfeeding. People who previously enjoyed fish at the coast when the boats were unloaded, now had to change to eating meat. Supper consisted of samp and beans, served once a week with offal and cooking fat. Chicken and vegetables were eaten only on Sunday.

Typical Diet of Middle-Income Group

After the father had left for work, the family, for breakfast, had bread, maize meal cooked with sugar and milk, also bread and leftovers, sometimes with eggs. Schoolchildren might be given a few cents for 'tuck'. In addition, there was schoolfeeding. Supper started with a thick soup in winter, which was made using meat bones; the soup included beans and split peas, which was served 3 times a week. This course was followed by beef brisket, sausages or mince, rice or potatoes. For Sunday, lunch there was brisket, beans, samp, cabbage or rice and potatoes.

Well-To-Do Families

Their pattern of meals was similar to that of the white population, save that cheese was rarely eaten. Cooking oil and peanuts were the main source of unsaturated fat. Margarine was seldom eaten.

Nutrient Intake

Carbohydrates provided between 62 and 70% of total energy intake; that, provided by protein was 11–13%. Fat supplied 15–20% of the total daily energy in the poorer segments, and 30% in well-to-do families. Crude fibre intake was 4–6 g, i.e. approximately 12–18 g dietary fibre per person in all groups, save among bachelors whose intake was about 10 g crude fibre, i.e. about 30 g dietary fibre. Calcium intake was low (range 169–391 mg/day), but no detectable deficiency was apparent. Whereas the intake of vitamins was satisfactory among persons in households in good socioeconomic circumstances, there were low intakes in the poorer families. Nutrition education was recommended at the time.

Nutrition/Health Study in 1990

A survey carried out recently on the urban African population (BRISK study) [28, 29] in Cape Town included 983 men and women. The study was undertaken primarily because of major current interest in the relationship between progressive urbanization/industrialization and changes in mortality and morbidity. Healthwise, it was noted that while frequencies of infectious diseases were declining, those of chronic disorders/diseases, namely, dental caries, obesity in women, hypertension, diabetes, and accidents as well as other trauma, were increasing. Although previous studies have indicated that the traditional food of Africans is low in fat, high in complex carbohydrates and in dietary fibre, with urbanization, it has become apparent that there is an increased consumption of energy, fat, animal protein, salt and sugar, but a decrease in dietary fibre.

The investigation showed milk intake to be low, less than half of the recommended portions of milk per day. Cheese intake was negligible; indeed, 42% took no dairy products during the previous 24 h. Meat intake was adequate for men and women, 2.6 and 1.9 portions daily as compared to the 2 portions that are recommended. Meat provided more total fat than the fat group of foodstuffs. Only about half of the recommended 4 portions of fruit and vegetables were eaten daily; indeed, 29% of the subjects had none at all. Understandably, there were low intakes of vitamin C and of carotene. Indeed, in a subsample of 169 subjects, deficiency, on biochemical grounds, of riboflavin, thiamin, vitamin B_6, vitamin C and folic acid were recorded in a significant proportion of the subsample [30].

Regarding cereals, white bread was favoured over brown. A fifth of white bread was homemade. Men and women respectively had 11 and 8 portions daily which exceeds the recommended minimum of 4 portions. Legumes, which are popular in the traditional African diet, were now low in consumption. As to fat, the added fat did not exceed the recommended number of portions.

Meal Patterns

While the composition of daily meals in general, and their timing followed the patterns described earlier [27], this more recent evidence clearly indicates the groups' tendency towards the diet and practices of the white population.

Dietary Intake

Mean energy intake fell below the RDAs for all groups; 53% of respondents had an intake below 67% of RDAs. Total fat contributed 27% to the total daily energy. Cholesterol intake averaged 241 mg daily. Protein, half of plant and half of animal origin, contributed 14% of the total energy. Total carbohydrate contributed 62% and sugar intake 10% of the daily energy. Alcohol contributed 2.8% of the daily energy for men, and 0.8% for women. Dietary fibre averaged 21 and 16 g for men and women, respectively.

Health/Ill-Health Changes

Accumulating evidence indicates that these dietary changes are associated with rises in serum cholesterol level. Also revealed are rises in weight, especially among women, in mean blood pressure and prevalence of hypertension, in smoking practices in men, not women, and a trend to lesser physical activity in men at work. Low fruit and vegetable intakes indicated low intakes of vitamins A and C. The 1974 study [27] also commented on the inadequate intake of vegetables. Actually, market research has shown a further decrease since then, for the drought has forced prices to rise. As comparisons of intakes elsewhere, in Glasgow in 1990, there was a poor consumption of vegetables and fruit, 200 g/day [31]. In the USA, consumption was 340 g/day/capita in the NHANES study; only 10% consumed 5 servings [32]. A WHO report recommends a daily intake of 400 g of vegetables (excluding potatoes) and fruit [33].

Johannesburg

Meal Patterns of Africans in Dobsonville, Soweto

In another recent survey [34] conducted in 1993 in Dobsonville, Soweto, it was found that there were three distinct classes of urban Africans:

The *professional class* ate a westernized diet, but retained their traditional likings for mealie meal porridge (hard) or pap (soft). This class included university lecturers, teachers, and businessmen. Breakfast consisted mainly of soft porridge with fresh milk, and sugar, or cornflakes. A cooked breakfast consisted of eggs and bacon, polony or cheese, bread with margarine, jam, peanut butter or fishpaste. Tea was taken with milk and sugar. At midday, a light meal was consumed made up of sandwiches, or stiff porridge, with tinned fish, bread, eggs, polony and salad. In the evening, a cooked meal of rice, meat, vegetables, macaroni, sausages or fish was eaten. At weekends, the Sunday midday meal was more special and included meat, vegetables, rice, pasta, fruit or fruit juices, jelly and custard.

The *middle class* included people with a regular salary such as police officers, post office workers and machine operators. Their breakfast consisted of maize or maltabella porridge, with milk and sugar, bread, peanut butter, jam or marmite; tea with milk and sugar. At midday, bread rolls, with any spread available, or tinned fish or polony was eaten. The evening meal consisted of sour porridge, meat (offal), sausage, cabbage, mealie rice, samp and beans, tinned fish, pap and cabbage, tomato and gravy. At weekends, the meal was similar to that on weekdays, but sometimes included soup or fish and chips.

The *poor class* included people with intermittent employment, workers on daily contracts, or those delivering goods. Breakfast was mostly tea with sugar and bread with morogo and cabbage, sometimes, margarine, no milk, occasionally condensed milk, soft porridge. The midday meal included pap and cabbage or tinned fish, bread, or any leftovers. In the evening, pap with a variety of accompaniments, tomato, dumplings, offal or potato were eaten. At weekends, perhaps rice with chicken livers, cabbage and potato were included in the meals.

African Informal Settlement (Squatter) Populations

'Squatter' is a name given to those who have lately arrived in the urban areas from rural areas or from neighbouring countries, in search of better living conditions than what they were experiencing, yet who are finding work and living accommodation almost non-existent. Consequently, such people have built shacks on any vacant ground, as near as possible to established residential areas. They usually have little or no running water, no proper sanitation, and hygienic conditions are, in general, very poor.

In 1991, a survey was undertaken [35] in a 'squatter' camp, Malukazi, near Durban (fig. 1). Average temperature in this coastal area is 21 °C, but during summer can often reach 30 °C or more. No family possessed a refrigerator; there was no electricity, nor cupboards, nor a cool place for storing food. A communal tap provided water for many. Very few owned the dwelling they were living in. The mother was the chief person to decide on the food purchased, and similarly she prepared the food, but the grandmother took her place in some cases. Very few grew any food; no space, was the reason given. Although Durban is a high fruit-producing area, only 16.9% had a fruit tree. According to custom, many believed that pork should not be given to children. Of the infants, 25.5% were exclusively breastfed, 17.0% bottlefed, and 54.4% breast and bottlefed.

Meals and Food Intake

The common foodstuffs eaten by preschool children were as follows: maize and maize products, condensed milk, sugar, jam, tea or coffee. Less commonly consumed foodstuffs included potatoes, vegetables, meat, white bread and saturated fats. Infrequent additions were fruit, curry and brown bread, and very rarely fish, rice, eggs, cow's milk, or fats such as butter and margarine. About 30% of the young children were underweight for age, according to NCHS reference standards, and 2–5% were stunted and wasted. While acute protein energy malnutrition was not common, chronic malnutrition was a problem.

Many factors were identified as contributory to the occurrence of malnutrition of the young child. These included socioeconomic status, availability of water and food, education of parents, particularly that of the mother, food distribution within the family, beliefs and traditional beliefs and taboos, methods of purchasing, preparation and storage of food and other health practices such as mother's time spent at home.

The older preschool child was the one most at risk for malnutrition, since a new baby may take priority in the family circle and, in the African community, the older child is not given any special place. For food availability, the father comes first and the children take second or third place in priority. These are the children, deprived in varying measure, who are most prone to infections, parasitic infestation, and accidents, especially in hot unhygienic conditions. While no detailed information on health/disease patterns was given in this survey, other studies have shown that common causes of admission of children to hospital in a similar area are gastroenteritis, pneumonia, nutritional deficiency diseases and trauma.

In 1994, a study on preschool children was reported [36], at Besters, another squatter area near Durban. The population was very poor, half of the men were unemployed. Unfortunately, little information was given on the diet consumed, although it is likely that it was much the same as that described in a squatter township [35] relatively nearby. The point of major interest was the finding that the numerous laboratory parameters which were determined lay within normal limits apart from low serum retinol levels, half of which values were <20 µg/dl. Of haemoglobin levels, 20% were <11 g/dl. Anthropometrically, while 27% were below the 5th centile of NCHS reference standards of height for age, 13% were below the weight for age level. No information was given on the clinical state or well-being of the children.

Pica Habits of African Women

Geophagy is the term given to the ingestion of soil, termite clay or other 'unnatural' food sources. The practice is very widespread throughout southern Africa, and has been excellently recorded after travels through five southern African countries [37]. Early explorers and missionaries reported the unusual practice of clay eating (pica) during pregnancy. It is certainly still widespread today, among both country and town expectant mothers. In a study in South Africa, made in 1985 [38], it was noted that 44% of the rural African women questioned regularly practised pica eating. Of the urban community, 39% did the same. The habit was not so widely practised among the Indian and Coloured mothers, 2 and 4%, respectively, while only 2% of white mothers partook of pica. The clay is only taken by pregnant women, and is discarded between pregnancies. In Malawi, it was reported that it would be very surprising if a pregnant woman did not eat clay; apparently, that is how you know you are pregnant. It has been claimed that the taste of clay can reduce the nausea, discomfort and vomiting of 'morning sickness'. Geophagy may continue throughout pregnancy and in some cases even afterwards.

In many parts of Africa, a lucrative trade exists among urban women, who sell the clay and termite soil in the city, having travelled to the rural areas to fetch it. Women wholesalers in Lusaka, Zambia, make a 500-mile round trip to the copper belt of Chingola, to buy clay. A woman will purchase up to four 50-kg sacks. White clay is more popular than the brown variety, but both command the same price. The clay is broken up into smaller pieces, to make a ready sale at retail stalls in big cities in southern Africa. The extent of the practice is not widely known by white physicians although they treat many African patients [37].

Some impression of the mineral benefits can be estimated by assuming a pregnant woman consumes 40–100 g clay/day, not an uncommon intake. White copper belt clay of this amount contributes 15 mg calcium, 48 mg iron, 42 µg zinc, as well as small amounts of copper, chromium, nickel, molybdenum. These amounts are nutritionally significant where dietary needs exist. For females, the white clay, at an upper consumption rate of 100 g/day, would supply 322% of RDA for iron, 70% copper and 43% of manganese [37].

Comment on Urban Africans

The urbanization of Africans has been accompanied by a number of major health/disease changes. In certain areas, reductions in the morbidity and mortality patterns among the very young were reported in 1980 [39]. Although many shortfalls from NCHS reference standards remain common and are indeed a cause for great concern in both rural and urban populations, their significance in terms of greater risk to ill-health has been questioned [40, 41]. The major changes which appear to be associated with alterations in diet and other environmental factors, concern the rises in dental caries [42], obesity in women [43], hypertension [44], diabetes [45], and of certain cancers, breast and prostate [46]. In this regard, it is interesting that the adverse transitional changes described, relating to increased proneness to diseases of prosperity, are particularly marked in some populations, such as Micronesian Nauruans. These people now have very high prevalences of obesity, 34% for women, and 35% for men; moreover, their prevalence of non-insulin-dependent diabetes is 13 times that of white Australians [47].

White Population

'Poor Whites', 1900–1950

The 'Poor White Problem' in South Africa [48] began to attract attention at the turn of the present century. The term was used to denote principally the economic and social regression of a considerable part of the white rural population. The groups included principally poor 'bywoners' or hired men on farms, owners of small holdings or of small undivided holdings of land, impoverished settlers, and the growing group of unskilled or poorly trained labourers and workers outside of farming. By the 1930s, of the total white population in the country at the time, 1,800,000, it was estimated that at least 300,000 were 'very poor'. Socioeconomically, 14% of families were in good circumstances, 24% in fair, 30% in poor and 34% 'very poor', i.e. the large majority were indigent. Their level of education in general was low. General health surveys showed a high birth rate, an average of 7 children per family, and a high mortality rate, an average of 1 in 7 children mentioned.

As to the diet consumed, it was found that in only a small proportion of the population was the *quantity* insufficient. Certainly, the food was monotonous and lacking in variety, especially with regard to vegetables. It was composed principally of cereals, potatoes, and sweet potatoes. The daily patterns of diets were reported as follows:

Good diet: Breakfast: porridge made from oatmeal or mealie meal, bread, wholemeal or white, butter, jam, some meat or tinned fish or egg, coffee with milk and sugar. Midday: soup, meat daily, three vegetables of the following – potatoes, cabbage, peas, green beans, carrots or pumpkin, and pudding or fruit. Evening: meat, cheese or egg, bread, butter, jam, coffee or tea with milk and sugar. Between meals: tea or coffee, milk and sugar, cake or biscuits, sweets or fruit.

Fair diet: Breakfast: porridge usually mealie meal, bread with butter or dripping, egg or jam, coffee, milk, sugar. Midday: meat most days, two vegetables – rice and potatoes, or sweet potatoes or pumpkin, fruit in season. Evening: usually soup, bread with butter or dripping, coffee or tea, milk and sugar. Between meals: tea or coffee, milk and sugar, biscuits, sweets occasionally.

Poor diet: Breakfast: 'Boer' bread – usually dry but occasionally with dripping or butter, coffee 'mixture' without milk but with sugar. Midday: meat once weekly, soup, dry bread, rice, sweet potatoes, or pumpkin, rarely green vegetables. Evening: as at breakfast. Between meals; dry bread or with dripping, black tea or coffee with sugar.

Very poor diet: Breakfast: dry 'Boer' bread, black coffee 'mixture', sugar. Midday: dry bread, sweet potatoes or pumpkin or mealies. Evening: as at breakfast. Between meals: often nothing; maybe fruit.

Health/Ill-Health

Concerning teeth, from the survey made, it was stated that 'careful inspection of the teeth revealed them to be not as a rule worse, but often showed a surprising lack of caries compared with the teeth of well-to-do children in the same schools'. However, there was a huge regional variation, e.g. in Karoo secondary schools 67% were caries-free, whereas at Langkloof schools, only 2.9% were caries-free. Undoubtedly, in some areas, a higher than average fluoride concentratioin in the drinking water contributed a measure of protection. From the heights and weights measured, it was not altogether surprising that the mean values for pupils aged 9–14 years were not significantly different from those depicted in the US NCHS reference values. However, boys of 15 years averaged 6.0 cm shorter and 4.6 kg lighter than NCHS reference values; in the case of girls, the data averaged 3.0 cm shorter but 4.0 kg heavier. Gastroenteritis and respiratory diseases were the primary causes of deaths of very young children. No data were given on the morbidity/mortality patterns in adults.

Present-Day Whites

The dietary habits, nutritional intake, anthropometry and associated biochemical parameters have been well documented in major investigations undertaken on the health/ill-health pattern of town dwellers in the Cape Province, the CORIS study [49, 50]. The general picture closely resembles that delineated in corresponding studies reported on populations in the UK and USA. It would appear from local investigations that few attempts are being made to conform to a 'prudent' diet, by lessening the intake of energy and of fat, and by increasing the consumption of cereal foods, vegetables and fruit.

Comment

The current diet of the white population and the non-dietary practices which concern smoking practice, alcohol consumption, and physical inactivity, could all be improved upon in order to avoid, or restrain, the chronic diseases of lifestyle. However, among all western populations, generally, there is a similar reluctance to conform to a 'prudent' diet [51]. That benefits can certainly result from dietary and non-dietary changes is well demonstrated by the better-than-average health scenarios of vegetarians [52], Seventh-Day Adventists [53], and Mormons [54].

Coloured Population

The Coloured people originated from four stocks: (1) slaves brought from East India to the Cape in the early 17th and 18th centuries; (2) Hottentots;

(3) Bushmen, and (4) whites. Populations 1 and 2 made the greatest contribution. Additionally, in recent times there has been interethnic group mixing with the African population. The Coloured people, evolving over a period of 250 years, while still being modified by outside influences, are now a relatively stabilized population. For many generations these people have lived in distinct residential areas mainly in the Cape Peninsula (fig. 1), but there are also small communities living in relatively distinct residential areas scattered throughout South Africa.

Dietary Patterns

Unfortunately, very little has been published regarding the meals and food habits of past generations of the Coloured population.

In 1990, an investigation on the anthropometric status and food intake of schoolchildren in the Richtersveld was reported [55]. This is an isolated semidesert mountainous area with few basic health facilities and where poverty is general. Goat farming is the major agricultural activity with the majority of the population owning these animals. As to foodstuffs, white sugar was the food item most frequently consumed by the participants. This was generally consumed with either tea or coffee and with a small amount of milk. Bread and margarine were the staple foods consumed frequently during the day, with goat's meat and rice being the most popular items at the main meal. No fruit and/or vegetables appeared among the most frequently consumed food items. Other sweet items such as jams, sweets, and cold drinks, were popular. A third to a half of the pupils, boys and girls, had heights and weights for age below the 5th centile of US NCHS reference standards. However, it is of importance that the low intake of most nutrients was not, in general, reflected by low values in biochemical blood investigations. Only in respect to red cell folate were levels abnormally low.

A study on various groups of 11-year-old children, including Coloured children, in the Western Cape was reported in 1989 [56]. In about a quarter of pupils, anthropometric measurements were below the 5th centile of US NCHS reference standards. The diet of the Coloured pupils was adequate in macronutrients, but for most mineral and vitamin intakes, levels were less than 67% of RDA.

In 1988, data on meals and nutritional intakes of a series of adult Coloured people in the Western Cape was reported [57]. The mean pattern indicated very little or no breakfast, midday consisting mainly of bread, a cooked supper, and heavy snacking between meals. The snacks frequently comprised sandwiches with meat balls, Vienna sausages, polony, eggs or cheese, or commercially fried fish and chips. Snacks also tended to supply large quantities of sugar and fat together with the more nutrient-rich foods. Of the foodstuffs, the main source of energy was the meat group which supplied 30%, followed by the cereal group, 24%, sugar 16%, and alcohol 4% of the total daily intake. The high animal protein and fat intake, supplying 37% of energy, reflects a typical western diet, despite the high polyunsaturated:saturated fatty acid ratio of 0.85. Sugar consumption was high and fibre intake low. An assessment of micronutrient intake revealed a low intake of all minerals (excluding iron and phosphorus in males) and vitamins (excluding nicotinic acid).

In a cross-sectional study of risk factors for coronary heart disease in a random sample of 976 urban Coloured adults, of the risk factors (hypercholesterolaemia, hypertension and smoking) one or more were present in 80% of men aged 45 years and older [58]. Smoking was the most common risk factor for both sexes. Almost 30% of women aged 45 years and older were hypertensive. Hypertension and smoking was the most common combination for men and hypertension and hypercholesterolaemia the most common for women.

Comment

In terms of nutrient intake, the Coloured population in measure are increasingly approaching the white population. With changes in diet, principally, with an increased intake of energy and fat, and with a rise in smoking practices among both men and women, also alcohol consumption, diseases such as diabetes and coronary heart disease and certain cancers, are now apparently as common as prevail among the white population.

Indian Population

Emigration of Indians to South Africa took place mainly before or soon after 1900, principally from south and south-east India, United Provinces, and around Bombay. Indians were brought in primarily as workers on sugar plantations. At present, about 70% of local Indians are Hindu, 20% Moslem, and 10% Christian. Most of these people live in cities or small towns. Of the approaching 1 million population, the majority live in Natal (fig. 1), particularly in the region of Durban [59].

Dietary Patterns and Intake
Unfortunately, there is no publication which described the dietary habits and meals of the early settlers, save that they tenaciously sought to retain their previous habits as far as possible. At present the diet varies. Broadly, Moslems usually are non-vegetarian, and eat all common foods, save pork. Some Hindus are vegetarian. Carbohydrate is supplied largely by rice, roti, white bread, potatoes and sugar. Fat is derived from *ghee* (produced by heating butter or

margarine and removing the sediment by filtering through cloth), although nowadays more from vegetable oils and fat spreads. Milk, pulses and cereals are chief sources of protein for Hindu vegetarians. For Hindu non-vegetarians, mutton, chicken, fish, eggs, pulses and cereals are the main sources of protein. Consumption of beef is forbidden by their religion. Additionally, for all populations, spices, chillies, garlic, ginger, and other flavourings are used as ingredients in everyday dishes [60, 61]. A more recent survey on Indian adolescents yielded similar information [62].

As to dietary intake, in a group of Indian male students in Durban [60], mean daily intake was: energy 8,600 kJ (2,043 kcal), protein 64 g, and fat 67 g. Speaking generally, carbohydrate foods contributed about 55–65% of energy, fat 25–30% and protein 10–12%.

The general patterns of meals among Indians in Lenasia, Johannesberg, are as follows:

Upper class: Breakfast includes tea/coffee with whole milk and sugar, toast (white) with butter or margarine, jam, peanut butter, biscuits, cakes, cereals; at midday, sandwiches (cheese, butter, polony), whereas the evening meal usually includes meat (mutton), vegetables particularly peas, beans, brinjals, tomato, onions, potatoes, roti (mainly white flour), salads, rice (white), fruit, apples, bananas and oranges. A high consumption of mangoes are also eaten (in season). Vegetarians would have pulses instead of meat.

Middle class: Their breakfast consists mainly of tea with whole milk and sugar, toast bread (white) with butter or margarine, jam, cereal. Midday sandwiches include cheese and tomato, polony or leftover curry with roti or bread. Housewives and schoolchildren would reheat left-over food. In the evening, roti, meat (mutton, chicken), fish, rice, vegetables particularly tomato, onions, potatoes, fruit 2–3 times per week, mainly apples, bananas make up the meal. Vegetarians would have pulses in tomato and onion gravy.

Lower class: Breakfast takes the form of tea with milk and sugar, bread and margarine. At midday, butter and jam sandwiches or leftovers in bread or roti are eaten. The evening meal consists of roti, meat (chicken) occasionally, onions, peas, beans, potatoes and brinjals; fruit is seldom eaten. A high intake of high fat maas (sour milk) is consumed.

Additionally, on Sundays most have their main meal at noon, rice dish 'biryani' with sour milk, salad, and dessert (seldom); on Saturdays, light snacks are eaten. The upper and middle class would buy convenience fast foods. Vegetarians, who are mainly Hindus, would eat the same foodstuffs as above, but include dahls, spinach and fruit, instead of meat. Savouries, such as pies and samoosas, are eaten by all, particularly on special occasions (the filling includes chicken, mutton, or vegetables; vegetarians would have a vegetable, potato, or cheese filling).

Most curries have a high amount of oil, and foods are highly spiced and overcooked. Yellow vegetables are seldom eaten. During Diwali and Eid (religious days), large amounts of fried foods, sweetmeats and savouries are consumed.

Health/Ill-Health

Among preschoolers, a number of studies have reported a high prevalence of low height-and-weight-for-age. Among school pupils, this lesser growth has also been reported [63]. Among older pupils, aged 17–18 years, when growth has ceased, shortfalls in height and weight are very common. Since this phenomenon also occurs among pupils in high socioeconomic circumstances, it is judged that a genetic element is in operation. The latter has also been observed among Indian immigrants in the UK [64].

Among adults, obesity in women is very common [65]. Diabetes is more common than it is among the white population [45]. The same applies regarding mortality from coronary heart disease [66]. This high rate, which also prevails among Indian immigrants in the UK, is not explicable on the basis of known risk factors [67]. All of the disorders/diseases mentioned are far more common than among people living in India and Pakistan.

Comment

Indians, when they first migrated to South Africa, strongly retained their previous dietary habits and practices. This retention has continued to a large extent. However, major changes have been rises in the intake of energy, fat, and protein, changes which, as described, have been associated with rises in the frequency of disorders/diseases of prosperity.

Discussion and Conclusions

In developing countries a marked population shift from rural to urban areas is seen. This transition has vast dietary implications with a shift from the traditional rural diet, high in fibre and low in cholesterol and animal fat, to an urban diet, characterized by the typical 'western' eating pattern of low fibre and high saturated fat and sugar. This is associated with an increased prevalence of chronic and degenerative diseases [68, 69].

The available evidence in South Africa indicates on the one hand that among African rural dwellers, traditional diets with varying modifications are still consumed, although more so in some regions than in others. On the other hand, among urban dwellers, changes have been proceeding relatively rapidly, such that even in Cape Town in 1978, both the food and nutrient composition

Table 5. Vital statistics of South African populations in 1980 and 1985

	Crude birth rate per 1,000 population		Infant mortality rate/1,000		Expectation at birth	
	1980	1985	1980	1985	1980	1985
Whites	16.5	16.3	13.1	9.3	70	71
Indians	24.0	22.5	24.4	16.1	65	67
Coloureds	27.8	27.6	60.7	40.7	58	61
Africans	40.0	39.5	70.0	61.0	55	62

in the somewhat small upper socioeconomic class were closely approaching that of the white population. As it was also shown in subsequent studies, the proportion consuming a near western diet has increased considerably. In brief, in urban areas and to a slight although varying extent in rural areas, the diet is changing from one, which, in pattern, could be regarded as a 'prudent' diet, to one which, in composition, is rapidly approaching a western diet.

The magnitude of the health/disease changes in African populations is often insufficiently appreciated [70]. It will be noted that with transition, the primary changes which have occurred have been (1) considerable improvements in vital statistics (table 5) [71]; (2) decreases in diet-related diseases in the poorer populations, particularly protein-energy malnutrition (PEM) and gastroenteritis, especially among the very young [39, 72], and (3) falls in birth rate as well as increased life expectancy (table 5), and simultaneously, increased occurrences, especially in urban dwellers, of the chronic diseases of prosperity [70, 73, 74].

However, despite these desirable changes, dental caries scores of 10- to 12-year-old urban African children, very low in the past, now *exceed* those of corresponding white children (table 6) [46, 70, 75]. Obesity, previously uncommon, has increased considerably in women, although not in men. Almost half of urban African women now have a BMI $\geq$ 30. As to blood pressure, although in rural areas levels have risen little, in urban areas the frequency of hypertension, 28% (WHO criteria), is now higher than that in the white population, 25%. As to diabetes, previously rare, in a survey made on rural elderly, the disease was detected in 7.5% [73]. In a recent study, at Hillbrow Hospital, Johannesburg, 6% of admissions of African adults was for diabetes [74]. As to diet-related cancers, while they were near absent in rural areas, rises are occurring in breast and prostate cancer, although not colon cancer [76, 77]. Yet even in urban areas, rates remain lower than those in the white

Table 6. Frequencies of some diseases of prosperity in South African populations

	Rural Africans	Urban Africans	Coloureds	Indians	Whites
Dental caries	+	+ + +	+ + +	+ + + +	+ + +
Femoral fractures	+	+	+ +	+ +	+ + + + +
Obesity (females)	+ +	+ + + +	+ + +	+ + +	+ + +
Hypertension	+	+ + + +	+ + + +	+ + +	+ + +
Diabetes	+	+ + +	+ + + +	+ + + + +	+ + +
Coronary heart disease	− [a]	+	+ + + +	+ + + + +	+ + + +
Stroke	+	+ +	+ + +	+ + +	+ +

[a] Implies that occurrence is rare.

population. Despite rises in serum cholesterol level, cases of coronary heart disease are extremely rare, indeed absent in villagers; and even in town dwellers, cases are few [78].

Non-dietary changes, particularly in the big cities, include diminished physical activity, and in men, increases in smoking practice [79] and alcohol consumption [80]. Hence, it is near certain that the disease pattern of the more prosperous of local Africans, especially urban dwellers [81], will shortly resemble that now manifest among transitional African immigrants in the UK, and, in time, approach the pattern displayed by Afro-Americans.

Can anything be done, by way of education, to control the adverse trend of changes? It is considered that it is near impossible to preach the 'prudent' lifestyle to African populations in transition – who are eager to attain, in all respects, the enjoyments of the white population. In a recent questionnaire survey carried out on the dietary choices of young African men in Johannesburg, it was revealed that the huge majority would love to have eggs, bacon, sausages, for everyday breakfast; they wish for more butter and other fats, and for far more sugar and carbonated drinks. The desire for more fruit and vegetables, while certainly present, was secondary to these choices. Scarcely any wished to eat more legumes (beans (previously widely consumed), peas, and lentils). So intense were the selections expressed that educational attempts directed in schools and by the media to encourage consumption of a 'prudent' diet would seem non-starters. African medical and other students at universities enjoy to the full their access to unlimited western-type meals. In the course of research studies carried out in the field, no African helper has ever asked for a 'continental' breakfast when staying at hotels! Clearly, the impact of the 'prudent' lifestyle message is likely to be minimal for rural Africans, and near nil for the urban dwellers [82]. Even in the USA, it appears that the response of the African population to dietary and non-dietary guidelines for the avoidance of diseases such as cancer, has been negligible [83, 84].

In western populations, despite strong encouragement from the time of 'Dietary Goals' [85] onwards, energy intake has fallen little or not at all. Fat intake has decreased by 15% in the USA, but only by 5% in the UK. Consumption of vegetables and fruit has not significantly increased in either country [86], although doubling the intake is advocated [51]. Certainly, mortality rates from stroke and coronary heart disease have fallen markedly [87]. Yet, since total mortality remains unchanged, it has been considered that cancer will now account for an increasing proportion of deaths.

Not least of the problems of adopting a 'prudent' diet is the increased cost. A recent study in the UK asked 'What can people eat to meet the dietary goals, and how much does it cost' [88]? The answer was that a 'prudent' diet, meeting dietary guidelines, costs more. It was considered that certain groups of the population could not afford to eat a diet that meets the goals recommended.

This then is the scenario now being faced in measure by huge proportions of populations in transition, in big cities not only in South Africa, but in other African countries. On the positive side, in the public health sense, as mentioned, there have been significant advantages. To re-iterate, in South Africa, in big cities such as Soweto, changes of tremendous importance, regarding birth rate, infant mortality rate, and survival, have occurred (table 5). Additionally, immunization rates are high and increasing [89]. Severe malnutrition is less common [39, 72]. However, on the negative side there are the increases described in certain western diseases (table 6); moreover, tuberculosis is a huge national problem, and AIDS is rising rapidly [90]. In brief, in the transitional situation described, there are major health gains as well as losses. As a comparison, it would seem that the transitional behaviour and responses of Africans in southern Africa, have been perhaps more orderly than those exhibited by Aboriginals in Australia [91–93].

As to the future, dietarily, the crusade for increased consumption by all of a variety of plant foods must continue. While warnings must be strongly continued against smoking and excessive drinking, such practices are now restrained only because of their cost. Although it will be difficult to maintain the previous high level of physical activity, increasing present-day activity levels should be strongly encouraged.

Regarding the far future, because of the projected inexorable population increase, and because land available for cultivation is limited, inevitably there will be greater reliance on plant foods. For it requires far more land, as much as 10 times, to produce foods from animals compared with foods from the soil [94]. Hopefully, in rural areas, as in Vendaland, there will be continued perhaps even increased consumption of 'spinaches' and other wild plants, which are known to make a significant contribution to micronutrient intake [17].

Regarding the other South African populations, transitions in food consumption follow a common pattern. The changes which have taken place are similar to those which occurred in many western populations during the last two or three generations. In the White, Indian and Coloured populations, there have been rises in intakes of energy, fat and protein, with varying falls in intakes of plant foods. The changes have been associated with rises in socioeconomic status. Broadly, for all of the populations under discussion, on the one hand, mortality rates in the very young have lessened and average survival time has increased. On the other hand, there have been rises in the occurrence of chronic disorders/diseases linked with increase in socioeconomic status. In our view, there would seem little hope, despite recommendations, of any of the populations returning in measure to diets of lower energy and fat content and with greater representation of plant foods.

Acknowledgements

The authors would like to thank Mrs. Katja Rossouw for providing considerable information regarding early literature and Miss Fatima I. Sookaria for typing the manuscript.

References

1   Coetzee R (ed): FUNA Food from Africa. Durban, Butterworth, 1982, p 3.
2   Fox FW, Norwood Young EC: Food from the Veld. Johannesburg, Delta Books, South African Institute for Medical Research, 1982.
3   Oliveira JFS, de Carvalho JP, de Sousa RXFB, Simao MM: The nutritional value of four species of insects consumed in Angola. Ecol Food Nutr 1976;5:91–97.
4   Truswell AS: Diet and nutrition of hunter-gatherers. Health Dis Tribal Soc 1993;49:213–226.
5   Lee RB: The subsistence ecology of !Kung Bushmen, PhD thesis, University of California, Berkeley 1965.
6   Lee RB, Mongongo: The ethnography of a major wild food source. Ecol Food Nutr 1973;2: 307–321.
7   Mitchener JA: The Covenant. Secker and Warburg. Reader's Digest Condensed Book, 1980, p 335.
8   Truswell AS, Hansen JDL: Medical research amongst the !Kung; in Lee RB, Devore I (eds): Kalahari Hunter-Gatherers. Cambridge, Harvard University Press, 1976, p 166–195.
9   Hansen JDL, Dunn DS, Lee RB, et al: Hunter-gatherer to pastoral way of life: Effects of the transition on health, growth and nutritional status. S Afr J Sci 1993;89:559–564.
10 O'Keefe SJD, Lavender R: The plight of modern Bushmen. Lancet 1989;ii:255–257.
11 Bishop W, Laubscher I, Labadarios D, et al: The effect of nutrified SASKO bread on the micronutrient status of an isolated rural community. In preparation.

12 Franz HC: The traditional diet of the Bantu in the Pietersburg District. S Afr Med J 1971;45: 1232–1233.

13 Quin PJ (ed): Foods and Feeding Habits of the Pedi. Johannesburg, Witwatersrand University Press, 1959.

14 Leary PM: The diet of Pedi schoolchildren. S Afr Med J 1969;43:792–795.

15 Recommended Minimum Daily Ration Scale for Farm Labourers. Pretoria, Department of Health, 1970.

16 Lubbe AM: Dietary evaluation. S Afr Med J 1971;45:1289–1297.

17 Vorster HH, Venter CS, Menssink E, et al: Adequate nutritional status despite restricted dietary variety in adult rural Vendas. S Afr J Clin Nutr 1994;7:3–16.

18 Recommended Dietary Allowances, ed 10. Washington, National Academy of Sciences, National Academy Press, 1989.

19 Report of an Expert Committee: Arterial Hypertensioin and Ischaemic Heart Disease Preventive Aspects. Tech Rep Ser No 231. Geneva, WHO 1962.

20 Walker ARP, Walker BF: Helminthiasis, nutritional status and health in Africa. S Afr J Food Sci Nutr 1994;6(4):153–158.

21 Rose EF: Some observations on the diet and farming practices of the people of the Transkei. S Afr Med J 1972;46:1353–1358.

22 Groenewald G, Langenhoven ML, Beyers MJC, et al: Nutrient intakes among rural Transkeians at risk for oesophageal cancer. S Afr Med J 1981;60:964–967.

23 Richter MJC, Langenhoven ML, Du Plessis JP, et al: Nutritional value of diets of Blacks in Ciskei. S Afr Med J 1984;65:338–345.

24 Ndaba N, O'Keefe SJD: The nutritional status of black adults in rural districts of Natal and Kwazulu. S Afr Med J 1985;68:588–590.

25 Bembridge JJ: Some aspects of household diet and family income problems in Transkei. S Afr Med J 1987;72:425–428.

26 Hamill PVV, Drizd TA, Johnson CL, et al: Physical growth: National Center for Health Statistics percentiles. Am J Clin Nutr 1979;32:607–629.

27 Manning EB, Mann JI, Sophangisa E, Truswell AS: Dietary patterns in urbanised Blacks. S Afr Med J 1974;48:485–498.

28 Bourne LT, Langenhoven ML, Steyn K, et al: The food and meal pattern in the urban African population of the Cape Peninsula, South Africa: The BRISK Study. Cent Afr J Med 1994;40: 140–148.

29 Bourne LT, Langenhoven ML, Steyn K, et al: Nutrient intake in the urban African population of the Cape Peninsula, South Africa. Cent Afr J Med 1993;39:238–247.

30 Labadarios D, et al: Biochemical evaluation of vitamin status and its relationship to dietary intake in urbanised black South Africans. In preparation.

31 Wrieden WL: Fruit and vegetable consumption in north Glasgow: Some results from the MONICA study of 1986 and 1989. Proc Nutr Soc 1993;52:12A.

32 Block G, Lanza E: Dietary fiber sources in the United States by demographic group. J Natl Cancer Inst 1987;79:81–91.

33 WHO Study Group: Diet, Nutrition and the Prevention of Chronic Diseases. Tech Rep Ser No 797. Geneva, WHO, 1990.

34 Walker ARP, Walker BF, Lelake A: Diets of three social classes of urban Africans living in Soweto, Johannesburg. In preparation.

35 Peberdy CN: The nutritional status of preschool children in Malukazi, MSc thesis, University of Natal, 1991.

36 Coutsoudis A, Jinabhai CC, Coovadia HM, Mametija LD: Determining appropriate nutritional interventions for South African children living in informal urban settlements. S Afr Med J 1994; 84:597–600.

37 Hunter JM: Macroterm geophagy and pregnancy clays in southern Africa. J Cult Geogr 1993;14: 70–92.

38 Walker ARP, Walker BF, Jones J, et al: Nausea and vomiting and dietary cravings and aversions during pregnancy in South African women. Br J Obstet Gynaecol 1985;92:484–489.

39 Stein H, Rosen EU: Changing trends in child health in Soweto. S Afr Med J 1980;58:1030–1032.

40 Walker ARP, Walker BF, Walker AJ: The significance of deficits in growth and other variables in rural South African black children aged 12 years. Int Clin Nutr Rev 1989;9:76–83.

41 Walker ARP, Walker BF, Vorster HH: Functional significance of mild to moderate malnutrition. Am J Clin Nutr 1990;52:178–179.

42 Walker ARP: Nutritional and dental implications of high and low intakes of sugar. Int J Food Sci Nutr 1995;46:161–169.

43 Walker ARP, Badenhorst CJ: Obesity revisited. S Afr J Sci 1995;91:25–30.

44 Seedat YK, Seedat MA: An inter-racial study of the prevalence of hypertension in an urban South African population. Trans R Soc Trop Med Hyg 1982;76:62–71.

45 Omar MAK, Seedat MA, Motala AA, et al: The prevalence of diabetes mellitus and impaired glucose tolerance in a group of urban South African blacks. S Afr Med J 1993;83:641–643.

46 Walker ARP: Cancer outlook: An African perspective. J R Soc Med 1995;88:5–13.

47 Hodge AM, Dowse GK, Zimmet PZ: Association of body mass index and waist-hip circumference ratio with cardiovascular disease risk factors in Micronesian Nauruans. Int J Obes 1993;17:399–407.

48 Murrary WA: The Poor White Problem in South Africa: Report of the Carnegie Commission. Stellenbosch, Pro Ecclesia-Drukkery, 1932, vol 4.

49 Rossouw JE, Jooste PL, Steenkamp HJ, et al: Socio-economic status, risk factors and coronary heart disease: The CORIS baseline study. S Afr Med J 1990;78:82–85.

50 Rossouw JE, Thompson ML, Jooste PL, Swanepoel ASP: Choice of coronary heart disease risk factor variables in a cross-sectional study of white South Africans. S Afr Med J 1990;78:570–577.

51 Bingham S: Dietary aspects of a health strategy for England. Br Med J 1991;303:353–355.

52 Knutsen SF: Lifestyle and the use of health services. Am J Clin Nutr 1994;59(suppl 5):1171S–1175S.

53 Snowdon DA: Animal product consumption and mortality because of all causes combined, coronary heart disease, stroke, diabetes, and cancer in Seventh-Day Adventists. Am J Clin Nutr 1988;48:739–748.

54 Enstrom JE: Health practices and cancer mortality among active California Mormons. J Natl Cancer Inst 1989;81:1809–1814.

55 Steyn NP, Pettifor JM, van der Westhuyzen J, van Niekerk L: Nutritional status of school children in the Richtersveld. S Afr J Food Sci Nutr 1990;2(3):52–56.

56 Steyn NP, Wicht CL, Rossouw JE, et al: Nutritional status of 11-year-old children in the Western Cape. I. Dietary intake. II. Anthropometry. S Afr J Food Sci Nutr 1989;1(1):15–20, 21–27.

57 Langenhoven ML, Wolmarans P, Groenewald G, et al: Nutrient intakes and food and meal patterns in three South African population groups. Front Gastrointest Res. Basel, Karger 1988, vol 14, pp 41–48.

58 Steyn K, Rossouw JE, Joubert G: The coexistence of major coronary heart disease risk factors in the coloured population of the Cape Peninsula (CRISIC study). S Afr Med J 1990;78:61–63.

59 Walker ARP: Nutritional, biochemical and other studies on South African populations. S Afr Med J 1966;40:814–852.

60 Booyens J, de Waal VM: The food intake, activity pattern and energy expenditure of male Indian students. S Afr Med J 1969;43:344–346.

61 Desai ID, Lee Pai C, Wright ME: Food habits and nutritional status of Hindu Indian families in British Columbia. Ecol Food Nutr 1983;13:87–90.

62 Walker ARP, Walker BF, Kadwa M: Dietary intakes of South African Indian adolescents. S Afr J Clin Nutr 1993;6:18–20.

63 Walker ARP, Walker BF, Jones J, Kadwa M: Growth of South African Indian schoolchildren in different social classes. J R Soc Health 1989;102:54–56.

64 Ulikaszek S, Evans E, Mumford P: Anthropometric survey. Lancet 1979;i:214.

65 Seedat YK, Mayet FGH, Khan S, et al: Risk factors for coronary heart disease in the Indians of Durban. S Afr Med J 1990;78:447–454.

66 Walker ARP, Adam A, Küstner HGV: Changes in total death rate and in ischaemic heart disease death rate in interethnic South African populations, 1978–1989. S Afr Med J 1993;83: 602–605.

67 Bhatnagar D, Anand IS, Durrington PN, et al: Coronary risk factors in people from the Indian subcontinent living in West London and their siblings in India. Lancet 1995;345:405–409.

68 Popkin BM: The nutritional transition in low-income countries: An emerging crisis. Nutr Rev 1994; 52:285–298.

69 Solomons NW, Gross R: Urban nutrition in developing countries. Nutr Rev 1995;53:90–95.

70 Walker ARP: Disease patterns in South Africa as related to dietary fiber; in Spiller GA (ed): CRC Handbook of Dietary Fiber in Human Nutrition (updated). Boca Raton, CRC Press, 1993, chapt 7.8, pp 491–496.

71 Kale R: Impressions of health in the new South Africa: A period of convalescence. Br Med J 1995; 310:1119–1122.

72 Walker ARP, Dunn MJ, Dunn SE, Walker BF: Causes of admissions of rural African patients to Murchison Hospital, Natal, South Africa. J R Soc Health 1994;114:33–38.

73 Walker ARP, Walker BF: Diabetes prevalence in elderly blacks in South Africa. S Afr J Food Sci Nutr 1991;3(4):68–71.

74 Dean MPG, Gear JSS: Medical admissions to Hillbrow Hospital, Johannesburg, by discharge diagnosis. S Afr Med J 1986;69:672–673.

75 Walker ARP, Labadarios D, Glatthaar II: Diet-related disease patterns in South African interethnic populations (epidemiological perplexities and future prospects); in Temple N, Burkitt DP (eds): Western Diseases: Their Dietary Prevention and Reversibility. Totowa/NJ. The Humana Press, 1994, pp 29–66.

76 Metz J, Livni N, Simson IW, Uys CJ: Cancer Registry of South Africa, 1986. Johannesburg, South African Institute for Medical Research, 1987.

77 Sitas F, Pacella R: Cancer Registry of South Africa, 1989. Johannesburg, South African Institute for Medical Research, 1994.

78 Steyn K, Jooste PL, Bourne L, et al: Risk factors for coronary heart disease in the black population of the Cape Peninsula. The BRISK study. S Afr Med J 1991;79:480–485.

79 Steenkamp HJ, Jooste PL, Jordaan PCJ, Swanepoel ASP, Rossouw JE: Changes in smoking during a community-based cardiovascular disease intervention programme. The Coronary Risk Factor Study. S Afr Med J 1991;79:250–253.

80 Seftel HC: Southern African perspective: Alcohol and alcoholism. Med Int 1985(June):1377–1378.

81 Molleutze WF, Moore AJ, Steyn AF, et al: Coronary heart disease risk factors in a rural and urban Orange Free State black population. S Afr Med J 1995;85:90–96.

82 Walker ARP: Letter from Johannesburg. Dietary trends in emerging city Africans: Is urging a 'prudent' lifestyle a non-starter? Nat Med J India 1995;8:83–84.

83 Anonymous: Nutrition and cancer, facts, fallacies and ACS activities. Cancer News 1987(summer): 18–19.

84 Cotugna N, Subar AF, Heimendinger J, Kahle L: Nutrition and cancer prevention knowledge, beliefs, attitudes and practices: The 1987 National Health Interview Survey. J Am Dietet Assoc 1992;92:963–968.

85 Dietary Goals for the United States: Prepared by the Staff of the Select Committee on Nutrition and Human Needs, United States Senate. Washington, United States Government Printing Office, 1977.

86 Patterson BH, Block G: Improving the American diet. Am J Publ Health 1992;82:465–466.

87 Davis DL, Diuse GE, Hoel DG: Decreasing cardiovascular disease and increasing cancer among whites in the United States from 1973 through 1987: Good news and bad news. J Am Med Assoc 1994;271:431–437.

88 Kingman S: Children eat poorly on state benefits. Br Med J 1992;305:1178.

89 Küstner HGV: National review of the expanded programme on immunization in South Africa. Epidemiol Comments 1994;21:203–218.

90 Bobat R, Coutsoudis A, Moodley D, Coovadia HM: Moving from AIDS to symptomatic HIV infection. S Afr Med J 1995;85:495.

91 O'Dea K: The therapeutic and preventive potential of the hunter-gatherers lifestyle: Insights from Australian Aborigines; in Temple NJ, Burkitt DP (eds): Western Diseases: Their Dietary Prevention and Reversibility. III. Totowa/NJ, Humana Press, 1994, pp 349–380.
92 O'Dea K, White NG, Sinclair AJ: An investigation of nutrition related task factors in an Aboriginal Community in Northern Australia: Advantages of a traditionally orientated life-style. Med J Austr 1988;148:177–180.
93 Harringan P: Bid to improve Aboriginal health in Australia. Lancet 1995;345:852.
94 Fox FW: The agricultural foundations of nutrition. Introduction. S Afr Med J 1954;28:97–98.

Demetre Labadarios, Department of Human Nutrition, Faculty of Medicine,
University of Stellenbosch and Tygerberg Hospital,
PO Box 19063, Tygerberg 7505 (South Africa)

Simopoulos, AP (ed): Metabolic Consequences of Changing Dietary Patterns.
World Rev Nutr Diet. Basel, Karger, 1996, vol 79, pp 109–132

Cultural and Nutritional Aspects of Traditional Korean Diet

Sook Hee Kim[a]*, Se-Young Oh*[b]

[a] Department of Food and Nutrition, Ewha Women's University, Seoul, Korea
[b] Department of Food and Nutrition, Kyunghee University, Seoul, Korea

Contents

Introduction

The history of Korean diet dates back to the Paleolithic Age when people began to settle down in the Korean Peninsula. Koreans started cultivating crops in the late Neolithic Age. Millet was the oldest grain found in Korea in the third millennium BC, and rice cultivation did not appear in Korean history until the 13th century BC [1]. Hunting/gathering/fishing remained important subsistence activities along with agriculture for a long time. The present type of diet, which includes rice as a staple and side dishes originated from the prehistoric period. However, it is said that Korean's traditional dietary pattern was not established until the *Chosun* period (chronologically from 1392 to 1909 AD) [2–4].

The focus of this paper is to discuss the traditional Korean diet from a nutritional and cultural perspective. In particular, it will concentrate on the *Chosun* period since the traditional Korean diet was fully developed in this period. The *Chosun* period is chronologically divided into two parts. The first part covers from 1392 AD to the period when Korea and Japan were at war (1592–1598 AD) and the second part spans the period from after the war to 1909 AD [5].

The dietary pattern of certain individuals or groups is affected by the interactions of biological, social, economic and cultural factors. It is very necessary to examine how the traditional dietary pattern of a certain cultural group was developed in order to understand what it is. Therefore, before presenting the traditional foods of Korea, we will examine the significant environmental factors that affected traditional diet in the *Chosun* period.

Social Factors Related to the Development of the Traditional Korean Diet

In human societies, many social factors exert influences on 'eating', either directly or indirectly. There were five important social factors related to the formulation of the traditional Korean dietary patterns. These were social status, agriculture and fishing development, introduction of foreign crops, and frequent natural disasters and wars [6].

Social Status

Korea was a strictly stratified society, particularly in the first part of the *Chosun* period. This means that the social status inherited from birth determined one's socioeconomic status, which affected what people had. There were four social classes: the gentry (*yanban*), the 'middle people', 'the common people' and 'the low born' [5]. The common people were engaged in agriculture, and the low born in trade, manufacturing of goods and other lesser occupations such as butchery. The *yanban* formed the educated and land-owning class of the *Chosun* period, and they occupied all high-ranking government positions. The middle people occupied government positions of middle and lower rank. Only those who passed the civil service examination were qualified to be government officials [5].

Since social and economic powers were provided entirely by an inherited social status in the first part of the *Chosun* period, one's meal pattern depended mainly upon one's social status. Various and abundant foods were available for those from the gentry class, who comprised only a small proportion of the total population. Meanwhile, the diet of the majority of people (the common people and the low born) barely satisfied their biological needs [6].

In the latter period of *Chosun*, the social stratum was disturbed to some degree by unfavorable natural and social conditions, such as droughts, floods, political rivalries and wars [5]. Some people from the gentry class lost their land mainly due to political reasons and became poor peasants while some rich peasants accumulated wealth by commercial activities. This disorder among social classes brought in a situation where inherited social status no longer guaranteed the quality of one's diet in some cases. Rather, dietary patterns of people were determined more by income or wealth. Social status, of course, revealed wealth in many cases, but not always. Rich peasants were able to enjoy the kind of diet that only the gentry people could enjoy in the former period of *Chosun* [6]. This has been one of the characteristics of the Korean dietary culture; that is, the kind of food that you have is determined by wealth rather than by social status.

Agricultural Development

Rice transplantation and two-crop farming became widely practiced in the latter period of *Chosun* owing to the development of agricultural technology [7]. In particular, technological improvement during this period increased the yields of staple foods such as rice, barley and millet. This had a favorable effect on the food situation for some poor petty farmers. The increase of food production also made some rich farmers become richer as they were engaged in commercial enterprises with farm surplus, which played an important role in developing the market economy in the *Chosun* period.

Even though there was an increasing yield of rice in the latter period of *Chosun*, rice was the most expensive grain. Only rich people could have it as a staple. The typical staple foods of the majority were barley in the south of Korea and millet in the north during that period [6].

Snacks and alcoholic beverages were refined in this period owing to the increase of staple food production. Traditional Korean snacks and alcoholic beverages are made of grains. Lee [8] indicated a variety of rice cakes as one of the features of the royal banquet in the latter period of *Chosun.* Various kinds of recipes for alcoholic beverages were also found in this period [9].

It is important, however, to note that the increase of food production was not evenly beneficial for people in the latter *Chosun* period. As compared to the former period of *Chosun,* the gap between the haves and the have-nots was greater in the latter period. The haves,. the beneficiaries of the higher yield of staple food production, enjoyed more diverse foods while many of the have-nots suffered from a shortage of provisions.

Development of Fisheries

Historically, fishery was practiced on a small scale in Korea since agriculture was dominant. Fisheries were not supported by the government in the *Chosun* period [5]. In the former *Chosun* period, freshwater fishing was practiced. In the latter period, due to a change of fishing technology, net fishing was widely practiced. Net fishing provided higher yield than freshwater fishing. Therefore, there was a noticeable increase of seafood production in the latter period of *Chosun* (18th–19th century) [10].

Although seafood production increased, seafood was so expensive that only rich people could afford to buy it. In general, the diet of the majority of people was not affected by the increase of seafood production. From this period, however, seafood came to be included as a significant component of the traditional Korean diet.

Natural Disasters and Wars

In the *Chosun* period, success of agriculture was determined by weather conditions, especially by rainfall. The *Chosun* people faced unfavorable weather in the latter period. There were 72 floods concentrated in July and August in the latter period of *Chosun* [11]. This constituted 87% of the total floods in the entire *Chosun* period. Twenty-one droughts accounting for 78% of the total droughts in the *Chosun* period were recorded at the same period. Besides frequent natural disasters, man-made disasters frequently occurred. There were the Japanese and Chinese invasions as well as frequent revolts. Frequent natural disasters and wars resulted in economic loss and a shortage of manpower. Thus, famine became a chronic and serious problem in the latter period of *Chosun* [12].

Because poor peasants suffered from a shortage of food, searching for something edible became an important part of their lives. Since there were many mountainous areas in Korea, various kinds of wild vegetables were exploited by the poor peasants [6]. Consequently, the chronic state of famine in the latter period of *Chosun* led Koreans to include various wild vegetables in their diet, which influenced modern vegetarian dietary habits. However, the wild vegetables did not considerably contribute towards the relief of famine at that time, probably due to their low energy content.

Kim [13] reported 341 kinds of famine-relief foods available in the late 17th century in Korea. Among those, the ten most frequently recorded were pine needles, elm tree skin, soybeans, wax, jujubes, black beans, glutinous millet, turnip seeds, white-pine mushrooms and chool (*Atractylodes japonica*). Some of the famine-relief foods exploited during the latter *Chosun* period are still used widely by modern Koreans, and these include acorn, lotus root, perilla, mugwort, aralia shoots, burdock, parsley, Indian millet, ginkgo nut, stems of sweet potatoes, bamboo shoots, mushrooms, sea lettuce, gelidum jelly, Chinese dates, pine nuts, black beans, walnuts, persimmon, ballon flower and chestnuts. The wild vegetables were used in porridge which was the poor people's diet. This resulted in a number of vegetable porridges available in the traditional Korean diet.

The use of various wild vegetables appeared to influence the ways in which vegetable dishes were prepared. In Korea, most vegetable dishes are cooked as follows: either boiled or steamed, and then mixed with seasonings such as garlic, soy sauce, salt, red pepper, green onions, sesame oil. Koreans might have been more willing to accept unfamiliar wild vegetables into their diet as they could prepare them with familiar seasonings. Since wild vegetables had aromatic compounds in many cases, strong seasonings were likely to be required to get rid of unfamiliar tastes and flavors. Frequent eating of hot and salty vegetable dishes might have resulted in Korean's taste for hotter and saltier foods.

Introduction of Foreign Crops

During the 17th–19th centuries, many foreign crops were introduced to Korea mainly through China and Japan [2]. Among those, the foods which considerably influenced the Korean traditional diet were peppers, water melon, tomatoes, corn, peas, cowpeas, peanuts, potatoes, sweet potatoes and squash. Red pepper, squash and sweet potatoes were introduced through Japan, while the others were through China [6].

Except for tomatoes, all these foods were readily accepted by Koreans in face of the chronic famine situation [6]. A distinct feature of these foreign crops is that their energy content is high, except for a few of them (red pepper, water melon, tomatoes). Particularly high carbohydrate foreign foods such as potatoes, sweet potatoes and squashes contributed to alleviate the famine situation.

The use of red pepper is particularly important since it led Koreans to create many hot and spicy dishes. Consequently, Koreans increasingly developed a taste for hot and spicy food.

Traditional Meal Patterns

The Korean meal includes steamed rice, hot soup, *kimchi*, and a number of meat, fish and/or vegetable side dishes with fruit as an after-meal refresher. As for serving, all the food dishes except for hot soups are generally set at the same time. Chopsticks and spoons are used for eating.

These days, it is common for each person to have his/her own bowl of rice and soup, but other dishes are set on the table for all to reach. However, the traditional manners of serving a regular meal was to set a dining table for each person, which seemed to be related to the structure of the traditional Korean house. Rooms in the traditional Korean house are small, where people sit, sleep and eat. There is a yard between the kitchen and the rooms, thus, dining tables have to be carried at each mealtime. Small individual dining tables were likely to be easily carried by one person.

Usually, generous portions of food were served. Individual dining tables were served first to the head of the household, son and elderly. When they finished their meals, other members of the family ate the leftovers from those tables [4]. This traditional way of serving meals is associated with one of the Korean customs, that is not to eat up all the food served at a meal.

People had different table settings according to their social status. Table settings were classified into the 3 *chop*, the 5 *chop*, the 7 *chop*, the 9 *chop* and 12 *chop* settings according to the number of side dishes [4]. Here *chop* means a side dish served in a vessel with a cover [14]. The number of *chop* increased as one's social status became higher. A 3 *chop* table setting was practiced by the common people, 5 *chop* and 7 *chop* by the gentry class, and 9 *chop* and 12 *chop* in the royal court. The compositions of different *chop* table settings are presented in table 1. For example, a 7 *chop* table includes 7 side dishes along with steamed rice, soup, three seasoning sauces, and two stews. The hot radish kimchi can be replaced with vegetable salad, and one of the stews with raw meat.

Not only the number of dishes served but also meal ingredients and cooking methods differed greatly by social status. The peasants' diet mostly comprised of vegetable foods, and this barely satisfied their biological needs. Often in classical Korean literature, it is not unusual to find a yearning desire for food among the poor. On the other hand, a regular meal of the gentry class included both vegetable and animal sources, which had at least 5 side

Table 1. Composition of different *chop* table settings [adapted from 4]

3 chop	Steamed rice, soup, *kimchi*, cooked vegetable,[1] fermented vegetable,[1] roasted meat or fish (or hard boiled tofu),[1] soy sauce
5 chop	Steamed rice, soup, whole cabbage *kimchi*, radish *kimchi*, soy bean paste stew with meat and vegetables, cooked vegetable,[1] fermented vegetable,[1] roasted meat,[1] thinly sliced sautéd fish,[1] salted dry fish,[1] soy sauce, seasoned soy sauce
7 chop	Steamed rice, soup, whole cabbage *kimchi*, radish *kimchi*, soy bean paste stew with meat and vegetables, pickled fish stew, cooked vegetable,[1] fermented vegetable,[1] roasted meat,[1] thinly sliced sautéd fish,[1] salted dry fish or fermented fish,[1] hard boiled tofu,[1] slices of boiled meat,[1] soy sauce, seasoned soy sauce, seasoned red pepper bean paste
9 chop	Steamed rice, soup, whole cabbage *kimchi*, radish *kimchi*, cucumber *kimchi*, soy bean paste stew with meat and vegetables, pickled fish stew, cooked vegetable,[1] fermented vegetable,[1] vegetable salad,[1] roasted meat,[1] thinly sliced sautéd fish,[1] salted dry fish or fermented fish,[1] hard boiled tofu,[1] slices of boiled meat,[1] raw fish (sashimi),[1] soy sauce, seasoned soy sauce, seasoned red pepper bean paste
12 chop	Steamed rice, steamed rice with red beans, two kinds of soup, whole cabbage *kimchi*, radish *kimchi*, cucumber *kimchi*, red pepper bean paste stew, pickled fish stew, cooked vegetable,[1] fermented vegetable,[1] vegetable salad,[1] roasted meat,[1] thinly sliced sautéd fish,[1] salted dry fish or fermented fish,[1] hard boiled beef,[1] slices of boiled meat,[1] raw fish (sashimi),[1] beef casserole,[1] steamed fish,[1] raw meat,[1] soy sauce, seasoned soy sauce, seasoned red pepper bean paste

[1] Side dish counted as *chop*.

dishes besides steamed rice, soup and *kimchi*. The diet for the gentry more than satisfied their biological needs, and sometimes what they ate was considered as a symbol of their prestige. Many expensive and precious foodstuffs were used for preparing their meals [6].

In the royal court, more diverse and extravagant meals were provided. Two hundred and ten various dishes were found in the cookbooks used in the royal court in the 18th century [15]. During royal families' birthday parties, 46–74 different kinds of foods were served to the King [16].

Mean frequencies differed in terms of social class in the *Chosun* period. In general, the gentry class had 3 Meals a day including breakfast, lunch and dinner. Hong [17] described the *yanban's* having porridge before breakfast in addition to the regular 3 meals. However, it is not clear whether this was commonly practiced by all *yanbans* – the gentry class.

The common people had 3 meals a day when there was enough food and 2 meals otherwise. During the year, 3 meals were provided for 7 months (from March to September) and 2 meals for 5 months (from October to February) [6]. Between meals, light meals named *gyutmuri* were served [14], which might be related to the type of work they were doing. Since most of the common people were peasants, they might have needed a high amount of energy to perform agricultural work, especially in the farming season. However, the vegetarian diet of the common people would not be able to satisfy their energy needs with only 3 meals a day.

These days, the majority of Koreans have 3 meals per day regardless of their social status. Sometimes, Korean farmers have light meals between regular meals, especially in the busy farming season.

Indigenous Korean Foods

In this section, we will discuss the nutrient values of several important indigenous foods, along with how they became important parts of the Korean diet.

Kimchi

Kimchi is a pickled and fermented vegetable and is the side dish without which no Korean meal is complete. It is the complement to all other foods, and the substitute if no other is available. The taste of *kimchi* varies according to vegetables and spices used. There are more than 200 varieties of *kimchi*, each prepared in an infinite number of subtly different ways.

Red pepper, garlic, green onion and ginger are the principal ingredients of *kimchi*. The most basic and widely encountered variety calls for heads of fresh cabbage to be sliced, salted, and placed in a brine with red pepper and garlic, and other seasonings as necessary, then set to ferment in big pots. In the summer, when fermentation is rapid and cabbages plentiful, *kimchi* is made fresh almost daily. Prior to the onset of winter, *kimchi* pots are packed in straw and buried up to their necks on the ground to prevent freezing, then left to ferment for months.

Kimchi appeared in Korean history 1,600–1,700 years ago [18]. This ancient *kimchi* was prepared by mixing vegetables with rice gruel, spices, dried fermented beans, or a mixture of vinegar, soy sauce and other spices. The ingredients used in ancient *kimchi* were Korean cabbage, Korean radish, mallow, mustard leaves, wild plants, rice gruel and spices such as garlic, vinegar, sesame oils, tangerine rind, dried fermented beans and soy sauce [19]. A distinct feature of the ancient *kimchi* was that no red pepper was used.

The present form of *kimchi* with red pepper appeared in the 17th century [4]. Korean use of garlic goes back to prehistoric times, but red pepper is a relative newcomer, having arrived in Korea during the late 16th century [9]. From this time on, Korean cabbage and radish were the major ingredients for

Table 2. Nutrient content of different types of *kimchis* (per 100 g) [data from 20]

Nutrient	Whole cabbage kimchi	Cubed radish kimchi	Juicy kimchi	Salted radish kimchi
Energy, kcal	19	31	9	14
Walter, g	88.4	87.0	93.6	89.7
Protein, g	2.0	2.7	0.7	0.9
Fat, g	0.6	0.8	0.2	0.1
Carbohydrates, g	1.3	3.2	1.1	2.2
Fiber, g	7.2	5.6	4.2	0.9
Calcium, mg	28	5	1	43
Phosphorous, mg	NA	NA	NA	24
Iron, mg	NA	NA	NA	1.0
Vitamin A, IU	492	946	0	0
Vitamin B_1, mg	0.03	0.03	0.01	NA
Vitamin B_2, mg	0.06	0.06	0.03	0.02
Niacin, mg	2.1	5.8	1.0	0.2
Vitamin C, mg	12	10	7	NA

NA = Not available.

kimchi. Besides red pepper and previously used spices, other newly introduced spices such as green onions, sea staghorn, pomegranate, citron and pears were also used [19].

The following presents the four main categories of *kimchi* found today: (1) whole cabbage *kimchi;* (2) juicy *kimchi – nabak, dongchimi;* (3) *kimchi* with a high content of salt – *janmookimchi,* and (4) *kimchi* with various extra ingredients such as fish, meat, abalone, pomegranate, tangerine rinds, pine nuts, chestnuts – *sobaki, sukbakchikimchi, bossamkimchi.*

The nutrient content of *kimchi* varies in terms of the ingredients used, and the duration of fermentation. *Kimchi* is a good source of vitamins and minerals. Table 2 shows the nutrient content of common types of *kimchi* per 100 g [20]. The National Nutrition Survey conducted in Korea in 1991 indicates that daily consumption of *kimchi* ranged from 100 to 200 g depending on regions [21]. *Kimchi* provides considerable amounts of vitamin A and C. For centuries, *kimchi* has been the major source of vitamin C for Koreans, especially during winter when fresh vegetables are not easily available. There are 492–496 IU of vitamin A in 100 g of *kimchi* depending on the kinds of vegetables used.

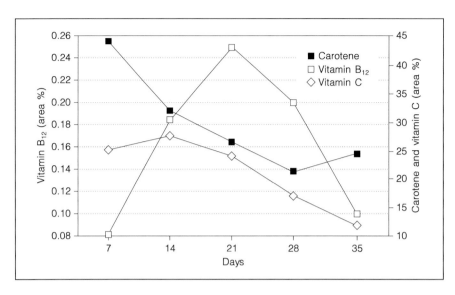

Fig. 1. Changes of nutrient values in *kimchi* by the length of fermentation (vitamins A, B₁₂ and C). Fermentation temperature 2–7 °C; salt concentration 3.25%.

The nutrient content of *kimchi* changes as fermentation proceeds. Changes of nutrient values were observed in terms of duration of fermentation over a 5-week period [22]. The nutrient content of *kimchi* was analyzed weekly. Vitamin C content was high at the first and second weeks of observation and then gradually decreased until the fifth week (fig. 1). Vitamin A was highest at the first week and decreased gradually. On the other hand, vitamin B₁₂ content of *kimchi* sharply increased until the third week and rapidly decreased afterwards.

In addition, B vitamins (B₁, B₂, B₁₂ and niacin) in *kimchi* increased remarkably in fermentation at low temperature (2–7 °C) [23]. The B vitamins reached their highest level after 3 weeks of fermentation. At that time, the amounts of B vitamins were twice those before fermentation. This suggests that fermenting *kimchi* is a good way of preserving vitamins during the winter.

At temperatures of 2–7 °C, the taste of *kimchi* is the most desirable after 2–3 weeks of fermentation. It is interesting to note that the time for maximum B vitamins coincides with the time for attaining the optimum taste of this fermented food [23].

The formation of nitrate and secondary amines during *kimchi* fermentation was examined by Yim et al. [24] and Yang and Kwon [25]. The amounts of nitrate and secondary amines were very low as compared to sausages and fish (table 3). The nitrate content in *kimchi* decreased rapidly during 4 days of fermentation

Table 3. Nitrite and secondary amines in different foods

	Nitrate, ppm	Secondary amines, ppm
Sausages	3.5–18.7	0.0–1.0
Fish	0.8–2.1	0.2–5.6
Canned fish	0.5–2.7	3.3–19.4
Salted fish	0.7–1.4	2.6–21.8
Kimchi, liquid	0.1–0.7	0.1–2.5
Kimchi, solid	0.2–1.2	0.1–2.7

at 20 °C, while the contents of nitrite and secondary amines increased slightly. Based on these results, it is assumed that fermentation reduced the nitrate level by the action of microorganisms, without increasing the concentrations of nitrite and secondary amines to any significant level (fig. 2).

Chang (Fermented Bean Products)

Typical Korean fermented bean products refer to soy sauce, soy bean paste and red pepper bean paste, and as a whole these are called *chang.* In Korea, the use of fermented beans dates back to 700 AD [4].

To make *chang,* fermented soy bean lumps are made first. Soaked soy beans are boiled thoroughly, drained well and pounded to a fine pulp while still hot. The pounded soy beans are shaped into square lumps while being tamped tightly. The soy bean lumps are fermented in a sealed box then covered with white mold. Soy sauce is made of fermented soy bean lumps, coarse salt, clean water, and some amounts of jujubes, red peppers, sesame seeds and charcoal. The major ingredients of soy bean paste are fermented soy bean lumps and coarse salt. Red pepper powders, glutinous rice powder, coarse salt and malts, in addition to fermented soy bean lumps, are needed for the preparation of red pepper bean paste. These bean products are set to ferment in a big jar [26]. Every home and restaurant has its own recipe for fermented bean products, and each batch comes out differently.

Fermented bean products are principal condiments of Korean cooking. Even though the sodium content is high in fermented bean products, they have been important sources of protein for many Koreans (table 4).

Before 1970, Koreans consumed about 50 g of fermented bean products per day (20 g of soy sauce, 20 g of soy bean paste and 10 g of red pepper bean paste) [27]. Since then, there has been a decrease in the consumption of fermented bean products. In 1991, the average consumption of fermented bean products was 20–30 g/day [21]. The lower consumption of fermented bean products at present can be explained by the popularity of less traditional

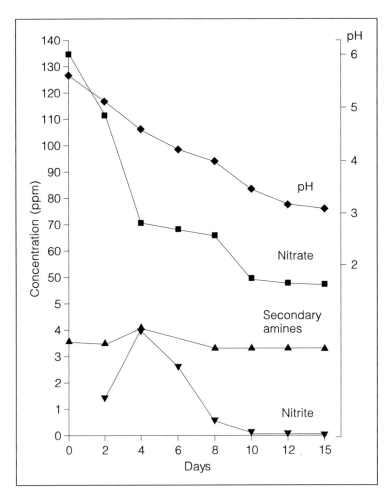

Fig. 2. Nitrites and secondary amines of kimchi by the length of fermentation (when stored at 20 °C) [from 25].

foods among Koreans, especially among youngsters. People living in rural areas consume more fermented bean products than those in urban areas. During 1973–1986, on average, rural people consumed 20% more soy sauce, 44% from soy bean paste, and 61% more red pepper bean paste than urban people [27].

Jeot or Jeotgal (Fermented Fish and Shellfish)

Fermented seafood, called *jeot* or *jeotgal* in Korea, is important in terms of providing the very taste of Korean foods. *Jeotgals* are made of shellfish or

Table 4. Nutrient values of fermented bean products (per 100 g) [data from 20 and 46]

Nutrient	Soy sauce	Red pepper bean paste	Soybean paste
Energy, kcal	38	136	128
Protein, g	4.3	8.9	12.0
Fat, g	0.4	4.1	4.1
Carbohydrates, g	4.4	15.9	10.7
Fiber, g	0.0	3.5	3.8
Calcium, mg	62	126	122
Iron, g	5.2	13.6	5.1
Vitamin B_1, mg	0.03	0.35	0.04
Vitamin B_2, mg	0.10	0.35	0.20
Niacin, mg	1.2	1.5	NA
Salt, %[1]	19–26	7.3–13.5	11

NA = Not available.

[1] Indicates coarse salt, thus the amounts of NaCl in the fermented bean products are lower than the values presented.

small fish such as tiny shrimps which are fermented whole with salt and other seasonings as necessary. In case of big fish, not their flesh but their intestines, organs, roe and branchia are used to make *jeotgals*. Since only very small amounts of fermented seafood are consumed as compared to other foods, the nutritional contribution of these foods would be negligible.

In Korea, fish is traditionally fermented in two ways: the jeotgal process where only salt is added, and the *sikhae* process where cooked cereals, garlic and red pepper powder are added [28]. When fish and fish products are fermented by the *jeotgal* process, their original shapes are not changed even after 2–3 months of fermentation, and these are served as side dishes. Fish sauces are made by keeping these products for a longer period (over 6 months). Protein hydrolysates produced during fermentation provide the very taste of *jeotgal* [28].

Fermented Foods in the Korean Diet

Fermentation is a good way of preserving food. One cannot discuss Korean indigenous foods without mentioning fermented foods. One reason for this is the characteristics of the Korean climate which consists of four seasons with long summer days. Another reason is having rice as a staple. Since rice tasted plain, people who ate enormous amounts of rice at a meal needed salty foods to compensate for the plain taste of rice. Most traditional Korean fermented foods are very salty. Salt is indispensable for fermented foods. Even though sweet or fatty foods could be consumed with rice, historically, these foods were too expensive to be consumed by common people in Korea. There was no locally grown sugar cane or sugar beets, and expensive malt was the only source for sweet taste [4].

During the last three decades, Korea has experienced rapid industrialization and urbanization, which has brought economic growth, as well as an increase in female employment and a change in living environments. Now, more people are living in apartment buildings. These changes negatively affect ones's ability to prepare indigenous fermented foods at home. In the future, the consumption of the fermented bean products will depend more on commercial products.

There are growing export markets for *kimchi,* thus the expansion of industrial production is considered inevitable. The major obstacle for mass production, however, is the inherent short shelf-life of *kimchi.* A number of attempts were made in the past to preserve *kimchi* for a longer period, but none of them were satisfactory. For example, canning, although considered to be a relatively good way to preserve *kimchi,* usually brings softening of texture and odd flavors [23].

These days, Koreans have more commercially produced *kimchi* mostly by small factories than ever before, yet many Koreans think *kimchi* has to be homemade. A survey noted that Koreans rated homemade *kimchi* much higher than commercially produced *kimchi* due to the better taste of the former. The taste of *kimchi* was considered to reveal a family dietary culture [27].

Cereals

Korean's major energy sources are starch foods such as rice, porridge and rice cake. For 5,000 years, with the exception of the last 30 years, these cereals constituted more than 80% of the total food consumed.

Steamed Rice

Rice plays a vital role in Korean diet and is the primary staple. 'Have you eaten rice yet?' is a common greeting in Korean, roughly equivalent to the English 'Hi, how are you?' The implication is that if you have rice, then you must be feeling all right; and if you have not, you should be offered some forthwith.

Steamed rice in Korea is comparable to bread and potatoes in the West. Throughout Korean history, when people could not afford rice, they had other grains such as barley, millet and wheat. Therefore, having these grains as staples meant living in distress. Nowadays, however, rice with these grains is gaining popularity as health food.

Porridge

Porridge is basically made of rice and water. Its carbohydrate content is about one fourth of that in steamed rice. Porridge was a precious food in the *Shilla* period (300–700 AD) and considered as a symbol of luxury, pleasure and indulgence [3, 4]. The porridge in the *Shilla* period contained apricot aroma powder, ground nuts and sesame seeds [4]. In the *Chosun* period, porridge was used as the poor man's rice due to its bulky effect. It was also served as a light meal for the rich [4]. In these two cases, of course, the ingredients of porridge were different. These days, porridge is served as a snack, an appetizer, a light meal, and as a special diet for patients recovering from illness. In Korea, one can find more than 150 different kinds of porridge depending on the ingredients used [29].

Rice Cake (*Dduk*)

Dduk is gelatinized by steaming, whereas steamed rice and porridge are by boiling. For steamed rice and porridge, intact grains are used, but for *dduk*, pulverized grains are used. Until the 7th century, Koreans had grains mainly in the form of *dduk*. But later on, *dduk* became a festive and ceremonial food while boiled rice became the staple [4].

Dduk is a sine qua non in all kinds of ceremonies from birth to death, such as the 'three-seven day' (a baby's 21st day of life), the 100th day, birthday, wedding day, the 60th birthday, funerals, etc. *Dduk* is made either only of rice or of the mixture of rice and other ingredients including dried fruits, legumes, pumpkins, red bean, etc. More than 200 kinds of *dduk* are available these days [30].

Based on the cookbooks found in the 19th century [30], one can assume the importance of *dduk* in the traditional Korean diet. The cookbooks classified *dduk* into four groups according to cooking methods: *tchin dduk* (steamed), *chin dduk* (struck), *chijin dduk* (fried) and *salmun dduk* (boiled). Among 198 kinds of *dduk* described in the old cookbooks, 99 were *tchin dduk, 45 chin dduk,* 30 *chijin dduk* and 14 *salmun dduk*. Ninety-five different ingredients were found. Thirty-four measuring units were reported, 13 for volume, 4 for weight, 9 for quantity, 4 for length and 4 for others. Fifty-five cooking utensils were presented, but at present many of them are not used owing to the development of food technology. There were 143 cooking terminologies of which 49 were for preparing ingredients, 25 for mixing, 27 for forming, 10 for preparing to cook, 14 for heating, 10 for cutting, 5 for setting, 3 for soaking in sugar or honey [30]. The above descriptions suggest that the cooking methods of *dduk* were well developed in the 19th century.

Since *dduk* is made of a variety of ingredients, nutrients complement each other. When rice (which lacks lysine) and beans (which lack methionine) are mixed, the biological value of protein in the mixture is improved.

Vegetables

According to the American Heritage Dictionary, herb is defined as 'an often aromatic plant used as medicine or as seasoning', and vegetable is defined as '(1) a usually herbaceous plant cultivated for an edible part, as roots, stems, leaves, or flowers. (2) The edible part of such a plant.' Based on these definitions, it is unlikely to distinguish vegetables from herbs in Korean diet. Traditionally, food and medicine were considered to have the same roots in Korea [4]. Therefore, some vegetables or herbs are used as both food and medicine. As a matter of convenience, in this paper, we use the term vegetables although it includes herbs in some cases.

One of the characteristics of Korean diet is that it has a number of vegetable dishes. As noted earlier, chronic famine situations in the later *Chosun* period introduced various wild vegetables into the Korean diet [6]. There are approximately 280 different edible vegetables available in the Korean diet [31].

Bean Sprouts

Bean sprouts are the most frequently used vegetable followed by *kimchi* [32]. The popularity of bean sprouts in the Korean diet is associated with the fact that they easily germinate and grow well even during the winter months. Bean sprouts were considered as a self-supplying vegetable in the past.

It is not exactly known when Koreans began to grow bean sprouts, although it is said that they did so in prehistoric times [33]. In the *Hyan yak ku eu bang,* published at the beginning of the 13th century, sun-dried germinated bean sprouts were described as medicine [34]. From this, it seems reasonable to assume that fresh bean sprouts were also used for food at that time. The books written after the 13th century presented two kinds of bean sprouts: dried bean sprouts (*dau du hwang*) as medicine and fresh bean sprouts (*du chae ah* or *du ah*) as food [35]. In addition, step-by-step instructions for growing bean sprouts were described in these books. The instructions were as follows: 'Soak selected bean seeds for 2 days and then wash swollen seeds with fresh water. Pour them over the moistened reed screen on the soil and cover with a jar. Water them twice a day and cover with damp strawstacks.' In a book written in the 18th century, temperature control in bean sprouts growing was noted, 'Grow bean sprouts in a warm room with warm water during the winter' [35].

The fact that bean sprouts appeared frequently in the old documents suggests its significance in the traditional Korean diet. Today, bean sprouts are still widely used and are one of the most inexpensive vegetables. People used to have home-grown bean sprouts, but at present, bean sprouts are mostly produced in small factories. In Seoul, there are more than 800 factories that produce bean sprouts [34].

Table 5. Nutrient values of Korean wild vegetables (per 100 g) [data from 20]

Nutrient	Shepherd's purse	Bud of aralia	Wild plant matari	Herb mulssuk	Amaranth	Mugwort	Sow thistle	Chang chwi	Herb hotlp	Red pepper leaves
Energy, kcal	45	39	37	26	37	56	42	29	48	48
Water, g	81.5	85.8	85.4	87.0	85.7	81.4	82.7	87.5	81.9	79.4
Protein, g	7.3	5.6	2.1	5.4	2.9	5.2	3.0	2.3	7.5	4.1
Fat, g	0.9	1.2	0.1	3.0	0.4	0.8	0.6	0.1	0.8	1.0
Carbohydrate, g	5.6	3.4	8.8	2.9	7.4	6.9	8.4	6.3	6.5	8.2
Fiber, g	2.0	2.5	2.1	2.7	1.5	3.7	1.7	2.3	2.1	3.8
Ash, g	2.7	1.5	11.5	1.7	2.1	2.0	3.6	1.5	1.2	3.5
Calcium, mg	116	50	8	106	126	93	76	8	187	364
Phosphorus, mg	104	150	80	99	46	55	34	80	124	62
Iron, mg	2.2	5.2	0.2	21.1	5.4	10.9	3.7	0.5	2.1	–
Sodium, mg	–	–	–	–	4	8	–	–	–	4
Potassium, mg	–	–	–	–	416	670	–	–	–	850
Vitamin A, IU	2,315	3,240	6,570	5,685	4,210	7,940	11,630	3,504	7,959	15,000
Vitamin B_1, mg	0.51	0.09	0.02	0.12	0.08	0.44	0.35	0.03	0.14	0.53
Vitamin B_2, mg	0.06	0.42	0.28	0.13	0.12	0.16	0.09	0.27	0.20	0.34
Niacin, mg	0.5	0.8	0.1	2.6	–	4.5	0.1	0.2	2.6	–
Vitamin C, mg	40	5	11	15	30	20	8	4	64	80
Refuse, g	14	17	–	–	–	5	–	–	–	–

Other Vegetables

Table 5 indicates the nutrient values of indigenous Korean vegetables which are mostly wild vegetables. As expected, their energy contents are not significant, but their micronutrient values are noticeable. Vitamin A contents of these vegetables are quite remarkable as well as vitamin C. For example, 100 g of red pepper leaves contain 15,000 IU of vitamin A and 80 mg of vitamin C. In particular, calcium/phosphorus ratios of the indigenous vegetables are noteworthy (tables 5, 6). Ca/P ratios were much higher in these vegetables as compared to animal foods such as beef and mackerel.

Spices
Sesame and Perilla Oils

Sesame and perilla oils are traditional Korean cooking oils and they are sine qua non for many Korean vegetable and meat dishes. Sesame seeds originated from the tropical regions of Africa. Sesame seeds were introduced to ancient Korea around the birth of Christ via China. At that time, sesame seeds were known as barbarian seeds in China [4].

Table 6. Calcium and phosphorus in Korean wild vegetables (per 100 g) [data from 20]

Nutrient	Shepherd's purse	Mugwort	Sow thistle	Chang chwi	Red pepper leaves	Milk	Beef	Mackerel
Calcium, mg	116	93	76	8	364	100	11	26
Phosphorus, mg	104	55	34	80	62	90	142	232
Ca/P ratio	1.12	1.69	2.24	0.10	10.23	1.11	0.08	0.11

Table 7. Fatty acids in dietary oils (in %)

Fatty acid	Sesame oil	Perilla oil	Beef tallow
14:0	–	–	2.6
1	–	–	–
16:0	10.1	7.4	25.1
1	–	–	–
18:0	3.7	1.6	23.1
1 (ω–9)	28.5	11.5	42.4
2 (ω–6)	37.9	14.5	3.6
3 (ω–3)	1.5	62.7	–
20:0			1.8
Unknown	2.8	2.3	1.4
P/S ratio	3.1	8.6	0.07

Cooking oils are important fat sources in the Korean diet. Yu [36] indicated that rural Koreans had one third of total fat from cooking. These days, the consumption of soy bean and cotton seed oils exceeds that of sesame and perilla oils in Korea due to the low price and long shelf life of the former. However, sesame and perilla oils are considerably consumed. A study noted that rural Koreans had, on average, 8.5 g of soy bean oil, 2.9 g of perilla oil and 1.8 g of sesame oil per day [36]. In this report, the consumption of perilla oil appeared higher than that of sesame oil. On the other hand, in urban areas, sesame oil was consumed more than perilla oil according to the National Nutrition Survey conducted in 1989 [37].

Sesame and perilla oils are similar regarding the ratios of polyunsaturated/saturated fatty acids (P/S ratio), but different in terms of the composition of polyunsaturated fatty acids (table 7). There is twice as much oleic (ω–9 fatty acid) and linoleic (ω–6 fatty acid) acids in sesame oil as compared to perilla

Table 8. Serum lipid composition and antithrombotic effect of dietary oils

	Perilla oil		Sesame oil		Beef tallow	
	mean	SD	mean	SD	mean	SD
Total lipid, mg/dl	200.7	16.9	227.6	9.1	315.2	20.1
Triglyceride, mg/dl	96.8	9.8	93.2	9.2	124.1	6.0
Total cholesterol, mg/dl	73.6	5.6	78.9	8.1	88.6	2.8
HDL cholesterol, mg/dl	53.2	5.7	40.3	5.9	39.8	5.7
Platelet number, 10^9/ml	200.7	16.9	227.6	9.1	720.0	51.5
Bleeding time, s	250.0	36.8	90.1	6.3	160.9	5.8

Note: The perilla and sesame oil groups were fed for 12 weeks while the beef tallow group was fed for 4 months.

oil. On the other hand, the amount of α-linolenic acid (ω–3 fatty acid) in perilla oil was 43 times greater than that in sesame oil. Thus the (ω–3)/(ω–6) ratio of perilla oil was much higher than that of sesame oil [38, 39].

Table 8 presents serum lipid compositions, platelet numbers and bleeding time in rats fed diets consisting of sesame oil, perilla oil, and beef tallow [38, 39]. Since the table combined the results of two different studies, further statistical analysis was not conducted. Both the sesame and perilla oil groups were fed for 12 weeks while the beef tallow group were fed for 4 months. Total lipid, triglyceride, total cholesterol and platelet counts were lower in the sesame and perilla oil groups than in the beef tallow group (table 8). The level of high density lipoprotein (HDL) cholesterol was the highest in the perilla oil group. In terms of bleeding time, the perilla oil group showed the longest time, followed by the beef tallow and sesame oil groups. The sesame and perilla oil groups presented similar effects regarding platelet number and serum lipid compositions, but the latter showed better effects on bleeding time and HDL cholesterol.

Immune responses of the traditional Korean cooking oils were examined with concanavalin A (Con A) and phytohemagglutinin (PHA) [40]. When the high fat diet (30% by weight) was provided, there were decreases of immune responses in all three experimental groups (table 9), but no differences of immune responses in terms of fat sources. At the low concentration (7% by weight), the sesame oil group responded better than the other two groups. On the other hand, the perilla oil group received the highest values at the medium concentration (15% by weight) (table 9).

Table 9. Mitogen responses of rats fed different types of oil (stimulation index/2.5 × 10⁵ spleen cell) [adapted from 40]

	Concanavalin A		Phytohemagglutinin, 10 µg/10 µl	
	mean	SD	mean	SD
7% sesame oil	174.74	63.54	93.39	29.49
7% perilla oil	101.39	24.50	62.28	14.18
7% beef tallow	70.89	9.44	34.20	9.94
15% sesame oil	88.64	22.95	69.62	15.17
15‰ perilla oil	105.36	19.45	70.87	18.96
15% beef tallow	68.49	15.97	53.31	18.44
30% sesame oil	52.47	12.00	38.31	7.65
30% perilla oil	74.17	16.85	62.01	18.87
30% beef tallow	60.30	13.22	45.15	9.79

Note: All groups were fed diets for 54 days.

Other Important Spices

Aside from cooking oils, basic seasonings of Korean cooking included garlic, red pepper, ginger, green onion, black pepper, sesame, mustard, soy bean paste, red pepper bean paste, soy sauce, vinegar and wine. There is a regional difference in terms of seasoning combinations – some hotter, some spicier – and each family also has its own particular seasoning pattern. Among all the seasonings, garlic and green onion are the most frequently used. Since small amounts of spices are used for cooking, their energy effect is small. However, special functions of the spices deserve our attention.

Antioxidant and anticarcinogenic effects of garlic and red pepper have been recently recognized. Volatile compounds and allicin in garlic have shown to suppress tumor growth. Water-soluble fractions of garlic, on the other hand, suppressed L5178 Y cell and sarcoma 180 cell which induced tumors in mice [41, 42]. Red pepper was reported to help calcium absorption. The diet with 2.5% of red pepper by weight increased calcium digestibility up to 11% as compared to the diet without red pepper [43]. Garlic and red pepper consumptions were affected by economic conditions in Korea. As the GNP went up, garlic consumption increased, while this pattern was not distinct for red pepper (fig. 3). The consumption of red pepper at present is similar to that in the early 1970s when the GNP reached USD 500 in Korea. According

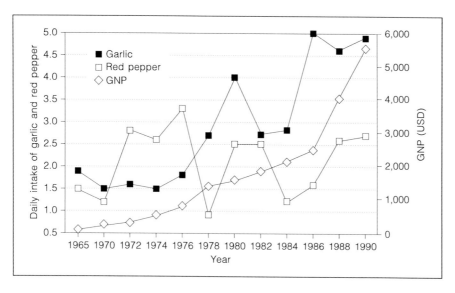

Fig. 3. Consumption of garlic and red pepper in terms of the GNP.

to figure 3, the national average consumption of garlic was 4.9 g and that of red pepper was 2.7 g/day in 1990. Rural people appeared to consume more garlic and red pepper than urban people. In a recent study on rural Koreans, the average garlic and red pepper consumptions were 9.9 and 4.8 g, respectively [36]. The higher consumptions of garlic and red pepper were likely to be associated with the fact that rural people consumed more rice than their counterparts in urban areas. Rice was eaten with spicy foods.

Conclusion

This paper addresses the traditional Korean meal pattern and foods in terms of a nutritional and cultural perspective. The eating pattern is determined by social, cultural, economic and nutritional factors which are interwoven in an intricate net. The ways in which the traditional Korean diet has developed is not exceptional as noted above. The traditional eating pattern of Koreans reveals not only their cultural identity but also how Korean ancestors maintained a balance between their biological needs and the foods available in their historical context.

In Korea, the rate of environmental change in the past was much slower as compared to in the recent 30 years. The rapid industrialization that has occurred during the last 30 years has brought increasing changes in the foods available as well as in eating behavior. Western-style fast-food restaurants have grown in popularity in Korea, and many studies indicate that nontraditional Korean foods, such as hamburger and pizza, are widely liked, especially by the younger Koreans [44]. The change of food consumption pattern is also noticeable, that is the increasing consumption of animal products (i.e. meat, milk) and the decreasing amount of energy from rice [21].

When it is assumed that traditional and modern are two ends of a unidimensional continuum, in which the addition of modern features generally occurs at the expense of traditional content [45], it can be said that today's Koreans are eating a less traditional diet. This may also imply that traditional components are losing their importance in the the modern Korean diet and will do so even more in the future as long as the process of industrialization or urbanization is irreversible. However, the meaning regarding the change of dietary pattern of present-day Koreans should not be interpreted in a simple way.

The Korean's increasing intake of animal foods (i.e. meat, milk) in recent years is referred to as evidence showing that their diet becomes more 'westernized' because traditionally they used to eat less meat. This is not a correct statement. There is no need to say that higher animal food intake is positively associated with better economic conditions, and this is also applied to the case of Korea. Koreans regard meat dishes positively, but they especially like those from Korea's traditional cuisine [44]. Therefore, the higher intake of animal food does not necessarily mean 'westernization of the Korean diet' although most Koreans used to have a vegetarian diet throughout history. Traditional foods are those that people have eaten for a long time, although there remains an unanswered question, that is: How long is long enough for a certain food to be qualified as being traditional? Traditional foods referred to in the previous sections continue to represent a major element of diet for present-day Koreans and they do not seem to prevent the adoption of new cultural food components. Understanding the traditional diet is important not only culturally but also nutritionally because it exerts a strong influence on the present eating patterns.

References

1   Choi ML, Yi SB: Subsistence pattern of prehistoric Korea: Archaeological perspective. Res Rep Miwon Res Inst Korean Food Diet Cult 1988;1:3–31.
2   Yoon SS: Food History in Korea. Seoul Shin Gwang Publishing, 1985.
3   Kang IH, Lee KB: The Customs of Korean Dietary Life. Seoul, Sam Young Sa, 1985.
4   Yoon SS: Korean Food: History and Cooking. Seoul, Soo Hak Sa, 1980.
5   The Committee on Korean History: The Korean History, 1977.

6   Kim HS: A study on the influences of socio-economic changes on dietary life in the later half of Chosun period, thesis, Ewha Woman's University, 1987.

7   Kim YS: The Agricultural History in the Latter Period of Chosun. II. Seoul, Il Cho Gak, 1971.

8   Lee HJ: Analyses of the royal feast in the latter period of Chosun, diss, Jung Ang University, 1985.

9   Lee SW: The Social History of Food in Korea. Seoul, Gyo Moon Sa, 1984.

10 The Fisheries Agency: The History of Fisheries in Korea. Seoul, The Fisheries Agency, 1985.

11 Kim YO: Climate and Culture of Korea. Seoul, Ewha Woman's University, 1985.

12 Lee KB: New Perspective on Korean History. Seoul, Il Cho Gak, 1975.

13 Kim SM: A study of relief food of the famine victims in the Chosun dynasty. Res Rep Miwon Res Inst Korean Food Diet Cult 1993;4:77–97.

14 Kang IH: Korean Food History. Seoul, Sam Yong Sa, 1979.

15 Kim SD, Chang KS, Kim MJ: Nutritional studies on the royal court dietary life of Chosun dynasty. Res Rep Miwon Res Inst Korean Food Diet Cult 1993;4:189–216.

16 Han BJ, Lee SW: An analytical study on the royal family birthday party menu of Chosun period. Korean J Diet Cult 1989;4:21–37.

17 Hong MH: Lim Gguk Jong I. Seoul, Four Seasons, 1991.

18 Chang JH: A study on the origin of Korean vegetable pickles. Thesis Collection of Sung-Shim Women's University 1975;6:149–174.

19 Yoon SS: The historical study on Korean kimchi. Korean J Diet Cult 1991;6:467–477.

20 Rural Nutrition Institute, Ministry of Agriculture and Fishery. Food composition table, 1991.

21 Ministry of Health and Social Affairs: National Nutrition Survey Report, 1991.

22 Kim SH: The meaning of kimchi in the modern Korean diet. Korean J Diet Cult 1991;6: 521–526.

23 Lee CH: Kimchi: Korean fermented vegetable foods. Korean J Diet Cult 1986;1:395–402.

24 Yim TK, Yoon MC, Kwon SP: Study on nitrosamines in foods. 1. The distribution of secondary amines and nitrites. Korean J Food Sci Technol 1973;5:169–173.

25 Yang HC, Kwon YJ: Study on the nitrite and nitrate in various kimchi in fermentation. Thesis Collection of the College of Agriculture, Chon Buk University 1982;13:111–120.

26 Chu WY: Traditional Korean Cuisine. Los Angeles, Jai Min Chang The Korea Times, 1985.

27 Lee SR, Chun HS: A study on the indigenous fermented foods in Korea: Consumption pattern and future prediction. Res Rep Miwon Res Inst Korean Food Diet Cult 1988;1:137–156.

28 Lee CH, Lee EH, Lim MH, Kim SH, Chae SK, Lee KW, Koh KH: Characteristics of Korean fish fermentation technology. Korean J Diet Cult 1986;1:267–278.

29 Ahn MS: Cultures of rice and porridge. Korean J Diet Cult 1992;7:195–202.

30 Lee HJ: A bibliographic study of dduk (Korean rice cake) in Yi dynasty. Res Rep Miwon Res Inst Korean Food Diet Cult 1988;1:45–113.

31 Kim SH, Lee JM, Park OJ: Nutrient values of indigenous foods in Korea. 15th International Congress of Nutrition, Adelaide 1993.

32 Korea Advanced Food Research Institute: Balanced Meal for Koreans, 1992.

33 Shin HK: Origin and importance of protein and oil of Korean soybean. Korean J Food Sci Technol 1972;4:158–161.

34 Lee Kim MS: A historical research on native foods of Korea. Korean J Diet Cult 1986;1:163–166.

35 Lee SW: Studies on the literature of dietary history. Han-Kuk Shik-Kyung Dae-Chun. Seoul, Hyang Moon Sa, 1981.

36 Yu JY: Development and assessment of food frequency questionnaire estimating dietary intake of the adults in rural areas of Korea, thesis, Seoul National University, 1993.

37 Ministry of Health and Social Affairs: National Nutrition Survey Report, 1989.

38 Jung HR, Han YN, Kim SH: Hypolipidemic and antithrombotic effects of increasing intakes of linolenic acid derived from perilla oil in rats. Korean J Nutr 1993;26:839–880.

39 Hong MY, Kim SH: The changes of body fat accumulation, serum lipids and platelet functions in rats fed the diet containing different common oils in Korea: Sesame oil, perilla oil and rice bran oil and mixed oil. Korean J Nutr 1993;26:513–523.

40 Kim WK, Kim SH: The effect of sesame oil, perilla oil and beef tallow on body lipid metabolism and immune response. Korean J Nutr 1989;22:42–53.

41   Moon JJ: Studies on the effect of the garlic supplementation to diet on sarcoma 180-induced skin cancer in mice, thesis, Donk-Guk University, 1984.

42   Son HS, Hwang WI: A study on the cytotoxic activity of garlic (*Allium sativum*) extract against cancer cells. Korean J Nutr 1980;23:135–140.

43   Lee KY, Lee-Kim YC: An analysis of traditional Korean diet practices in nutritional aspects. Proc 14th International Congress of Nutrition, Seoul, 1989, pp 998–1001.

44   Oh S-Y: Bicultural aspects of Korean's eating behaviour during the last 50 years. Korean J Diet Life 1993;8:373–380.

45   Grivetti LE, Paquette MB: Nontraditional ethnic food choices among first-generation Chinese in California. J Nutr Educ 1978;10:109–112.

46   Lee SR: Formented Food in Korea. Seoul, Ewha Women's University, 1986.

Se-Young Oh, PhD, Department of Food and Nutrition, Kyunghee University,
I, Hoiki-dong, Dongdaemoon-ku, Seoul 130–701 (Korea)

Simopoulos, AP (ed): Metabolic Consequences of Changing Dietary Patterns.
World Rev Nutr Diet. Basel, Karger, 1996, vol 79, pp 133–153

....

Historical Development of Chinese Dietary Patterns and Nutrition from the Ancient to the Modern Society

J.D. Chen [a], *Hong Xu* [b]

[a] Research Division of Sports Nutrition and Biochemistry, Institute of Sports Medicine, Beijing Medical University, and
[b] Department of Sports Medicine, Beijing University of Physical Education, Beijing, PR China

Contents

Introduction

China is an old nation with a long history. The ancestors of several hundred thousand years ago, in order to seek a livelihood and to be prosperous, had strived for food variety and quality. In this article, we will briefly introduce the characteristics of food, diet patterns, nutritional problems and their development from the ancient Xian-Qin (ca. 21st–16th century BC) to Qin Dynasty (1644–1911) according to the recorded history. We will also provide information of both the main achievements and problems of nutrition of present-day China.

Although every country has its own characteristics and patterns of diet and nutrition, there also exist many common aspects, such as promotion of a nutritionally balanced diet, encouragement of breast-feeding, etc. In addition, there might be more common trends in dietary and nutritional development such as advocating 'natural' fresh fruits, vegetables, and freshly prepared foods.

The History of Food and Dietary Patterns in China

Xian-Qin Dynasty (ca. 21st–16th Century BC). The first story recorded that a famous person named Shen-Nong had tasted 100 kinds of grass to identify whether they were suitable as foods, pharmaceuticals or contained toxins [1]. The second legend tells that another person named Sui produced sparks by rubbing very hard stones (flint found in lumps like pebbles, steel-gray inside and white outside, to make fire). From that time on, people started to cook (prepare) raw foods in order to improve their quality and composition. Before the invention of fire, people ate bird and animal meat raw, and diseases and death threatened people's lives. Henceforth, gastrointestinal diseases decreased significantly which led to both prosperity and longevity of human beings [1].

Xia-Yu Dynasty (ca. 21st–16th Century BC). Chinese people began to make wine and ferment foods. Soy sauce, sauce and vinegar were invented at that time, and these foods have continued to be in use today [2].

Shang Dynasty (ca. 16th–11th Century BC) – The Slave Society. Production developed faster during this period. One of the officers, Yi-Yin, reformed the cooking utensils, and he was the first to produce liquid food (a kind of thick soup) to maintain good health [3].

Zhou Dynasty (ca. 11th–5th Century). During this period it was recognized that some foods also possess therapeutic effects, which was also the beginning of the establishment of the first dietician, whose work was to be in charge of the diet, drinks, and banquets, etc., for the King of Zhou [3].

The Spring and Autumn Period (770–476 BC). A series of plants were used both as foods and remedies, e.g., *Fructus lycii* (fruit of the Barbary wolfberry), *Radix glycyrrhizae* (liquorice root) and *Fructus mume* (smoked plum) [2]. A famous book entitled 'Ben-Wei-Pian' recorded the effectiveness of ginger and cassia bark (laurel). Another medical monograph, 'Nei-Jing', advocated that foods should be comprehensive and blended adequately, and eating be moderate [1]. The monograph also introduced a number of recipes of diet therapy, some of which are still in use to day, e.g., stir-fried egg with fragrant flowered garlic; stew baby pig and fruit of the Barbary wolfberry, etc. 'Nei-Jing' also recorded the food principles and the relation between foods and health which was the first theory of balanced diet as follows [1, 3]: 'Five grains support one's health'; 'Five fruits are helpful'; 'Five animals are beneficial' and 'Five vegetables are for fullness'.

The Spring and Autumn (770–476 BC) and the Warring States Period (475–221 BC). During this period [4], game such as wild fowl, hare, tail of deer, and bear's paw, etc. contributed a rather large proportion of the diet. Besides, edible wild herbs as brake (fern) and natural fruits (mulberry, wild jujube) were used as food and were considered nutritious and delicious. In the late period of the Warring States, fish farming and planting of melons and vegetables began. Thereafter, the Chinese learned to steam rice, boil gruel, and add salt to foods. Records indicate that people knew about producing salt from sea water and that salt added flavor to foods [4]. People strived to provide many varieties of food and to improve the quality.

Han (206 BC–220 AD) and Tang (618–907 AD) Dynasties. One of the characteristics of this period was that people began to study the physiological and clinical effects of traditional Chinese foods. Another characteristic was to introduce a number of new varieties of food through the Silk Road. In the book 'Sheng-Nong Ben Cao Jing', herbal classics recorded the tonic effects of Chinese dates (jujube), yam, honey, lotus root and Job's tears, etc. The excavated 'Fifty-Two Prescriptions' from 'Ma-Wang Dui' in Hunan Province stated that one third of medicines or herbs were to be found in daily foods, e.g. milk, honey, lard and butter. Among the herbs, people boiled black soy beans for treatment to produce diuresis.

The Kingdom of Wei (220–265 AD) and Jin Dynasty (265–420 AD). The book 'Shi-Jin' (food classics) was representative of more than 40 book catalogues which illustrated systematically the efficacy of diet therapy. Ge-Hong in the book 'Zhou Hou Fang' explained that marine algae (sea weed) was used to treat goiter, pancreas of pig was adopted to cure diabetes, and pig's liver was employed for nyctalopia (night blindness). The book written by Sun Si-Miao was the earliest and most special monograph of diet therapy e.g., he suggested to boil grain skins and rice together as a medicine to prevent beriberi [2].

The cultural exchange between China and western countries through the Silk Road was not only the earliest exchange of silk, but also an exchange of food culture as well. New varieties of foods, e.g. European grapes, sesame seed cake, were introduced to China as well. At that time, exchanges were not only carried out between China and foreign countries, but also between northern and southern provinces within China. Fruits such as dried longan pulp, *Fructus litchi*, coconut palm, sugarcane and some seafood from Taiwan were transported to the inner land and thus enriched Chinese food [4].

In the Han-Tang dynasty period (206 BC–907 AD), people started to pay attention to vegetarian food and used vegetable oil. Bean products, such as bean curd, were already used in recipes, indicating the development of fermented foods. Another progress during this period was the use of iron pans to cook, leading rapidly to developments in cooking skills [4].

The Song (920–1279), Yuan (1271–1368), Ming (1368–1644) and Qing (1644–1911) Dynasties. Characteristics of this period were as follows [4]: Wheat and beans became the staple food, as did meat from domestic fowls and animals instead of game. It was widespread to adopt diet therapy to prevent and cure diseases, e.g., a group of herbs including *Fructus amomi, Fructus tasoko, F. mume* (smoked plum), *R. glycyrrhizae, Dolichos lablabl* and *Radix puerariae* were used to invigorate the function of spleen, stomach, acid digestion and to kill pathogens. Besides, people paid much more attention to the color, flavor and taste of foods. Flowers and herbs were added to teas or wines, such as jasmine in tea, osmanthus flowers in wine and day lily to cooked food [2].

The study and application of mushroom and algae also started [4] during the Qin Dynasty, e.g., black edible fungus, mushroom, hedgehog hydnum (Hydnuerinaceus), Chinese caterpillar fungus, *Cordyceps sinensis*, laver, etc., were all used in cooked food and soup.

As regard to the meal patterns, it was recorded that people usually had 3 meals a day. Snacks were only arranged for children, the aged and rich people. A famous saying has been handed down from the ancient times to the present day among the masses namely: 'Breakfast should be eaten well, lunch must be in one's fill, and food for dinner should be little.' Generally, people ate porridge or millet gruel (but poor people usually had steamed bread made of corn) for the main food for breakfast; soy bean milk, salted vegetables, eggs (boiled or fried), deep-fried twisted dough sticks, and cakes were the commonly eaten foods for breakfast as well. Steamed rice, boiled noodles, cake (in a round flat shape) were the main foods for both lunch and dinner. Meat, fish, eggs, chicken, duck, and vegetables as nonstaple foods; the dishes were usually prepared by stir-frying. Salt or soy sauce were often added during cooking, but people living in the southern part of China usually preferred to add some sugar and sometimes vinegar in preparing the dishes. Some of the dishes were steamed in clear soup (usually without soy sauce) instead of being stir-fried, such as steamed fish with some Chinese onions and ginger, etc. The majority of people had three dishes and one soup for lunch or dinner.

Development of Nutrition Studies before the Establishment of the People's Republic of China to the Present Day

The importance of a close relation between diet and health had been recognized already in ancient China, yet the study of nutrition was not able to develop in the feudal society.

After the 1911 revolution (the Chinese bourgeois democratic revolution led by Dr. Sun Yi-Xian which overthrew the Qing Dynasty), traditional Chinese medicine and western medicine developed simultaneously. Publication of books on diet and diet therapy increased in 1937–1938 (before World War II) [5].

Along with the development of chemistry and medicine, modern nutrition sprouted in the 19th century. Studies were carried out on requirements of protein, fat, carbohydrate, minerals, energy, and vitamins; however, the study of nutrition was only gradually perfected after microbiology, chemistry and food industry were developed and people attained a deeper understanding about food toxins, food preservation and food additives. Thus, rational nutrition and food health made up the base and main contents of modern nutrition in China [5, 7].

At the beginning of 20th century, the natural sciences expanded in China. Scholars did enormous work on nutritional investigations and nutritional composition of foods, but nutritional science was not fully developed due to limitations of prevailing conditions. After the establishment of the People's Republic of China, the study of modern nutrition and food science and health gradually developed and came into being. In 1950, health and antiepidemic stations were established, and nutrition work groups were set up as departments in the stations. The Institute of Nutrition and Food Hygiene of the Chinese Academy of Preventive Medical Science was founded as well. At the same time, nutrition and food health departments were set up for teaching in medical schools, universities or colleges. Since then, teaching, training, practicing and research activities continue in China [5–7].

Main Achievements of Diet and Health

Chinese Food Composition Table
The first edition of the 'Food Composition Table' was published in 1963 [8]. After being reprinted several times, a new composition table was completed and published in 1991 with the support of the China National Foundation of Natural Sciences. This new table contains 28 categories with 1,358 kinds of foods; every food has 26 nutritional profiles. Information is included for the amino acid content of 456 kinds of food, for the fatty acid content of 356

kinds of food, and the cholesterol content of 400 kinds of food. Thus, this food composition table serves as a very useful tool and nutrition guide for regulating food composition, and it also provides precise data as a reference for food production [9].

Nationwide Nutrition Survey

This survey was carried out under the organization of the Institute of Nutrition and Food Hygiene of the Chinese Academy of Preventive Medical Science [10, 11]. The first survey was carried out in 1959, and the second survey was finished in 1985 which included 27 provinces and 256 places. 250,000 people were investigated about diet, 50,000 people underwent physical examinations, about 40,000 people had blood and urinary tests, and the main results were announced in the China People's Daily. The data of the nutrition survey results were presented as averages since the data from peasants accounted for 80% of the total population studied, i.e., the average data represent mostly the data of peasants. It was shown that the average energy intake was 2,060 kcal/day in 1959, which meant that in recent years China basically provided enough food for people to eat. Average protein intake was 67 g/day (RDA is 70 g/day). Calcium intake was insufficient especially for preschool children and students of primary and middle schools. Vitamin A and vitamin B_2 were insufficient (table 1). Calories from animal foods were fairly low which was only 4.2%, because diet was basically vegetarian for peasants. Calories from animal sources were 9.2% for middle school students. Intake of milk, eggs, meat, and seafood was 108 g/day for city residents, and only 40 g/day for peasants. Protein calorie was about 10% or a bit more for the majority of people investigated except for students of primary schools which was 11.9% (tables 2, 3).

Results of physical examinations showed that 5% of the investigated people were deficient in vitamin B_2 and 4.6% in vitamin C. The incidence of rickets of 2- to 6-year-old children was 3%, and it was 7.9% for 2- to 3-year-olds (tables 4, 5).

The above-mentioned results indicate that dietary improvements should be stressed to increase foods from animal and bean sources in order to improve protein, riboflavin, calcium and vitamin A nutritional status. As regard to rickets, more outdoor activities should be arranged for children. Patients should also take vitamin D_3, but care must be taken to avoid overdose-induced toxicity. China is an agricultural country. After the establishment of the People's Republic of China, the government adopted a number of policies to solve the problem of a large population to have enough to eat, such as grains, edible oils and clothing. Prices of the rationed grains, oil and cloth were under governmental control, and this policy guaranteed people adequate food and

Table 1. Daily nutrient intakes per person and the average data of the whole country [data from 1]

Category	Protein g	Fat g	Chol. g	Energy kcal	Cellulose g	Ca mg	P mg	Fe mg	Vit. A IU	Carotene mg	Vit. B$_1$ mg	Vit. B$_2$ mg	Vit. pp mg	Vit.C mg
Heavy industry	89.0	105.4	526.6	3,350	7.8	637	1,882	42.9	356	2.22	3.20	0.96	24.8	109.5
Light industry	76.1	85.3	438.6	2,842	6.2	576	1,787	38.3	632	1.84	2.66	0.80	20.2	93.5
Institutions	74.3	81.4	434.4	2,570	6.9	576	1,686	38.7	340	2.09	2.66	0.81	19.5	94.9
University	73.5	84.5	447.0	2,820	6.9	597	1,745	35.3	300	2.16	2.63	0.80	20.9	100.0
Middle school	68.5	54.1	457.0	2,581	6.9	522	1,717	34.0	106	1.61	2.45	0.70	20.6	87.1
Primary school	57.6	52.0	308.0	1,929	4.6	470	1,236	26.2	761	1.31	1.66	0.69	14.4	69.4
Nursery	35.2	44.7	187.3	1,292	3.0	318	752	15.4	402	0.90	1.10	0.40	8.8	33.8
City residents	66.7	68.2	401.0	2,446	6.8	561	1,571	34.1	346	2.60	2.20	0.80	17.9	109.4
Countryside residents	68.8	41.3	489.7	2,615	8.9	557	1,834	50.7	109	4.50	2.50	0.80	18.3	143.9
Average of whole country	66.8	49.3	444.0	2,485	7.7	540	1,685	43.1	253	3.48	2.33	0.77	17.8	121.8

Table 2. Total intakes of energy, protein, fat and their distributive percentage of sources [data from 11]

Category	Distribution of food calorie source						Distribution of nutrient calorie source		Distribution of protein source				Distribution of fat source	
	grains	pota-toes	beans	other plant foods	animal foods	net calorie foods	protein	fat	grains	beans	other plant foods	animal foods	animal	plant
Heavy industry	66.9	0.9	2.5	3.9	15.1	10.6	10.6	28.0	65.7	8.9	8.3	17.1	59.1	40.9
Light industry	66.8	1.1	2.8	4.0	13.6	11.5	10.7	26.8	64.9	10.9	8.7	15.9	57.6	42.4
Institutions	67.5	0.8	3.2	4.0	13.8	10.4	10.9	26.6	64.2	11.5	8.6	15.7	59.1	40.9
University	66.2	1.2	2.4	4.5	15.6	10.1	9.8	27.6	64.1	9.2	9.8	17.0	58.8	41.2
Middle school	74.8	2.3	2.2	3.8	9.2	7.6	10.5	19.6	72.5	8.3	10.3	9.9	47.2	52.7
Primary school	65.2	1.2	4.2	3.7	15.5	10.3	11.9	25.1	56.2	11.9	7.1	24.8	56.4	43.6
Nursery	53.8	0.9	4.5	5.6	21.6	13.6	10.9	31.0	50.1	15.4	8.4	25.9	57.8	42.2
City residents	65.0	2.3	3.2	5.9	12.4	11.8	10.9	25.0	60.3	10.8	11.9	16.9	46.6	53.4
Countryside residents	74.6	9.0	2.6	4.0	4.2	5.8	10.5	14.3	70.9	10.0	13.0	6.3	32.8	67.1
Average of whole country	71.3	6.2	2.9	4.2	7.9	7.7	10.8	18.4	66.6	10.7	12.8	11.4	40.3	59.6

Table 3. Intakes (in g) of various foods of resident family in different districts (per person per day)

District	Rice	Flour	Other grains	Pota-toes	Beans and bean products	Vege-tables	Fruit	Milk	Eggs	Meat	Aquatic pro-ducts	Animal and plant oil	Salt
North (Shan Xi)	11	179	357	331	18.5	282	11.8		1.1	1.4	0.1	8.2	16.1
Northeast (HeiLongJiang)	39	223	325	359	15.1	377	11.2	2.4	3.3	19.6	6.6	14.8	9.7
Northwest (Gan Su)	12	565	31	106	5.5	246	39.3	11.2	5.8	17.7	1.2	16.1	10.5
Middle (He Nan)	41	391	147	326	14.0	273	9.8	1.9	6.1	18.3	1.6	10.7	17.3
Southeast (GuangDong)	498	11		96	17.9	308	30.5	1.4	5.1	42.0	40.9	18.7	11.9
Southwest (Si Chuan)	304	133	83	111	23.3	490	7.2	11.8	4.9	38.8	2.0	16.8	15.5
Plateau (Qing Hai)	15	444		266	3.6	137	5.7	14.8		27.8	1.4	15.9	12.7
Pastoral area (NeiMengGu)	30	199	269	302	7.8	200	4.2	34.7	2.1	50.2	0.7	15.7	12.6
Northern City (Bei Jing)	101	311	103	38	9.9	440	94.1	20.6	18.3	40.7	9.8	20.7	14.7
Southern City (Shang Hai)	459	44		43	12.3	325	9.1	7.1	16.7	46.2	33.2	23.1	13.7

Table 4. Incidence of nutritional deficiency disease (% of the number investigated) [data from 11]

	Vitamin A	Thiamine	Riboflavin	Niacin	Vitamin C
Incidence of deficiency disease	0.9	1.1	5.0	0.3	4.6

Table 5. Disease rate of rickets [data from 11]

	Age group, years		
	2–3	4–6	2–6
Total number investigated	1,726	4,946	6,672
Number of rickets cases	136	67	203
Disease rate, %	7.9	1.4	3.0

clothing. However, nutritional insufficiencies and deficiencies still constitute a major concern and problems of overnutrition are developing in some of the Chinese people [12, 13]. According to statistics, the income of peasants was less than 500 Chinese Yuan in 1989. Energy intake was less than 70% of RDA in 7.1% of peasants.

Although the total trend of body height change has been increasing year after year, the height of city and rural area children still falls 5 and 10 cm respectively behind that of the WHO's standard. Examination of 90,000 0- to 6-year-old children revealed that about 10–20% were malnourished. 15,000,000 children had a low body weight. The incidence of rickets was 30–50% in children of less than 3 years of age. The average incidence of anemia was 30%. Besides, there had been 7,500,000 present illness patients of epidemic goiter. These susceptible and nutrient-deficient people were mainly distributed in rural areas. On the other side, fat intake of city residents of the whole country had already reached 30% of the total in 1988, but for rural areas, it was 16%. The incidence of overweight and obesity of middle- and old-aged women reached 50% in 1987. The onset of high blood pressure has shifted to an earlier age. The incidence of high blood pressure in 12- to 15-year-old adolescents was 110/100,000. The proportion of death rate due to cardiovascular disease increased from 12.07% in 1957 to 44,4% in 1985; 800,000 people died of cancer every year. According to predictive calculations, if the Chinese do not adopt

Table 6. Comparison of the dietary composition of Chinese people with those of the whole world, Asia, developed and developing countries [data from 11]

	Calories		Protein			Fat		
	intake kcal	animal source %	intake g	animal source %	calories provided %	intake g	animal source %	calories provided %
Average of whole world (1979–1981)	2,624	16	68.5	36.0	10.4	63.4	52.0	21.7
Average of Asian countries (1979–1981)	2,336	8	57.5	20.5	9.8	38.7	40.8	14.9
Average of developed countries (1979–1981)	3,385	30	98.9	56.8	11.7	120.4	66.5	31.9
Average of developing countries (1979–1981)	2,350	9	57.5	22.4	9.8	40.6	39.1	15.5
Average of whole nation (1979-1981)	2,485	8	66.8	11.4	10.8	49.3	40.3	18.4
Average of nationwide cities (1982)	2,446	12	66.7	16.9	10.9	68.2	46.6	25.0
Average of nationwide rural areas (1982)	2,615	4	68.8	6.3	10.5	41.3	32.8	14.3

preventive measures, the number of deaths due to cardiovascular disease will increase 3 times by the year 2025 [12, 13].

Since 1987, the Chinese government has instituted reform steps which promoted a further development of agricultural production which led to the improvement of the nutritional status of the people. The levels of food intake of city residents have approached the average of other parts of the world. The levels of energy intake of the whole nation were similar to other Asian countries (table 6).

In comparing the data with the Dietary Goals of WHO, the dietary intake of the Chinese is still below that of the WHO (tables 7–9), but data have shown that intake of calories from fat of Chinese city residents was near 30% of the total energy, saturated fatty acids accounting for <10%. The statistics of disease prevalence illustrate that mortality due to cardiovascular disease and cancer have become the first and second causes of death. Thus, measures of diet improvement should be closely connected with the monitoring of incidence of disease.

Table 7. Comparison between the diet goal suggested by WHO and diet status of various Chinese population groups [data from 11]

	Distribution of calorie source			kcal % from animal fat source
	protein	fat	carbohydrate	
Suggestion of WHO	12.0	30.0	58.0 (10% from sugar)	10
Average of whole nation	10.8	18.4	70.8 (<2% from sugar)	7
Average of nationwide city residents	10.9	25.0	64.1	12
Average of whole nation heavy industrial staff	10.6	28.0	61.4	17
Average of whole nation light industrial staff	10.7	26.8	62.5	15
Average of the whole nation institutions or office staff	10.9	26.6	62.5	16

Table 8. Recommendation of the Chinese diet composition in 1968–1990 (average kg intake/year/person) [data from 11]

	Grains	Pota-toes	Beans	Vege-tables	Fruit	Poultry and meat	Milk	Eggs	Fish and shrimps	Plant oil
1981–1985	180	36	12	144	–	12	–	6	6	3
1982	187	58	6	113	10	14	3	3	4	4
1986–1990	170	36	12	144	10	18	24	6	6	3

Table 9. Comparison between the recommended Chinese diet composition in 1986–1990 and the diet goal of WHO [data from 11]

	Distribution of calorie source, %			Distribution of protein source, %	Distribution of fat source, %
	protein	fat	Chol.	animal protein	saturated fat
WHO	12	30	58	–	33.3
Diet composition in 1986–1990	12	21	67	17	54.3
Result of nutrition survey in 1982	10.8	18.4	70.8	11.4	40.3

Recommended Dietary Allowances (RDA)

The results of the whole nation's diet survey provides references and information for programming of food provision and improvement for diet composition and it pushed forward the development of nutrition studies in China. The third nationwide nutrition investigation was carried out in 1992. The RDA of the Chinese were published in 1990 by the Chinese Nutrition Society (table 10) [14]. The RDA was worked out on the basis of the Chinese dietary characteristics: grains are the main food, consumption of animal food is insufficient, calcium from dairy products and heme iron are inadequate, etc. Thus, the RDA of some of the nutrients have been stipulated rather high, and it needs revision periodically through practice. The new revised RDA can not only be used as a reference for evaluating nutritional status of the Chinese, but also as a basis for mapping out the scheme of food development and production in China.

Dietary Goals and Guidance

The dietary goals and guidance for the Chinese are shown in table 11[12, 15]. Chinese scientists have put forward the dietary goal for the year 2000. The concrete RDA per person is as follows: energy, 2,400 kcal (10,045 kJ), in which 60% should be from carbohydrate, 14% from animal foods. Protein, 70 g, in which 30–40% should be from animal and bean foods. Energy from fat is 25–30% of the total, adequate plant oil should be used. Sodium chloride should be < 10 g.

On the basis of the revised RDA and the results of the nationwide nutrition survey, Chinese nutritional scientists proposed the dietary guidance as follows [15]:

(1) Diet should consist of a variety of nutritionally balanced foods including an adequate amount of grains, animal foods, beans and bean products, vegetables and fruits, net calorie as edible oil, sugar, etc. The energy source should be mainly from grains; stress plant food first and animal food as supplementary.

(2) Amount of food intake should be adequate and body weight should be monitored regularly.

(3) Fat makes up 20–25% of the total energy uptake. Plant oil is 0.75 kg/month which is about 25 g/day, and other fats are from various foods.

(4) Food rich in cellulose as coarse food and grains, beans, vegetables and fruit are recommended and encouraged.

(5) Salt should be restricted because the incidence of high blood pressure positively correlates with sodium intake. For prevention, < 10 g NaCl is recommended for daily intake.

(6) Decrease sweet foods because they are detrimental to dental health.

Table 10. Recommended dietary allowances of the Chinese Nutrition Society, revised in October 1988 [data from 14]

Category	Body weight kg		Energy kcal		Protein g		Fat, kcal of total %	Ca mg	Fe mg		
	M	F	No sex differences								
Infants											
New born											
–6 months	6.7	6.2	120/kg BW		2–4/kg. BW		45	400	10		
7–12 months	9.0	8.4	100/kg BW				330–40	600	10		
			M	F	M	F					
Children											
1 year	9.9	9.2	1,100 (4.6)	1,050 (4.4)	35	35		600	10		
2 years	12.2	11.7	1,200 (5.0)	1,150 (4.8)	40	40		600	10		
3 years	14.0	13.4	1,350 (5.7)	1,300 (5.4)	45	45		800	10		
4 years	15.6	15.2	1,450 (6.1)	1,400 (5.9)	50	45		800	10		
5 years	17.4	16.8	1,600 (6.7)	1,500 (6.3)	55	50		800	10		
6 years	19.8	19.1	1,700 (7.1)	1,600 (6.7)	55	55	→ 25–30	800	10		
7 years	22.0	21.0	1,800 (7.5)	1,700 (7.1)	60	60		800	10		
8 years	23.8	23.2	1,900 (8.0)	1,800 (7.5)	65	60		800	10		
9 years	26.4	25.8	2,000 (8.4)	1,900 (8.0)	65	65		800	10		
10 years	28.8	28.8	2,100 (8.8)	2,000 (8.4)	70	65		1,000	12		
11 years	32.1	32.7	2,200 (9.2)	2,100 (8.8)	70	70		1,000	12		
12 years	35.5	37.2	2,300 (9.6)	2,200 (9.2)	75	75		1,000	12		
									M	F	
Adolescents											
13 years	42.0	42.4	2,400 (10.0)	2,300 (9.6)	80	80	→ 25–30	1,200	15	20	
14 years	54.2	48.3	2,800 (11.7)	2,400 (10.0)	90	80		1,000	15	20	
18 years	63	53						No sex difference	M	F	
	(reference)										
Adults											
Very light work			2,400 (10.0)	2,100 (8.8)	70	65		800	12	18	
Light work			2,600 (10.9)	2,300 (9.6)	80	70		800	12	18	
Medium work			3,000 (12.6)	2,700 (11.3)	90	80		800	12	18	
Heavy work			3,400 (14.2)	3,000 (12.6)	100	90	→ 20–25	800	12	18	
Very heavy work			4,000 (16.7)	–	110	–		800	12	–	
Pregnant women	(4–6th months)		+200 (+0.8)		+15			1,000		28	
Pregnant women	(7–9th months)		+200 (+0.8)		+25			1,500		28	
Wet-nurse			+800 (+3.3)		+25			1,500		28	
45 years											
Very light work			2,200 (9.2)	1,900 (8.0)	70	65		800	12		
Light work			2,400 (10.0)	2,100 (8.8)	75	70		800	12		
Medium work			2,700 (11.3)	2,400 (10.0)	80	75		800	12		
Heavy work			3,000 (12.6)	–	90	–		800	12		
60 years							→ 20–25				
Very light work			2,000 (8.4)	1,700 (7.1)	70	60		800	12		
Light work			2,200 (9.2)	1,900 (8.0)	75	65		800	12		
Medium work			2,500 (10.5)	2,100 (8.8)	80	70		800	12		
70 years											
Very light work			1,800 (7.5)	1,600 (6.7)	65	55		800	12		
Light work			2,000 (8.4)	1,800 (7.5)	70	60		800	12		
Over 80 years			1,600 (6.7)	1,400 (5.9)	60	55		800	12		

Materials taken from documents of the Chinese Nutrition Society [15].

Recommended dietary allowances of nutrients were drawn up on the basis of the present Chinese diet model, i.e. provision of animal food is about 10% of the total calories. Protein from animal and soy bean is about 20% of the total.

Chen/Xu

Zn mg	Se mg	Iodine µg	Retinol EQ µg	Vit. D µg	Vit. E mg	Vit. B_1 mg (M)	Vit. B_1 mg (F)	Vit. B_2 mg (M)	Vit. B_2 mg (F)	Niacin mg (M)	Niacin mg (F)	Vit. C mg
		No sex differences										
3	15	40	200	10	3	0.4		0.4		4		30
5	15	50	200	10	4	0.4		0.4		4		30
10	20	70	300	10	4	0.6		0.6		6		30
10	20	70	400	10	4	0.7		0.7		7		35
10	20	70	500	10	4	0.8		0.8		8		40
10	40	70	500	10	6	0.8		0.8		8		40
10	40	70	750	10	6	0.9		0.9		9		45
10	40	70	750	10	6	1.0		1.0		10		45
10	50	120	750	10	7	1.0		1.0		10		45
10	50	120	750	10	7	1.1		1.1		11		45
10	50	120	750	10	7	1.1		1.1		11		45
15	50	120	750	10	7	1.2		1.2		12		50
15	50	120	750	10	8	1.3		1.3		13		50
15	50	120	750	10	8	1.3		1.3		13		50
						M	F	M	F	M	F	
15	50	150	800	10	10	1.6	1.5	1.6	1.5	16	15	60
15	50	150	800	5	10	1.8	1.6	1.8	1.6	18	16	60
No sex difference		No sex differences				M	F	M	F	No sex differences		
15	50	150	800	5	10	1.2	1.1	1.2	1.1	12	11	60
15	50	150	800	5	10	1.3	1.2	1.3	1.2	13	12	60
15	50	150	800	5	10	1.5	1.4	1.5	1.4	15	14	60
15	50	150	800	5	10	1.7	1.6	1.7	1.6	17	16	60
15	50	150	800	5	10	2.0	–	2.0	–	20	–	60
20	50	175	1,000	10	12	1.8		1.8		18		80
20	50	175	1,000	10	12	1.8		1.8		18		80
20	50	200	1,200	10	12	2.1		2.1		21		100
15	50	150	800	5	12	1.2		1.2		12		60
15	50	150	800	5	12	1.2		1.2		12		60
15	50	150	800	5	12	1.3		1.3		13		60
15	50	150	800	5	12	1.5		1.5		15		60
15	50	150	800	10	12	1.2		1.2		12		60
15	50	150	800	10	12	1.2		1.2		12		60
15	50	150	800	10	12	1.3		1.3		13		60
15	50	150	800	10	12	1.0		1.0		10		60
15	50	150	800	10	12	1.2		1.2		12		60
15	50	150	800	10	12	1.0		1.0		10		60

Data of body weight of 1- to 18-years-old children and adolescents was taken from the compilation on the physical development investigation of children and adolescents of nine cities.

Unit of calorie is expressed as kcal., data in parentheses are MJ (1,000 kcal. = 4.184 MJ).

Table 11. Schemes of food provision to achieve the Chinese diet goal (kg/person/year) [data from 12]

Food	First scheme		Second scheme	
	amount of supply	grain needed	amount of supply	grain needed
Unproceesed food grains	214	214	214	214
Pork	15	75	10	60
Poultry	7	18	12	30
Eggs	12	30	12	30
Fish	6		6	
Milk	15		15	
Soybean	15		15	
Plant oil	6		6	
Vegetables	120		120	
Fruit	18		18	
Sugar	6		6	
Total		352		339

(7) Wine drinking should be controlled and restricted. Pregnant women and children should abstain for drinking wine.

(8) Establish rational dietary regulations, avoid eating and drinking too much at one meal. Calorie distribution for 3 meals including breakfast 30%, lunch 40%, and dinner 30% of the total calories respectively is recommended. Meal patterns may be regulated according to lifestyle and working hours. However, breakfast should be encouraged and arranged nicely because most work is performed intensively in the morning, and people cannot work properly without having had a breakfast.

The habit of having 3 meals a day has been handed down from generation to generation, but there have been some changes in recent times. People often neglect breakfast and many students do not have breakfast at all. Lunch is simple for most professional persons; because the lunch break is short and the distance between home and workplace is too far, numerous people bring some simple food from home, and many just buy some convenient (fast) food for lunch. When people leave work and have plenty of time to prepare dinner at home, they usually eat more then. These changes are not considered to be very healthy, but that is the present trend.

In order to study the mutual relations between nutrition and environmental factors, the Chinese Academy of Preventive Medicine and the Chinese

National Statistics Office agreed and signed to bring the nutritional monitoring system into line with the national statistics investigation project in August 1988. This will be beneficial and provide information for government policy decision [16].

Nutrition-Related Epidemic Diseases

Nutrition-related epidemic diseases have been decreased and gradually controlled. According to the report of investigation on 16 provinces, 8,840,000 patients of epidemic goiter were found [17], an incidence of 6.89% of the people investigated. After 30 years of investigations and studies, iodine deficiency in both water and foods were considered as the causative factors. In 1983 it was reported that 320 million people were threatened by iodine deficiency, and 35 million patients were found. After the popularization of adding iodine to salt and muscular injection of iodine, about 60% (21 million patients) were treated. There had been 89.6% of the population of the epidemic goiter area using iodinized salt, but still about 50% of the goiter patients are waiting to be cured [17].

In the early 1980s, an experimental study showed that sodium selenite is effective in the prevention of Ke-Shan disease in China [18]. Results of a large number of investigations showed that selenium status of Ke-Shan disease and Non-Ke-Shan disease district people were significantly different. On the basis of the gathered materials, the Chinese Nutrition Society suggested that RDA of selenium be 40–240 µg/day. In 1989, the Chinese Academy of Science established a database on 'Selenium and Health' and used the model identification method for solving the problems of selenium bioecology-food chain and for food selenium contents in different districts.

Prevention and Control of Nutritional Deficiency Diseases in Children

Considerable progress has been made in the prevention and control of children's nutritional deficiency diseases [19, 20]. Since nutrition is the guarantee for growth and development of children and is also an important factor for the nation's prosperity and improvement of physique, the government has attached great importance to measures of improving the nutrition status of children. Besides, in 1980, the government implemented a policy of 'one family, one child' which makes families take great care of children's nutrition as well. The progress on the aspects of children's nutrition was as follows:

(1) RDA for children has been revised.

(2) Breast-feeding has been promoted. Since the establishment of the People's Republic of China, women take an active part in collective productive labor. In order to let more infants have adequate breast milk, the government set up a system on women labor worker production which stipulates that

women can have breast-feeding time during work to guarantee breast-feeding of their babies. Along with the development of industry, milk, milk products and milk substitutes increased, therefore the breast-feeding rate decreased during 1960–1970. In 1982, the Chinese Ministry of Health with the cooperation of WHO analyzed the situation of breast-feeding in China, and adopted measures such as affirming studies on breast-feeding to increase the rate of breast-feeding.

(3) Studies on milk production, milk substitutes and supplementary food for children have not ceased.

(4) Nutritional deficiency diseases obviously decreased through measures of prevention and treatment. Along with the improvement of people's living standards and extensively launching child care, infant malnutrition and nutritional deficiency diseases decreased significantly.

Infant malnutrition was very common before and during the initial period of establishment of the People's Republic, e.g., the number of patients in Shanghai Children's Hospital was 11,926 from January 1938 to December 1950; among the patients, 3,293 (27.6% of the total number) suffered from malnutrition and different kinds of vitamin deficiency. The incidence of malnutrition was even higher in rural, mountainous, and border areas.

In the early 1960s, infant malnutrition was still a common disease in pediatric departments of hospitals, and it gradually decreased in the mid-1970s. During the initial period of 1980, malnutrition was seen less often in hospitals. In 1979, the International Children's Year, the Ministry of Health selectively examined 100,000 children in different districts of China and found the incidence of malnutrition to be 4%; 90% of the malnutrition patients were unserious and induced by inadequate nursing of other diseases. The incidence of infant anemia (mainly iron-deficient anemia) in 16 provinces and cities in 1980 was 57.6%, i.e., 15,806 patients had been found among 26,177 children investigated. The incidence significantly decreased through taking great care on nutrition of pregnant women, advocating breast-feeding and application of iron-fortified supplementary foods. The anemia rate had been decreased to 8–10% in the experimental areas as the Shi-He region of Xing-Jiang and Tian-Jin City.

A general survey of rickets in 1950–1960 showed that the incidence was more than 70% in the northwest, 50% in the north, and 10% in the south of China. The Rickets Research Coordination Group had investigated 184,901 children of less than 3 years of age, and found 75,259 of the investigated patients had rickets, which meant that the average incidence was 40.7%. Results of studies on rickets showed that the etiology was not only attributed to vitamin D deficiency, but the metabolic processes including intestinal absorption, liver transformation, formation of more active $1,25(OH)_2D_3$ to $25(OH)D_3$ in kidney, metabolism of hormone, amino acid, enzyme effector, and calcification process were all involved. The incidence of rickets decreased to a great extent through measures of synthetic and energetic prevention and treatment. For example, the incidence of rickets decreased from 67.7 to 7.6% in 1981, and it decreased by 76.9% in He-Bei Province in 1986 as compared with the data of the incidence in 1982.

International Exchanges among Nutrition Scientists

The international exchange of nutritional scientists has developed rapidly. China has carried out the reform and open policy since 1976. Many nutritional scientists have had the opportunity to participate at international conferences, study abroad, or exchange experiences with international colleagues. Simultaneously, quite a number of foreign nutrition scientists have been coming to visit China, exchange academic ideas and even cooperate with Chinese scholars in studies involving nutritional research projects.

Under the approval of the Chinese Ministry of Health, the Chinese Nutrition Society organized the First International Nutrition Conference at Tian-Jin City in 1985 [21]. In the same year, the President and Secretary-General of the Chinese Nutrition Society were invited by the British Society of Nutrition to attend the 13th International Nutrition Conference in England. Seventeen Chinese nutritional experts with about 30 papers attended this conference. In 1987, an American group of the People International Exchange Association came on a visit and carried out lecture exchanges [22]. In September 1991, about 30 Chinese nutritional experts joined the 6th Asian Congress on Nutrition at Kuala Lumpur, Malaysia. China also hosted the 7th Asian Congress at Beijing in 1995. A number of international collaborative nutrition research projects are in progress. Frequent contacts between China and foreign countries have brought about a great advancement of nutrition work in China.

At present, the main aspects of nutrition work going on in depth is as follows [5]: (1) From the point view and methodology of molecular biology to approach the physiological functions of main nutrients (especially trace elements and vitamins). (2) To illustrate the relation among nutrition, aging, infectious disease, immunity, intelligence, behavior, psychic function, work efficiency, growth and development, cardiovascular disease, cancer, etc. (3) Make thorough studies on new additives, possible and natural toxic and pathogenic substances, and mold toxins in foods. (4) Explore nutrition value and food toxicology of new natural resources, and new food for human consumption.

Summary

Actually, food, diet and diet therapy germinated together with the change of meal patterns and traditional Chinese medicine from very ancient China; they appeared in an embryonic form till the Shang and Zhou Dynasties and received great importance from the governors who arranged officials to manage their diets and banquets. Moreover, food, diet and meal patterns were replenished through the Zhou, Qin, Han and Jin Dynasties and epitomized and reached thriving and prosperous standards till the Tang Dynasty. They then became perfected, developed, and formed a complete theory in the dynasties of Song, Jin, Yuan, Ming and Qing.

The basis of modern nutrition was made up until the end of 19th century and the beginning of 20th century, which was the time when natural science, including microbiology, chemistry, food industry, etc. were extended into China, yet it was not fully formed until the establishment of the People's Republic of China. Practicing, teaching, training and research activities started regularly in 1950. With a big population and poor economy basis, the first problem that the Chinese people and government had to face was to have enough food to eat; the problem has now been basically solved.

Chinese nutritional scientists worked hard to find out the nutritional problems and status of the people. Through the broad-scale 'Nationwide Nutrition Survey', we now understand our main problems. On this basis, RDA, dietary goal and dietary guidance have been put forward. Although the problem of adequate food and clothing has been basically solved, the Chinese are still facing both the problem of nutrition insufficiency and nutrition excess. However, although nutrition insufficiency and deficiency still extensively exist, nutrition excess and imbalance are emerging in other sections of the population. There is still a shortage of qualified nutritional scientists and technicians, and the training of nutritionists is urgent [23].

Food supplies, including milk, beef, green vegetables and fruit should be increased, especially for some rural and remote areas. The good traditional eating habits and meal patterns should be kept, e.g., breakfast and lunch cannot be neglected, and plant protein meals and Chinese medicinal diets should be promoted. Animals fat intake and fried foods should be reduced, and exercise and fitness programs should be recommended for the overweight population.

In the future, our meal pattern may take on a mixed form with the advantages of both the eastern and western diets. Chinese scientists are confident of solving the nutritional problems and improving the whole nation's physical fitness and physique under the situation of gradual improvements of the economy and nutritional status of people.

References

1   Weng WJ: Trace to the nutritionology of traditional Chinese medicine; in Thesis Collection in 30 Years of Beijing Traditional Chinese Medical College. Beijing, TCM Ancient Book Publishing House, 1986, pp 210–213.
2   Meng ZF, Gu YM: Developmental history of Chinese diet therapy; in Qian BW, Meng ZF (eds): Chinese Diet Therapy. Shanghai Science and Technology Publishing House, 1987, pp 9–12.
3   Zhen ZY, Fu WK: Practice of medicinal health in early stage; in Zhen EY (ed): Chinese Medical History. Shanghai Science and Technology Publishing House, 1984, pp 13–15.
4   Wang MD, Wang ZH: A glimpse of the primitive diet society: Raw material of the ancient diet; in Wang MD, Wang ZH (eds): Chinese Ancient Diet. Shan Xi People's Publishing House, 1988, pp 8–56.
5   Liu YG, Zhou YZ: Nutrition and food health volume; in Chinese Medical Encyclopedia. Shanghai Science and Technology Publishing House, 1987, pp 1–4.
6   Chen HF, Zhu C: Brief history of Chinese health protection; in Chen HF, Zhu C (eds): China Health Protection. Beijing, People's Health Publishing House, 1957, pp 16–38.
7   Xue GH: General situation of nutrition health: Nutritional investigation of the whole nation; in China Health Yearbook of 1983. Beijing, People's Health Publishing House, 1983, pp 114–115.
8   Institute of Nutrition and Food Health, Chinese Academy of Preventive Medicine: Food Nutrition Composition Table (Shiwu Chengfen Biao), ed 3. Beijing, People's Health Publishing House, 1981, pp 1–262.
9   Wang GY, Shen ZP, et al: Food Nutrition Composition Table. Nationwide Representative Data. Beijing, People's Health Publishing House, 1991, pp 1–183.
10 Xue GH: Nutrition health: Nutrition investigation of the whole nation; in China Health Yearbook of 1987. Beijing, People's Health Publishing House, 1988, pp 89–92.
11 Jing DX, Chen CM et al: Summary of the Whole Nation's Nutrition Investigation. Beijing, Institute of Nutrition and Food Hygiene/China Academy of Preventive Medicine, 1985, pp 53–76.
12 Ge KY, Shen TF: Perfecting food policies and improving people's health. Acta Nutr Sin 1991;13: 376–381.
13 Chen JS: Changes of disease model and the countermove direction of prevention and treatment. Chin Prev Med 1990;24:290–293.
14 Chinese Nutrition Society: Illustration of the recommended dietary allowances of the Chinese. Acta Nutr Sin 1990;12:1–10.
15 Chinese Nutrition Society: The dietary guidance of the Chinese. Acta Nutr Sin 1990;12:10–12.
16 Kong LZ: Food health monitoring: Bring the nutritional monitoring system into line with the national statistics investigation project; in Cui YL, Qian XZ (eds): China Health Yearbook of 1989. Beijing, People's Health Publishing House, 1990, pp 1–141.
17 Qian XZ (Ed): Endemic goiter and endemic cretinism; in Historical Experience of Preventive Medicine in New China. Beijing, People's Health Publishing House, 1988, pp 397–421.
18 Bai NB, Zhang KM: Selenium, health data, and nutrition study. Acta Nutr Sin 1989;11:60–61.
19 Xue XB, Liu XY: Children's health: Children's nutrition, prevention and treatment of nutritional disease; in Qian XZ (ed): Historical Experience of Preventive Medicine of New China. Beijing, People's Health Publishing House, 1990, pp 159–217.
20 Xue XB: Recent progress of children's health; in Recent Progress of Domestic and Foreign Medical Science; Children's Health. Shanghai Institute of Medical Science Information/Science and Education Department of Ministry of Health, 1984, pp 144–150.
21 Ding W: Chinese Nutrition Society: General work situation of 1985; in Cui YL, Chen MZ, et al (eds): China Health Yearbook of 1986. Beijing, People's Health Publishing House, 1987, pp 358–359.
22 Jin GZ: Chinese Nutrition Society; in Chen MZ, He JS (eds): China Health Yearbook of 1988. Beijing, People's Health Publishing House, 1989, pp 1–476.
23 Xue GH: Discussion of training of qualified nutritionists in China; in Chen MZ, He JS (eds): China Health Yearbook of 1987. Beijing, People's Health Publishing House, 1988, pp 1–92.

J.D. Chen, Research Division of Sports Nutrition and Biochemistry, Institute of Sports Medicine, Beijing Medical University, Beijing 100083 (PR China)

Simopoulos, AP (ed): Metabolic Consequences of Changing Dietary Patterns.
World Rev Nutr Diet. Basel, Karger, 1996, vol 79, pp 154–184

....

Tea Consumption and Cancer[1]

Santosh K. Katiyar, Hasan Mukhtar[1]

Department of Dermatology, Skin Diseases Research Center, University Hospitals of
Cleveland, Case Western Reserve University, Cleveland, Ohio, USA

Contents

[1] Original work from author's laboratory was supported by USPHS Grant ES-1900
and P-30-AR-39750, and American Institute for Cancer Research Grants 90A47 and
92B35.

Introduction

Ever-increasing epidemiological, experimental, and metabolic studies are providing convincing evidence that nutrition plays an important causative role in the initiation, promotion and progression stages of several types of human cancer [1]. It is also becoming clear that, in addition to substances that pose a cancer risk, the human diet also contains agents which are capable of affording protection against some forms of cancer [2–5]. This collective information strongly suggests that the occurrence of cancer can be prevented by dietary intake of substances that have the capacity to afford protection against cancer occurrence. Chemoprevention of cancer is a means of cancer control in which the occurrence of the disease, as a consequence of exposure to carcinogenic agents, can be slowed, completely blocked or reversed by the administration of one or more naturally occurring or synthetic compounds. Such chemopreventive compounds are known as anticarcinogens, and ideally they should be nontoxic. In this category of agents, phytochemicals present in a variety of food and beverages consumed by humans are receiving increasing attention.

For many reasons, next to water, tea (*Camellia sinensis*) is the most popular beverage consumed worldwide. Tea contains several polyphenolic components which are antioxidant in nature, and many studies have shown that tea possesses the ability to prevent oxidant-induced cellular damage.

In recent years, studies from several laboratories conducted in various organ-specific animal bioassay systems have shown that tea, specifically the polyphenolic constituents isolated from it, is capable of affording protection against cancer induced by both chemical as well as physical agents. The majority of the studies are based on green tea whereas a limited number of studies have been done with black tea. This review presents a critical examination of this topic. To introduce the subject we feel it is necessary to provide some discussion on the consumption, composition, basic chemistry of tea and epidemiologic studies of tea usage.

Consumption of Tea

The tea plant originated in Southeast Asia and is presently cultivated in over 30 countries around the globe and currently tea beverage is consumed worldwide, although at greatly varying levels. Consumption of tea is far from uniform. Large segments of the world's population virtually consume no tea. Not only does tea consumption vary from country to country, but also there is enormous variation in any given population. This ranges from none to as many as 20 or more cups per day [6]. Although no firm data are available, it appears universally accepted that next to water, tea is the most consumed beverage in the world; with a per capita worldwide consumption of approximately 120 ml/day [6].

Of the approximately 2.5 million metric tons of dried tea manufactured annually, only 20% is green tea and less than 2% is oolong tea. Green tea is produced in relatively few countries, and is consumed primarily in China, Japan, India, and a few countries in North Africa and the Middle East. About 78% of the world tea consumption is the beverage prepared from black tea, generally consumed in the Western countries and some Asian countries. Oolong tea production and consumption is confined to southeastern China, and Taiwan [7].

Composition of Various Teas

Normally the composition of tea leaf varies with climate, season, horticultural practices, variety of the plant, and age of the leaf, i.e. the position of the leaf on the harvested shoot. Three main commercial tea beverage varieties are available, and their composition varies according to the manufacturing processes involved. In table 1 the principal components present in typical green and black tea beverages are shown but variations may be considerable [6]. Oolong tea composition in general falls in between green and black teas.

Green Tea: In the process of green tea manufacture, the steps include plucking, rapid enzyme inactivation by steaming or pan firing, rolling, and air drying at high temperature. During the final drying step many new aromatic compounds are formed which provide tea its characteristic flavor.

Black tea: In the process of black tea production the steps are plucking, withering, maceration, and drying. Withering lowers the moisture level and renders the leaf more amenable to maceration. In this step, cell disruption takes place and polyphenol oxidase catalyzes oxidation of epicatechin derivatives. The oxidation is allowed to proceed for 45–90 min, during which catechins are converted to theaflavins and thearubigins, which give the characteristic color and taste of black tea.

Oolong tea: In the process of manufacture of oolong tea, oxidation for a short period of time is allowed. Normal oolong tea is considered to be about

Table 1. Principal components of green and black tea beverages (measured in weight % of extract solids)

Components	Green tea	Black tea
Catechins	30–42	3–10
Flavanols	5–10	6–8
Other flavonoids	2–4	–
Theogallin	2–3	–
Ascorbic acid	1–2	–
Gallic acid	0.5	–
Quinic acid	2.0	–
Other organic acids	4–5	–
Theanine	4–6	–
Other amino acids	4–6	13–15
Methylxanthines	7–9	8–11
Carbohydrates	10–15	15
Minerals	6–8	10
Volatiles	0.02	<0.1
Theaflavins	–	3–6
Thearubigins	–	12–18

half fermented compared to black tea. Oolong tea extracts contains catechins at a level of 8–20% of the total dry matter.

Chemistry of Tea

The chemical composition of green tea is approximately similar to that of the fresh leaf with regard to the major components. Green tea contains polyphenols, which include flavanols, flavandiols, flavonoids, and phenolic acids. These compounds account up to 30% of the dry weight of green tea leaves. Most of the polyphenols present in green tea are flavanols, commonly known as catechins. Some major catechins present in green tea are (–)-epicatechin (EC), (–)-epicatechin-3-gallate (ECG), (–)-epigallocatechin (EGC), and (–)-epigallocatechin-3-gallate (EGCG). The chemical structures of these compounds are given in figure 1. In addition, caffeine, theobromine, theophylline, and phenolic acids such as gallic acids are also present in green tea (table 1).

During the fermentation process involved in the manufacture of black tea, the monomeric flavan-3-ols undergoes polyphenol oxidase-dependent oxidative polymerization leading to the formation of bisflavanols, theaflavins, thearubigins, and some other oligomers. Theaflavins (1–2%, on dry weight basis) contain benzotropolone rings with dihydroxy or trihydroxy substitution systems. About 10–20% of the dry weight of black tea is due to thearubigens,

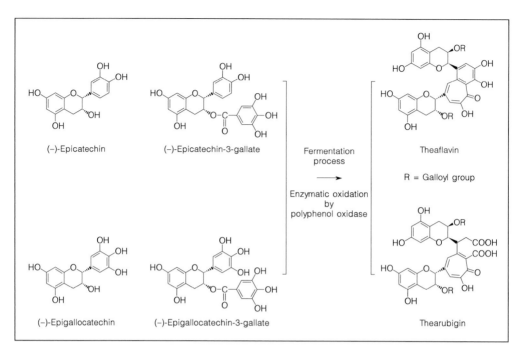

Fig. 1. Structures of major polyphenols present in green (left) and black (right) tea.

which are even more extensively oxidized and polymerized. The structures of theaflavins and thearubigins are shown in figure 1.

Oolong tea contains monomeric catechins, theaflavins, and thearubigins. In addition, epigallocatechin esters, theasinensins, dimeric catechins, and dimeric proanthocyanidins also occur as characteristic components in oolong tea.

Epidemiologic Studies on Tea and Cancer

The epidemiologic studies reviewed by the Working Group of the International Agency for Research on Cancer (IARC) on consumption of tea and its effects on cancer of various body sites, yielded inconsistent and inconclusive results [8]. This study concluded that there is inadequate evidence for the carcinogenicity of tea in humans (who drink tea), and also inadequate evidence for the carcinogenicity of tea in experimental animals [8]. Additionally, available epidemiologic data do not provide sufficient indication that tea consumption has a statistically significant causative effect on human cancers (table 2). However, possible harmful effects of the consumption of excessive amounts of tea, tea consumption at very high temperature, or salted tea, cannot be ruled out, and this is an area in which additional research is required. In this review we are providing a general overview of the pertinent epidemiologic studies on tea consumption and cancer causation and/or prevention at different sites.

Tea and Cancer of the Esophagus

Morton and co-workers [9–11] suggested that excessive consumption of tea may be a causative factor for the high incidence of esophageal cancer in the geographical zone between Iran to northern China. A geographical correlation study in the Caspian littoral of Iran [12] indicated that individuals in the high-incidence area consumed more tea than in low-incidence areas. A similar study by Segi [13] suggested that consumption of hot green tea-gruel is a causative factor for esophageal cancer in the Nara and Wekayama Prefectures in Japan. In China, most of the areas with higher esophageal cancer mortality rates are in the northern provinces where tea is not produced and is infrequently consumed. In the high-incidence area of Linxian in northern China, consumption of tea is rare and is believed not to be a contributing factor [14]. Two case-control studies in southern Brazil [15] and northern Italy [16] also indicated that there was no relationship between esophageal cancer risk and the frequency of tea consumption.

Several case-control studies [17–21] showed no association between drinking of tea at normal temperature (35–47 °C) and esophageal cancer, but ingestion of tea at hot temperature (55–67 °C) was associated with 2- to 3-fold increases in the risk for esophageal cancer. Case-control studies conducted in Kazakhastan [18, 19] revealed that only the consumption of very hot tea was associated with a 3-fold higher risk of esophageal cancer. A case-control study by Cook-Mozaffari et al. [20] indicated that only the ingestion of very hot tea had a statistically significant association with esophageal cancer. Yang and Wang [22] have suggested that the high temperature of tea or hot tea itself, rather than the components present in tea, is an important factor in human esophageal cancer. In a case-control study, Gao et al. [23] showed that consumption of green tea reduces the risk of esophageal cancer. This study concluded that 'the population-based case-control study of esophageal cancer in urban Shanghai, People's Republic of China, suggests a protective effect of green tea consumption. Although these findings are consistent with studies in laboratory animals, indicating that green tea can inhibit esophageal carcinogenesis, further investigations are definitely needed' [23]. Recently, Zheng et al. [24] have conducted a cohort study in postmenopausal women in Iowa which revealed inverse associations between tea consumption and cancer risk for oropharyngeal and esophageal cancers. Daily consumption of tea was found to be associated with an over 50% lower risk of these cancers.

Table 2. Summary of epidemiological studies conducted in relation to tea consumption and human cancer

Test organ	Association of tea drinking to cancer	Number and kind of studies	Ref.
Bladder and urinary tract	No relationship	1 ecological study	39
		2 cohort studies	33, 40
		16 case-control studies	16,36–38, 41–52
Breast	Enhanced risk	1 ecological study	39
	No relationship	5 case-control studies	12, 65–67
	Lower risk	1 ecological study	25
Colon and rectum	Enhanced risk	1 ecological study	39
		1 cohort study	40
		1 case-control study	16
	No relationship	1 cohort study	33
		5 case-control studies	27, 28, 60–62
	Lower risk	3 case-control studies	57–59
Esophagus	Enhanced risk	3 ecological studies	9, 13
		5 case-control studies (with high temperature tea)	18–21
	No relationship	1 ecological study	39
		4 case-control studies (with normal temperature tea)	18–21
		2 case-control studies	15, 16
	Lower risk	1 cohort study	24
		1 case-control study	35
Kidney	Enhanced risk	1 cohort study	33
	No relationship	5 case-control studies	16, 53–56
	Lower risk	1 cohort study	24
Liver	No relationship	1 ecological study	39
		1 cohort study	40
		1 case-control study	16
	Lower risk	1 ecological study	25
Lung	Enhanced risk	1 ecological study	39
		1 cohort study	33
		1 case-control study	63
	Lower risk	1 ecological study	25
Nasopharynx	No relationship	3 case-control studies	75–77
Pancreas	Enhanced risk	1 case-control study	74
	No relationship	3 cohort studies	33, 40, 70
		7 case-control studies	16, 66, 68, 69, 71–73

Table 2 (Continued)

Test organ	Association of tea drinking to cancer	Number and kind of studies	Ref.
Stomach	Enhanced risk	1 cohort study	33
		1 case-control study	34
	No relationship	7 case-control studies	16, 26–31
	Lower risk	1 ecological study	25
		1 case-control study	35
		1 cohort study	24
Uterus	Lower risk	2 ecological studies	25, 39

Tea and Cancer of the Stomach

Epidemiological studies conducted in Shizuoka Prefecture, Japan [25] indicated that the cancer death rate in this tea-producing area, especially from stomach cancer, was lower than the national average. Case-control studies conducted on stomach cancer and tea consumption in Buffalo [26], Kansas City [27], Nagoya, Japan [28], Piraeus, Greece [29], Milan, Italy [16], Spain [30], and Turkey [31] indicated that there was no statistically significant association between tea consumption and cancer of the stomach. However, a case-control study in Kyushu, Japan, showed that individuals consuming green tea more frequently or in larger quantities tended to have a lower risk of gastric cancer [32]. A cohort study conducted in London [33] showed a positive association between black tea consumption and stomach cancer. A case-control study in Taipei, Taiwan, also suggested that green tea consumption is a risk factor for gastric cancer [34]. A cohort study conducted in Iowa by Zheng et al. [24] showed inverse relationship between tea consumption and stomach cancer. A case-control study to evaluate risk factors of gastric cancer was carried out in areas with contrasting incidence rates in Sweden [35]. This population-based study confirmed that tea had a statistically significantly protective effect when it was consumed during adolescence [35].

Tea and Cancer of the Bladder, Kidney and Urinary Tract

Several case-control studies were conducted to find out the association of tea consumption and the cancers of bladder and urinary tract [16, 33, 36–53] but no positive relationship was observed. In a cohort study [33], a positive correlation was observed between tea consumption and cancer of the kidney. On the other hand, in five other case-control studies, no association was found between green tea consumption and renal cell cancer [16, 53–56].

A recently reported cohort study in Iowa revealed that daily tea consumption reduced the risk of kidney cancers in postmenopausal women [24].

Tea and Cancer of the Colon, Rectum and Uterus

Three studies [16, 39, 40] showed a positive association between tea consumption and colon and rectal cancer. Three other studies [57–59] indicated that consumption of black tea decreased the risk for rectal cancer, while six other studies [27, 28, 41, 60–62] showed no correlation. Two observations [25, 39] report the possible negative association between tea consumption and cancer of the uterus, but many more studies are required to draw a final conclusion.

Tea and Cancer of the Liver, Lung, Breast, Pancreas and Nasopharynx

A negative association between green tea consumption and liver cancer incidence was observed in Shizuoka Prefecture of Japan [25], while no relationship was observed in three other studies [16, 39, 40]. Both positive and negative associations with tea consumption and lung cancer have been reported [25, 39, 41, 63]. No association between tea consumption and breast cancer was observed in five case-control studies [12, 64–67]. These studies are believed to be more informative than the contradictory results from two ecologic studies [25, 39]. In ten individual studies, no relationship was found between pancreatic cancer and tea consumption [16, 40, 41, 66, 68–73], while only one positive association was observed in a case-control study [74]. In three case-control studies [75–77], no correlation between tea consumption and nasopharyngeal cancer was observed.

On the basis of available epidemiologic studies and careful recent observations made in laboratory animals, we believe that tea consumption is likely to have protective effects in reducing cancer risk and suggest that more case-controlled studies be undertaken.

Experimental Studies on Anticarcinogenic Effects of Tea

Protection against Chemical Carcinogen-Induced Skin Tumorigenesis
Protection against Skin Tumor Initiation

Utilizing several tumor bioassay protocols, studies from this and other laboratories [22, 78–80] have shown that topical application or oral feeding of a polyphenolic fraction isolated from green tea, hereafter referred to as GTP, to SENCAR, CD-1, and Balb/C mice results in significant protection against skin tumorigenesis (table 3). In a complete carcinogenesis protocol, topical application of GTP on the backs of BALB/C mice for 7 days prior to

Table 3. Summary of studies demonstrating chemopreventive effect of tea against tumorigenesis in mouse skin

Tumorigenesis protocol	Mouse strain	Carcinogen used	Promotor used	Treatment	Mode of application	Ref.
Complete						
	Balb/C	3-MC		GTP	Topical	81
	SKH-1 hr	UVB	UVB	GTP	Topical	92
	SKH-1 hr	UVB	UVB	GTP	Drinking water	92
Multistage (during initiation)						
	SENCAR	DMBA	TPA	GTP	Topical	81
	SENCAR	DMBA	TPA	GTP	Drinking water	81
	SKH-1 hr	UVB	TPA	WEGT	Drinking water	93
	CD-1	BP/DMBA	TPA	GTP	Topical	86
Multistage (during promotion)						
	SENCAR	DMBA	TPA	GTP	Topical	85
	CD-1	DMBA	TPA	GTP	Topical	86
	CD-1	DMBA	Teleocidin	EGCG	Topical	87
	SKH-1 hr	DMBA	TPA	WEGT	Drinking water	93
	SKH-1 hr	DMBA	UVB	WEGT	Drinking water	93
	SKH-1 hr	DMBA	UVB	WEGT/WEBT	Drinking water	94
Stage I	SENCAR	DMBA	TPA	GTP	Topical	88
Stage II	SENCAR	DMA	Mezerein	GTP	Topical	88
Multistage (during progression)						
	SENCAR	4-NQO[a]	–	GTP	Topical	90
	SENCAR	BPO[a]	–	GTP	Topical	90
	SKH-1 hr	DMBA	UVB	WEGT/WEBT	Drinking water	94
Chemotherapeutic effect						
	CD-1	DMBA/UVB	TPA	GTP/WEGT/ EGCG	Drinking water/i.p.	96

[a] Used as malignant enhancer.

that of 3-methylcholanthrene, was found to result in significant protection against the development of skin tumors [81]. Studies were also conducted to assess whether GTP possesses antitumor initiating effects. For these studies a two-stage skin carcinogenesis protocol in SENCAR mice was employed. Topical application of GTP for 7 days prior to the single application of 7,12-dimethylbenz[*a*]anthracene (DMBA) as the initiating agent followed by twice weakly applications of the tumor promoter 12-O-tetradecanoyl-phorbol-13-acetate (TPA) resulted in significant protection against tumorigenesis [81]. In this study, in GTP-treated animals considerable delay in the latency period for the appearance of the first tumor and subsequent tumor growth was also observed. Oral feeding of 0.05% (w/v) GTP in drinking water (this dose approximately corresponds to four cups of tea drinking per day by an adult human) for 50 days prior to the DMBA-TPA treatment or its continuous feeding during the entire period of the tumor protocol was also found to result in significant protection both in terms of the tumor incidence and tumor multiplicity [81].

EGCG is the major constituent (61–85%) present in GTP [82], and in a cup of green tea its concentration ranges from 10 to 30 mg. As such the intake of EGCG in individuals who habitually consume green tea is substantial. For this reason, it was of interest to examine the utility of this tea component as a cancer-chemopreventive agent. Topical application of 15 μmol EGCG/mouse for 7 days prior to initiation with DMBA followed by twice weekly applications with TPA as the tumor promoter resulted in a significant protection against skin tumor initiation in SENCAR mouse skin [82]. In these experiments, skin application of EGCG to the SENCAR mouse prior to that of carcinogen treatment was found to result in 30% inhibition in carcinogen metabolite binding to epidermal DNA suggesting that EGCG may be affording its inhibition by inhibiting the metabolism of the precarcinogen [82].

Protection against Skin Tumor Promotion

Since without promoting substances usually cancer does not result, the inhibitors of tumor promotion stage of carcinogenesis are most likely of value as chemopreventive agents for human population. Phorbol ester TPA is the most widely employed tumor promoter in two-stage skin tumorigenesis protocol [83, 84]. We investigated the effect of GTP on TPA-induced skin tumor promotion in DMBA-initiated SENCAR mouse. Topical application of varying doses of GTP prior to that of TPA resulted in highly significant protection against skin tumor promotion in a dose-dependent manner [85]. The animals pretreated with GTP showed substantially lower tumor body burden such as decrease in total number of tumors per group, number of tumors per animal, tumor volume per mouse and average tumor size, as compared to the animals which did not receive GTP [85]. In other studies, it was shown that topical application of GTP to CD-1 mice also inhibited TPA-induced tumor promotion in DMBA initiated skin [86]. Topical application of GTP or its major component EGCG has been shown to inhibit tumor promotion mediated by TPA [85, 86] and by other skin tumor promoters teleocidin and okadaic acid [86, 87].

Protection against Stage I and Stage II Skin Tumor Promotion

Skin tumor promotion is often divided in two operational stages known as stage I and stage II. We performed experiments to determine which of these two stages of tumor promotion is inhibited by GTP. Topical application of GTP concurrently with each application of either TPA (anti-stage I) or mezerein (anti-stage II) resulted in significant protection against tumor formation in DMBA-initiated SENCAR mouse, in terms of both tumor multiplicity (42–50%) and tumor growth (43–54%) [88]. Furthermore, sustained inhibition of tumor promotion by GTP required a continuous application of GTP in conjunction with each promotional treatment of TPA or mezerein. Under this treatment regimen, compared to non-GTP-treated positive controls, GTP application was found to inhibit significantly tumor growth/development. These data indicate that GTP is capable of inhibiting both stage I and stage II of skin tumor promotion, and that the inhibition of tumor promotion depends on the duration of GTP treatment [88].

Protection against Malignant Conversion of Chemically Induced Benign Skin Papillomas to Carcinomas

Progression of benign tumors to malignant cancer is the most critical step in carcinogenesis since malignant lesions are capable of metastatic spread and eventual death [89]. To assess the possible role of GTP in inhibition of conversion of chemically-induced benign skin papillomas to squamous cell carcinomas, SENCAR mice were initiated by topical application of DMBA following by twice weekly applications of TPA as tumor-promoting agent. Beginning at the 20th week, when papilloma yield was stabilized, enhancement of rate of malignant conversion was achieved by twice weekly topical applications of either free-radical generating compound, benzoyl peroxide or genotoxic agent, 4-nitroquinoline-N-oxide, whereas spontaneous malignant conversion was associated with topical application of acetone. In these protocols, preapplication of GTP 30 min prior to skin application of acetone, benzoyl peroxide or 4-nitroquinoline-N-oxide resulted in significant protection when assessed for the conversion of papillomas to carcinomas. This study suggests that green tea also possesses significant protective effects against tumor progression induced by free-radical generating compounds and genotoxic agents [90].

Protection against Ultraviolet B (UVB) Radiation-Induced Photocarcinogenesis

UVB radiation present in the solar spectrum is the major risk factor for skin cancer in humans [91]. We assessed the effect of oral feeding of GTP in drinking water as well as its topical application to SKH-1 hairless mice on UVB radiation-induced photocarcinogenesis [92]. Chronic oral feeding of 0.1%

(w/v) GTP in drinking water to mice during the entire period of UVB exposure was found to result in significantly lower tumor body burden as compared to non-GTP fed animals [92]. Topical application of GTP before UVB radiation exposure was also found to afford some protection against photocarcinogenesis; observed protection was, however, lower than that observed after oral feeding of GTP in drinking water. This observation was validated in terms of percentage of mice with tumors and number of tumors per mouse [92]. In another study [93] it was shown that infusion of green tea extracts as a sole source of drinking water (1.25%, w/v) to mice afforded protection against UVB radiation-induced intensity of red color and area of skin lesions, as well as UVB radiation-induced tumor initiation and tumor promotion.

Wang et al. [94] have shown that black tea consumption markedly reduced tumor formation in SKH-1 hairless mice initiated with DMBA and then exposed to multiple applications of UVB. Oral administration of 0.63 or 1.25% black tea, green tea, and decaffeinated black or green tea as the sole source of drinking water 2 weeks prior to and during 31 weeks of UVB treatment was found to reduce tumor risk in terms of number of tumors per animal, and also the tumor size. These studies suggest that consumption of tea as a sole source of drinking water may reduce the risk of some forms of human cancers induced by solar UV radiation. Liu et al. [95] have analyzed p^{53} and H-*ras* mutations in UV- and UV/green tea-induced skin tumors in SKH-1 mice, and found that mutations in exon 6 of the p^{53} gene are unique for tumors from UV/green tea group. They suggested that green tea may, somehow, select certain p^{53} mutations during the chemoprevention process.

Effect on Growth of Skin Tumors

Wang et al. [96] have demonstrated that consumption of water extracts of green tea (WEGT) or GTP in addition to resulting in decreased tumor formation and their multiplicity, also markedly reduced the tumor size. In this study it was also shown that feeding WEGT, or GTP or EGCG given intraperitoneally, inhibited tumor growth and caused partial regression of established skin papillomas in female CD-1 mice [96]. These observations suggest that green tea may also possess chemotherapeutic effects.

Protection against Forestomach and Lung Tumorigenesis

We assessed whether oral consumption of tea may result in anticarcinogenic effects in internal body organs [97]. In our laboratory, 2.5% (w/v) WEGT (when analyzed on HPLC showed ≈0.2% GTP) was fed to female A/J mice as the sole source of drinking water. Diethylnitrosamine (DEN) (20 mg/kg body weight of animal and benzo[*a*]pyrene (BαP) (2 mg/animal) were employed as test carcinogens. The mice were sacrificed 26 weeks after the first carcinogen challenge, and tumors were counted in lungs and forestomach. By modifying the tumorigenesis protocols, we assessed whether WEGT affords protection against tumor initiation, tumor promotion and complete carcinogenesis. Our data indicated that compared to DEN-treated group of mice, the animals fed with WEGT plus DEN show significantly lower tumor body burden both in lungs and forestomach. When data were considered in terms of appearance of total number of tumors per mouse, significant protection against tumorigenesis in forestomach (80–85%) and lung (41–61%) at all the stages of carcinogenesis was evident. In case of BαP-induced tumorigenicity, WEGT also resulted in 60–75 and 25–35% protection in total number of tumors per mouse against forestomach and lung tumorigenesis at all the stages of carcinogenesis [97]. In other studies, we and others have shown that treatment of A/J mice with 0.63, 1.2 or 1.25% WEGT protects against DEN and BαP-induced forestomach and lung tumorigenesis [98, 99]. Xu et al. [100] have also shown that 2% green tea infusion or 560 ppm EGCG feeding in drinking water for 13 weeks affords protection against 4-(methylnitrosamino)-1-(3-pyridyl)-1-butanone (a carcinogen found in cigarette smoke and tobacco which is highly specific for lung cancer induction in various laboratory animals and possibly in man) -induced lung tumorigenesis in A/J mice.

Utilizing the absolutely identical protocols as mentioned for WEGT [97], we also assessed the protective effects of GTP against DEN and BαP-induced tumorigenesis in forestomach and lung of female A/J mice. The results of these studies showed that oral feeding of 0.2% (w/v) GTP significantly affords protection against DEN-induced total number of tumors per mouse in forestomach (68–82%) and lung tumorigenesis (37–45%) during initiation, promotion and complete carcinogenesis. Comparable protective effects of GTP were also observed when BαP was used as a carcinogen in these studies. In further studies, we [101] have also demonstrated that administration of GTP (5 mg/animal) by gavage 30 min prior to challenge with carcinogen afforded significant protection against both DEN- and BαP-induced forestomach and lung tumorigenesis in A/J mice. In a subsequent study, Shi et al. [102] have shown that when decaffeinated green or black tea extracts were given to female A/J mice as the sole source of drinking water before an intraperitoneal injection of NNK (100 mg/kg body weight), a significant reduction in lung tumor multiplicity was observed. Wu et al. [103] reported that oolong tea, jasmine tea and green tea inhibited urethan-induced lung neoplasia in Kunming mice. Collectively, the data summarized in tables 4 and 5 suggest that polyphenolic compounds present in tea afford protection against chemical carcinogen-induced tumor initiation, and tumor promotion in lung and forestomach of A/J mice.

Table 4. Summary of chemopreventive effects of oral feeding of WEGT, and GTP in drinking water against chemical carcinogen-induced forestomach and lung tumorigenesis in A/J mice

Tumorigenesis protocol	Carcinogen administered	Treatment	Ref.
Complete	DEN	WEGT	98
Complete	BP	WEGT	98
Complete	DEN	WEGT	99
Initiation, promotion, and complete	DEN	WEGT	97
Initiation, promotion, and complete	BP	WEGT	97
Initiation, promotion, and complete	DEN	GTP	97
Initiation, promotion, and complete	BP	GTP	97

Protection against Esophageal Tumorigenesis

Chen [104] reported the chemopreventive effects of different varieties of Chinese tea including green tea against N-nitrosomethylbenzylamine (NMBzA)-induced esophageal tumorigenicity in Wistar rats. Oral administration of 2% tea infusion as the sole source of drinking water to rats during the entire experimental period resulted in inhibition of esophageal tumorigenesis induced by NMBzA. All five brands of green and black tea tested were effective; the tumor incidence was reduced by 26–53%, and tumor multiplicity was reduced by 58–75%. Oral feeding of green tea infusion also inhibited esophageal tumor formation induced by precursors of NMBzA [105] or by nitrososarcosine in mice [25]. Oral administration of 0.6% decaffeinated green or black tea extracts as the sole source of drinking water to Sprague-Dawley rats during the NMBzA (2.5 mg/kg) treatment period or after the NMBzA treatment period decreased the papilloma multiplicity and reduced the size of esophageal papillomas [106].

Table 5. Summary of chemopreventive effect of oral feeding of WEGT, GTP, and EGCG in drinking water against chemical carcinogen-induced tumorigenesis in different tumor models

Animal model	Tumor site	Carcinogen administered	Treatment	Ref.
A/J mice	Lung	NNK	WEGT	99
A/J mice	Lung	NNK	WEGT	100
A/J mice	Lung	NNK	EGCG	100
A/J mice	Lung	NNK	decaffeinated WEGT	102
A/J mice	Lung	DEN/BαP	GTP	101
C57BL/6 mice	Duodenum	ENNG	EGCG	107
Wistar rats	Esophagus	NMBzA	WEGT	104
Fisher rats	Colon	AOM	GTP	109
Sprague-Dawley rats	Mammary gland	DMBA	GTP	108, 115
F344 rats	Small intestine	_[a]	GTP	108
Rats, male Swiss mice	Liver	DEN	GTL	112, 113
Rat	Liver	Aflatoxin B$_1$	GTL	111
Syrian golden hamster	Pancreas	NBA[b]	WEGT	117

[a] In multiorgan carcinogenesis model, DEN, NNK, 1,2-dimethylhydrazine, N-butyl-N-(hydroxybutyl)nitrosamine, N-methylnitrosamine and 2,2'-dihydroxy-di-*n*-propylnitrosamine were used as carcinogens.

[b] N-nitroso-bis(2-oxopropyl)amine.

GTL = Green tea leaves.

Protection against Duodenum and Small Intestine Tumorigenesis

Fujita et al. [107] reported the chemopreventive effects of EGCG against N-ethyl-N′-nitro-N-nitrosoguanidine (ENNG)-induced duodenum tumorigenicity in C57BL/6 mice. In this study, compared to non-EGCG-fed animals, oral feeding of 0.005% EGCG in the drinking water after treatment with carcinogen resulted in significant protection against ENNG-caused tumor promotion in duodenum as observed by a decrease in tumor incidence and number of tumors per mouse. In multiorgan carcinogenesis model in which F344 rats were pretreated with combined administration of five carcinogens for the initial 4 weeks, Hirose et al. [108] demonstrated that the diet, supplemented with 1% GTP given during or after the carcinogen exposure period, inhibited adenoma and adenocarcinoma formation in the small intestine.

Protection against Colon Tumorigenesis

Yamane et al. [109] used a rat colon tumorigenicity model, and showed that 1 week after subcutaneous administration of azoxymethane to fisher rats, oral feeding of 0.01 or 0.1% GTP in drinking water for an additional 10 weeks resulted in the inhibition of azoxymethane-induced colon tumorigenesis as observed by decrease in tumor incidence, tumor number, and tumor size compared to non-GTP-fed control rats. However, in a multiorgan tumorigenesis model with rats, administration of 1% GTP in the diet was not found to inhibit tumorigenesis in the colon [108]. Narisawa and Fukaura [110] tested a very low dose of GTP against colon carcinogenesis in F344 rats. In this study a total of 129 female F344 rats were given an intrarectal instillation of 2 mg of N-methyl-N-nitrosourea 3 times a week for 2 weeks, and provided WEGT as a sole source of drinking water throughout the experiment. Autopsies at week 35 revealed significantly lower incidence of colon carcinomas in rats ingesting 0.05, 0.01 or 0.002% WEGT than in control rats which were not given WEGT [110].

Protection against Liver Tumorigenesis

Administration of 5% green tea leaf in the diet from 10 days prior to the test carcinogen aflatoxin B_1, treatment until 3 days after the treatment resulted in a significant inhibition of aflatoxin B_1-induced γ-glutamyltranspeptidase-positive foci in the rat liver [111]. It was also shown that 2.5% green tea leaf in the diet given to rats produced significant inhibition of DEN-induced hepatocarcinogenesis [112]. Decaffeinated black tea extract given by oral gavage to male Swiss mice was also found to decrease tobacco-induced liver tumors [113].

Protection against Mammary Carcinogenesis

The spontaneous mammary tumor formation was markedly inhibited in female C3H/HeN mice when fed GTP with 0.2% aluminum hydroxide from birth to the age of 330 days [114]. Hirose et al. [108, 115] reported the effect of 1% green tea catechins on mammary gland carcinogenesis in female Sprague-Dawley rats pretreated with DMBA. Although the final incidences and multiplicities of mammary tumors were not significantly different between tea drinkers and nontea drinkers, it was found that the number of survivors in the green tea catechins-fed group at the end of the experiment at week 36 were significantly higher than in the basal diet group. The average size of the palpable mammary tumor was significantly smaller in the green tea catechins-fed group. The results of this study indicate that green tea catechins also inhibit rat mammary gland carcinogenesis after DMBA initiation. Recently, Sakamoto et al. [116] have shown that GTP and BTP depressed the growth of canine mammary tumor (CMT-13) cells in culture when added at 25 ppm or more for 24 h or more. This study also showed that black tea polyphenols (BTP) are more effective inhibitors of mammary tumor cells than GTP.

Protection against Pancreatic and Prostate Carcinogenesis

In a carcinogenesis model in which Syrian golden hamsters were treated with N-nitroso-bis(2-oxopropyl)amine and then put on a protein-deficient diet consisting of *D,L*-ethionine and *L*-methionine for tumor promotion, dietary supplementation with GTP (500 mg/kg/day) during the promotion stage was found to reduce pancreatic tumorigenesis [117].

Recently, Mohan et al. [118] have shown that pretreatment of human prostate carcinoma cell line LNCaP for 1 h with GTP resulted in a significant inhibition, in a dose-dependent manner, of testosterone-induced ornithine decarboxylase (ODC) activity and mRNA expression. ODC is the rate-limiting enzyme in polyamine biosynthesis and plays an important role in cellular proliferation and differentiation, the steps involved in cancer induction. This study suggests that the consumption of GTP may be an approach for prostate cancer chemoprevention. Additional work is required to validate this suggestion.

Experimental Studies against Inflammatory Disorders by Tea

Protection against TPA-Caused Inflammatory Responses

Since edema and hyperplasia are often used as an early marker of skin tumor promotion, we assessed the effect of preapplication of GTP on these parameters. As described [85], skin application of GTP to SENCAR mice was found to result in significant protection against TPA-caused effects on cyclooxygenase and lipoxygenase activities. Lipoxygenase plays a role in inflammatory responses. Prior application of GTP to that of TPA onto the mouse dorsal skin was found to result in significant inhibition of TPA-induced epidermal edema and hyperplasia [85]. In further studies, we found that single or multiple application of GTP to SENCAR mouse ear skin prior to or after the application of TPA affords significant protection against TPA-induced edema [119]. Preapplication of GTP also afforded significant protection against TPA-induced hyperplasia in the ear skin. The percentage protection by GTP both in terms of epidermal thickness and vertical cell layers was 75 and 90% respectively. It was also found that GTP afforded protection against TPA-caused infiltration of polymorphonuclear leukocytes [119].

Protection against UVB Radiation-Caused Inflammatory Responses

Experiments were performed to assess whether GTP possesses protective effects against UVB radiation-caused changes in murine skin. Chronic oral feeding of 0.2% GTP (w/v) as the sole source of drinking water for 30 days to SKH-1 hairless mice followed by irradiation with UVB (900 mJ/cm^2) was found to result in significant protection against UVB radiation-caused cutaneous edema, and depletion of antioxidant-defense system in epidermis [120]. The oral feeding of GTP also afforded protection against UVB radiation-caused induction of epidermal ODC and cyclooxygenase activities in a time-dependent manner [120].

Inhibition of Tumor Promoter-Caused Induction of Cytokines

Cytokines play an important role in a variety of physiological and pathological processes including inflammation, wound healing, immunity, and hematopoiesis. One cytokine, interleukin-1α (IL-1α), is known to play an important role in both immune and inflammatory reactions, and it has been shown that IL-1α is induced in response to various skin tumor promoters [121]. We conducted studies to assess whether pretreatment of the animal with GTP can afford protection against tumor promoter-caused induction of IL-1α expression in the murine skin model system. Northern blot analysis of IL-1α gene expression in mouse skin reveals that topical application of GTP or black tea polyphenols prior to treatment with TPA resulted in significant inhibition of TPA-induced expression of epidermal IL-1α mRNA. These inhibitory effects were found to be dependent on the dose of GTP or black tea polyphenols used. GTP was also found to inhibit IL-1α gene expression, and IL-1α protein levels, induced by various other structurally unrelated skin tumor promoters like mezerein, benzoyl peroxide and anthralin [121]. In this study, EGCG and ECG showed maximum inhibitory effects at equimolar dose as compared to other ECDs [121].

Implications of Anti-Inflammatory Effects

The above outlined studies suggest that tea, and particularly green tea, may be used against inflammatory responses associated with the exposure of skin to UV solar radiation [120, 121]. The validity of these studies to humans exposed to low level of UV radiations chronically through solar radiation is an area for further study.

Mechanistic Studies regarding Anticarcinogenic and Anti-inflammatory Effects

Protection against Mutagenicity and Genotoxicity

Tea was found to suppress the mutagenicity of products formed in a model nitrosation reaction system [78]. GTP and WEGT were found to significantly inhibit the mutagenicity induced by BαP, aflatoxin B_1, 2-aminofluorene, and methanol extract of coal tar pitch in bacterial or mammalian cell test systems

[122]. Jain et al. [123] showed that tea extracts inhibited N-methyl-N'-nitro-N-nitrosoguanidine (MNNG)-induced mutagenicity in vitro as well as in intragastric tract of rats. It was also observed that pyrogallol-related compounds of green tea, such as EGCG, ECG and EGC are antimutagenic in nature in the *Escherichia coli* B/r WP_2 assay system [123–125]. Oral feeding of green tea or black tea extracts to rats was shown to inhibit chromosomal aberrations in rat bone marrow cells if the extracts were given 24 h prior to aflatoxin B_1 treatment [126]. Other studies showed that compared to other chemopreventive agents like ellagic acid, ascorbic acid, tocopherol and β-carotene, GTP afforded stronger inhibitory effects against mutagenicity of cigarette smoke condensate in the Ames test [127].

Heterocyclic amines (HCAs), formed during the cooking of meats and fish, are thought to be the genotoxic carcinogenes associated with important types of human cancer in meat-eating populations, such as cancer of the breast, colon or pancreas [128]. Weisburger et al. [128] studied the effect of black and green tea, and of the tea polyphenol theaflavin gallate (black tea) and EGCG (green tea) on the formation of typical HCAs, 2-amino-3,8-dimethylimidazo[4,5-f]quinoxaline, and 2-amino-1-methyl-6-phenylimidazo[4,5-b]pyridine, using the model in vitro systems of Jagerstad. This study revealed that the polyphenols were inhibitory in the production of HCAs, 2-amino-3,8-dimethylimidazo[4,5-f]quinoxaline or 2-amino-1-methyl-6-phenylimidazo[4,5-b]pyridine. It was suggested that the tea polyphenols represent another approach to lower the formation of HCAs and its associated cancer risk [128].

Inhibition of Biochemical Markers of Tumor Initiation: Cytochrome P_{450}-Dependent Metabolism

Cytochrome P_{450} (P_{450}) is the major enzyme system responsible for the metabolism of procarcinogens to their DNA binding metabolites [129, 130]. This binding to DNA is considered essential for tumor initiation [129, 130]. We studied the interaction of GTP and its constituent polyphenols EC, EGC, ECG, and EGCG with P_{450} and associated monooxygenase activities [131]. The addition of EC, EGC, ECG, EGCG, and GTP to microsomes prepared from rat liver resulted in a dose-dependent inhibition of P_{450}-dependent arylhydrocarbon hydroxylase, 7-ethoxycoumarin-o-deethylase, and 7-ethoxyresorufin-o-deethylase activities [131]. In this study it was also shown that epidermal arylhydrocarbon hydroxylase activity and epidermal enzyme-mediated binding of BαP and DMBA to DNA was inhibited by these polyphenols [131]. In recent studies, Sohn et al. [132] found significant increase in liver of rat drinking green tea or black tea of P_{450} 1A1, 1A2 and 2B1 activities, but no change in P_{450} 2E1 and 3A4 activities. Of the phase II enzymes, UDP-glucuronyltransferase was found to be increased, but glutathione S-transferase was not [132]. Shi et al. [102] have shown that EGCG inhibited the catalytic activities of several P_{450} enzynmes and was more potent against P_{450} 1A and 2B1 than 2E1.

We showed that topical application or orally administered GTP to SENCAR mice was found to inhibit carcinogen-DNA adduct formation in epidermis after topical application of [^{3}H]BP or [^{3}H]DMBA [81]. We also showed that chronic oral administration of GTP to mice for 4 weeks resulted in moderate to significant enhancement in glutathione peroxidase, catalase, NADPH-quinone oxidoreductase, and glutathione S-transferase (GST) activities in small bowel, lung and liver [133]. Enhancement of these enzymatic pathways that play a role in detoxification of carcinogenic metabolites formation by P_{450} and other enzymes by green tea and/or its ability to inhibit enzymatic pathways that are key determinant for cancer initiation may be expected to have protective functions against carcinogenesis [81, 102, 131–133]. These pathways alone or in combination may contribute to overall protective effects of green tea against cancer.

Inhibition of Biochemical Markers of Tumor Promotion

Topical application of phorbol esters like TPA on mouse skin results in induction of ODC activity followed by an increase in the levels of polyamines, epidermal hyperplasia, inflammation and increase in the number of dark basal keratinocytes [83–85]. It has not been possible to establish which of these parameters or many others are obligatory or sufficient for the process of tumor promotion. The induction of ODC activity is considered to be closely associated, though not sufficient, with the tumor-promoting activity of a variety of tumor promoters [83, 84]. ODC plays an essential role in cell proliferation and differentiation [83, 84]. The induction of inflammation in skin mediated by TPA is believed to be governed by cyclooxygenase- and lipoxygenase-catalyzed metabolites of arachidonic acid, specifically prostaglandins and hydroxyeicosatetraenoic acids respectively [83, 84, 134]. The importance of induction of epidermal ODC, cyclooxygenase and lipoxygenase activities in skin tumor promotion is evident from the fact that several inhibitors of these enzymes inhibit the tumor promotion in murin skin [134–136 and references therein].

Topical application of GTP to mouse skin was found to inhibit TPA-mediated induction of epidermal ODC activity in a dose-dependent manner [135]. The inhibitory effect of GTP was also dependent on the time of its application relative to TPA treatment. GTP application, to SENCAR mice was also found to inhibit the induction of epidermal ODC activity caused by several structurally different mouse skin tumor promoters [135]. Prior application of GTP to mouse skin was found to result in significant inhibition of TPA-induced epidermal edema and hyperplasia [85, 119]. As quantitated by the formation of prostaglandins and hydroxyeicosatetraenoic acids, metabolites from respectively cyclooxygenase- and lipoxygenase-catalyzed metabolism of arachidonic acid, skin application of GTP to SENCAR mice was also found to result in significant inhibition of TPA-caused effects on these two enzymes [85]. Inhibition of all of these pathways alone or in combination may contribute to overall antitumor-promoting effects of green tea.

Scavenging of Activated Metabolites of Carcinogens

Flavanols are group of chemicals that possess strong nucleophilic centers at two positions. This property provides an opportunity for the flavanols to react with electrophilic carcinogenic species to form flavanol-carcinogen adducts which may result in prevention of tumorigenesis. In general, the initial step in carcinogenesis is the metabolic activation of chemical carcinogens by the P_{450}-dependent biotransformation reaction. For example, the ubiquitous environmental pollutant BαP is known to cause cancer of the skin or other body site in experimental animals only after its metabolic activation to highly reactive molecules [119, 129, 134]. The ultimate carcinogenic metabolite of BαP is BαP diolepoxide-2 (BPDE-2), the formation of which is catalyzed by successive enzymatic steps catalyzed by P_{450} and epoxide hydrolase [129, 130]. We have shown that tea polyphenols interact with BPDE-2 and shown that topical application of GTP prior to BPDE-2 treatment resulted in inhibition of skin tumor initiation [137].

Antioxidant and Free Radical Scavenging Activity

The generation of reactive oxidants in biological systems, either by normal metabolic pathways or as a consequence of exposure to chemical carcinogens, has been extensively studied and it is clear that their generation contributes to the multistage process of carcinogenesis [5, 83]. Several reports suggest that peroxides and superoxide anion ($^\cdot O_2$-) produce cytotoxicity/genotoxicity in the cellular systems [136]. The source of hydrogen peroxide (H_2O_2) in cells/tissues is mainly through superoxide dismutase-mediated dismutation of $^\cdot O_2$-, which is generated in the cells/tissues by endogenous enzyme systems as well as by the nonenzymatic pathways [136]. In addition, the highly reactive hydroxide radical ($^\cdot OH$), generated from H_2O_2, is known to damage DNA to produce the pathological alterations [136]. The two electron reduction of the metabolic products of PAH such as quinones, catalyzed by NADPH quinone reductase (QR), has been considered to be a detoxification pathway, since the resulting hydroquinones may be conjugated and excreted through mercapturic acid pathway [140]. Phase II enzyme, GST, not only catalyzes the conjugation of both hydroquinones and epoxides of PAH with reduced glutathione for their excretion, but also shows low activity toward organic hydroperoxides for their detoxification from cells/tissue [140]. Since cancer chemoprevention studies have shown that following administration of chemopreventive agents, the levels of antioxidant enzymes are elevated in various organs of the test animals [141], we assessed the effect of oral feeding of 0.2% (w/v) GTP in drinking water for 30 days to SKH-1 hairless mice on the activities of antioxidant, glutathione peroxidase and catalase, and phase II detoxifying enzymes, GST and QR [133]. Compared to that observed in non-GTP-fed control group of mice, the oral feeding of GTP resulted in a significant increase in glutathione peroxidase, catalase and QR activities in small bowel, liver and lungs, and GST activity in small bowel and liver [133]. In another study, compared to DEN- or BαP-fed animals, feeding of 2.5% WEGT or 0.2% GTP in drinking water with DEN or BαP to female A/J mice resulted in significant enhancement in GST activity in liver and small bowel and QR activity in small bowel, lung and stomach [97]. The significant enhancement in the activity of the antioxidant and phase II enzymes in various organs of experimental mice orally fed with WEGT or GTP in drinking water suggest that it may contribute to the cancer-chemopreventive effects observed with green tea.

It is becoming clear that anticarcinogenic properties of tea may be due to the antioxidant effect of ECDs present therein. Katiyar et al. [138] found that EGCG, EGC and ECG from green tea significantly inhibits Fe^{3+}/ADP-supported spontaneous lipid peroxidation in mouse epidermal microsomes. Interestingly each of these ECDs was also effective in inhibiting photo-enhanced lipid peroxidation generated by incubating epidermal microsomes in the presence of silicon phthalocyanine and 650 nm irradiation. At equimolar basis, EGCG, which is also the major constituent in GTP, showed maximum inhibitory effects compared to other ECDs. This study provides the evidence for the antioxidant property of ECDs. The concept of antioxidative activities is also supported by the findings that EGCG inhibited the formation of 8-hydroxydeoxyguanosine in HeLa cells [139], oral administration of green tea inhibited the formation of 8-hydroxydeoxyguanosine in mice [100], and topically treated GTP inhibited TPA-induced hydrogen peroxide formation [140]. The mechanism of antioxidant property of these ECDs can be explained as follows: (1) Tea polyphenols such as EGCG, ECG and EGC are strong scavengers against superoxide anion radicals and hydroxy radicals – two major reactive oxygen species that can damage DNA and other cellular molecules and can initiate lipid peroxidation reactions. (2) Tea flavanols can react with peroxy radicals and thus terminate lipid peroxidation chain reactions. Reactive oxygen species play important roles in carcinogenesis through damaging DNA, altering gene expression, or affecting cell growth and differentiation [141].

Conclusion and Future Prospects for Human Cancer

Changing lifestyle, as reflected in dietary habits and culinary practices, has been recognized as a major factor for human cancer risk [1–5, 22, 78–80]. There is suggestive evidence in humans that diets rich in fruits, or containing reduced levels of fats, particularly those derived from animal sources, are less likely to lead to cancer than the current North American diet to which the population has got used to. For these reasons, changes in dietary habits with the intake of more cancer-chemopreventive agents appear to be a practical approach for cancer prevention. Because tea is one of the most popular beverages consumed worldwide, the relationship between tea consumption and human cancer incidence is an important concern. The available epidemiologic information does not indicate that tea consumption has a statistically significant causative effect on human cancers. However, possible harmful effects of the consumption of excessive amounts of tea, tea at very high temperature, or salted tea [22] cannot be ruled out. The epidemiologic studies reviewed by the working group of the IARC, on consumption of tea and its association with causation or prevention of cancer, have yielded inconsistent and inconclusive results [8]. The monograph published by IARC concluded that there is inadequate evidence for the carcinogenicity in humans of tea drinking and also inadequate evidence for the carcinogenicity of tea in experimental animals [8]. On the basis of many epidemiologic observations published following this monograph and numerous laboratory studies, we believe that tea consumption is likely to have beneficial effects in reducing certain cancers in certain populations.

Although a considerable body of information has accumulated on the causation and prevention effects of tea on cancer, a clear understanding of the mechanisms by which tea and tea components may affect the induction, growth, and subsequent progression of specific cancers is essential for examining the effect of tea on health. Black tea is the major form of tea consumed mostly in western countries. The chemistry, biological activities and chemopreventive properties of black tea and its components, however, are poorly understood. Research in these areas requires more extensive attention.

Since considerable experimental data on the protection of mouse skin carcinogenesis and inflammation by GTP and its constituents exists, an intervention study on human skin carcinogenesis and inflammatory responses would be of great importance. The dose-response effect is a key issue in such studies. However, there is only limited data on the bioavailability of tea components following its consumption by the human population. Therefore, studies on the absorption, distribution, and metabolism of key components from green and black tea in animals and humans are of great importance.

Definitive answers on the deleterious or beneficial effects of tea consumption will most likely come from studies with human populations.

In the light of the suggestive epidemiologic data from Japan and other places, an intervention study on gastric cancer with other high-risk populations should be valuable. Because the causative factors are different for different populations, tea consumption may affect carcinogenesis only in selected situations rater than to have a general effect on all cancers. Therefore, in future epidemiological studies, it is important to consider the etiologic factors of the specific cancers and to collect more specific information on the qualitative and quantitative aspects of tea consumption. More well-designed case-control and cohort studies are needed to address the issue of whether tea consumption enhances or inhibits the development of specific cancers in specific populations. Intervention studies may certainly provide useful information on the protective effects of tea on cancer. After completing additional studies, recommendations may be made to consume tea components by humans. Such agent(s) do not necessarily have to be consumed by tea drinking. They can be supplemented in other items, for example food items and vitamin supplements. This approach can be called 'designer items' for consumption by the human population.

References

1   Ames BN: Dietary carcinogens and anticarcinogens. Science 1983;221:1256–1262.
2   Stich HF: The beneficial and hazardous effects of simple phenolic compounds. Mutat Res 1991; 259:307–324.
3   Black HS, Mathews-Roth MM: Protective role of butylated hydroxytoluene and certain carotenoids in photocarcinogenesis. Photochem Photobiol 1991;53:707–716.
4   Hunter DJ, Manson JE, Colditz GA, et al: A prospective study of the intake of vitamin C, E, and A and the risk of breast cancer. N Engl J Med 1993;329:234–240.
5   Wattenberg LW: Inhibition of carcinogenesis by naturally occurring and synthetic compounds; in Kuroda Y, Shankel M, Waters MD (ed): Antimutagenesis and Anticarcinogenesis: Mechanisms. II. New York, Plenum Publishing, 1990, pp 155–166.
6   Graham HN: Green tea composition, consumption, and polyphenol chemistry. Prev Med 1992;21: 334–350.
7   Yaminishi T, Tomita I: Proceedings of the International Symposium on Tea Sciences. Tokyo, Kurofune Printing Co, 1992.
8   IARC monographs on the evaluation of the carcinogenic risk to humans: Coffee, tea, maté, methylxanthines and methylglyoxal. Lyon, International Agency for Research on Cancer Working Group, 1991, vol 51, pp 1–513.
9   Morton JF: The potential carcinogenicity of herbal tea. Environ Carcinog Rev (J Environ Sci Health) 1986;C4:203–223.
10 Morton JF: Tentative correlation of plant usage and esophageal cancer zones. Econ Bot 1970;24: 217–226.
11 Kapadia GJ, Rao S, Morton JF: Herbal tea consumption and esophageal cancer; in Stich HF (ed): Carcinogens and Mutagens in the Environment. Boca Raton, CRC Press, 1983, pp 3–12.
12 Lubin F, Ron E, Wax Y, et al: Coffee and methylxanthines and breast cancer: A case-control study. J Natl Cancer Inst 1985;74:569–573.

13   Segi M: Tea-gruel as a possible factor for cancer of the esophagus. Gann 1975;66:199–202.

14   Yang CS: Research on esophageal cancer in China: A review. Cancer Res 1980;40:2633–2644.

15   Victora CG, Munoz N, Day NE, et al: Hot beverages and oesophageal cancer in southern Brazil: A case-control study. Int J Cancer 1987;39:710–716.

16   La Vecchia C, Negri E, Franceschi S, et al: Tea consumption and cancer risk. Nutr Cancer 1992; 17:27–31.

17   International Agency for Research on Cancer: Coffee, tea, maté, methylxanthines, and methylgloxyal. IARC Monogr Eval Carcinog Risk Hum 1991;51:1–513.

18   Kaufman BD, Liberman IS, Tyshetsky VI, et al: Some data concerning the incidence of oesophageal cancer in the Gurjev region of the Kazakh SSR (Russ). Vopr Onkol 1965;11:78–85.

19   Bashirov MS, Nugmanov SN, Kolycheva NI: On the epidemiology of cancer of the esophagus in the Aktubinsk region of the Kazakhastan SSR. Vopr Onkol 1968;14:3–7.

20   Cook-Mozaffari PJ, Azordegan F, Day NE, et al: Oesophageal cancer studies in the Caspian Littoral of Iran: Results of a case-control study. Br J Cancer 1979;39:293–309.

21   De Long UW, Breslow N, Hong JGE, et al: Aetiological factors in oesophageal cancer in Singapore Chinese. Int J Cancer 1974;13:291–303.

22   Yang CS, Wang ZY: Tea and cancer. J Natl Cancer Inst 1993;85:1038–1049.

23   Gao YT, McLaughlin JK, Blot WJ, et al: Reduced risk of esophageal cancer associated with grean tea consumption. J Natl Cancer Inst 1994;86:855–858.

24   Zheng W, Doyle TJ, Hong CP, et al: Tea consumption and cancer incidence in a prospective cohort study of postmenopausal women. Proc Am Assoc Cancer Res 1995;36:278.

25   Oguni I, Chen SJ, Lin PJ, et al: Protection against cancer risk by Japanese green tea. Prev Med 1992;21:332.

26   Graham S, Lilienfeld AM, Tidings JE: Dietary and purgation factors in the epidemiology of gastric cancer. Cancer 1967;20:2224–2234.

27   Higginson J: Etiological factors in gastrointestinal cancer in man. J Natl Cancer Inst 1966;37: 527–545.

28   Tazima K, Tominaga S: Dietary habits and gastro-intestinal cancers: A comparative case-control study of stomach and large intestinal cancers in Nagoya, Japan. Jpn J Cancer Res 1985;76: 705–716.

29   Trichopoulos D, Ouranos G, Day NE, et al: Diet and cancer of the stomach: A case-control study in Greece. Int J Cancer 1985;36:291–297.

30   Agudo A, Gonzalez CA, Marcos G, et al: Consumption of alcohol, coffee, and tobacco, and gastric cancer in Spain. Cancer Causes Control 1992;3:137–143.

31   Demirer T, Icli F, Uzunalimoglu O, et al: Diet and stomach cancer incidence. A case-control study in Turkey. Cancer 1990;65:2344–2348.

32   Kono S, Ikeda M, Tokudome S, et al: A case-control study of gastric cancer and diet in northern Kyushu, Japan. Jpn J Cancer Res 1988;79:1067–1074.

33   Kinlen LJ, Willows AN, Goldblatt P, et al: Tea consumption and cancer. Br J Cancer 1988;58: 397–401.

34   Lee HH, Wu HY, Chuang YC, et al: Epidemiologic characteristics and multiple risk factors of stomach cancer in Taiwan. Anticancer Res 1990;10:875–881.

35   Hansson L-E, Nyren O, Bergstrom R, et al: Diet and risk of gastric cancer. A population-based case-control study in Sweden. Int J Cancer 1993;55:181–189.

36   D'Avanzo B, La Vecchia C, Franceschi S, et al: Coffee consumption and bladder cancer risk. Eur J Cancer 1992;28A:1480–1484.

37   Kunze E, Chang-Claude J, Frentzel-Beyme R: Life style and occupational risk factors for bladder cancer in Germany: A case-control study. Cancer 1992;69:1776–1790.

38   Nomura AM, Kolonel LN, Hankin JH, et al: Dietary factors in cancer of the lower urinary tract. Int J Cancer 1991;48:199–205.

39   Stocks P: Cancer mortality in relation to national consumption of cigarettes, solid fuel, tea and coffee. Br J Cancer 1970;24:215–225.

40   Heilbrun LK, Nomura A, Stemmermann GN: Black tea consumption and cancer risk: A prospective study. Br J Cancer 1986;54:677–683.

41   Morgan RW, Jain MG: Bladder cancer: Smoking, beverages and artificial sweeteners. Can Med Assoc J 1974;111:1067–1070.

42   Simon D, Yen S, Cole P: Coffee drinking and cancer of the lower urinary tract. J Natl Cancer Inst 1975;54:587–591.

43   Miller CT, Neutel CI, Nair RC, et al: Relative importance of risk factors in bladder carcinogenesis. J Chronic Dis 1978;31:51–56.

44   Howe GR, Burch JD, Miller AB, et al: Tobacco use, occupation, coffee, various nutrients, and bladder cancer. J Natl Cancer Inst 1980;64:701–713.

45   Hartge P, Hoover R, West DW, et al: Coffee drinking and risk of bladder cancer. J Natl Cancer Inst 1983;70:1021–1026.

46   Ohno Y, Aoki K, Obata K, et al: Case-control study of urinary bladder cancer in metropolitan Nagoya. Monogr Natl Cancer Inst 1985;69:229–234.

47   Jensen OM, Wahrendorf J, Knudsen JB, et al: The Cophenhagen case-control study of bladder cancer. II. Effect of coffee and other beverages. Int J Cancer 1986;37:651–657.

48   Claude J, Kunze E, Frentzel-Beyme R, et al: Life-style and occupational risk factors in cancer of the lower urinary tract. Am J Epidemiol 1986;124:578–589.

49   Iscovich J, Castelletto R, Esteve J, et al: Tobacco smoking, occupational exposure and bladder cancer in Argentina. Int J Cancer 1987;40:734–740.

50   Slattery ML, West DW, Robison LM: Fluid intake and bladder cancer in Utah. Int J Cancer 1988; 42:17–22.

51   Risch HA, Burch JD, Miller AB, et al: Dietary factors and the incidence of cancer of the urinary bladder. Am J Epidemiol 1988;127:1179–1191.

52   La Vecchia C, Negri E, Decarli A, et al: Dietary factors in the risk of bladder cancer. Nutr Cancer 1989;12:93–101.

53   Armstrong B, Garrod A, Doll R: A retrospective study of renal cancer with special reference to coffee and animal protein consumption. Br J Cancer 1976;33:127–136.

54   Goodman MT, Morgenstern H, Wynder EL: A case-control study of factors affecting the development of renal cell cancer. Am J Epidemiol 1986;124:926–941.

55   Yu MC, Mack TM, Hanisch R, et al: Cigarette smoking, obesity, diuretic use, and coffee consumption as risk factors for renal cell carcinoma. J Natl Cancer Inst 1986;77:351–356.

56   McCredie M, Ford JM, Stewart JH: Risk factors for cancer of the renal parenchyma. Int J Cancer 1988;42:13–16.

57   Kono S, Shinchi K, Ikeda N, et al: Physical activity, dietary habits and adenomatous polyps of the sigmoid colon: A study of self-defense officials in Japan. J Clin Epidemiol 1991;44:1255–1261.

58   Kato I, Tominaga S, Matsuura S, et al: A comparative case-control study of colorectal cancer and adenoma. Jpn J Cancer Res 1990;81:1101–1108.

59   Watanabe Y, Tada M, Kawamoto K, et al: A case-control study of cancer of the rectum and the colon. Nippon Shokakibyo Gakkai Zasshi 1984;81:185–193.

60   Miller AB, Howe GR, Jain M, et al: Food items and food groups as risk factors in a case-control study of diet and colorectal cancer. Int J Cancer 1983;32:155–161.

61   Dales LG, Friedman GD, Ury HK, et al: A case-control study of relationships of diet and other traits to colorectal cancer in American blacks. Am J Epidemiol 1979;109:132–144.

62   Phillips RL, Snowdon DA: Dietary relationships with fatal colorectal cancer among Seventh-Day Adventists. J Natl Cancer Inst 1985;74:307–317.

63   Tewes FJ, Koo LC, Meisgen TJ, et al: Lung cancer risk and mutagenicity of tea. Environ Res 1990; 52:23–33.

64   Rosenberg L, Miller DR, Helmrich SP, et al: Breast cancer and the consumption of coffee. Am J Epidemiol 1985;122:391–399.

65   La Vecchia C, Talamini R, Decarli A, et al: Coffee consumption and the risk of breast cancer. Surgery 1986;100:477–481.

66   Schairer C, Brinton LA, Hoover RN: Methylxanthines and breast cancer. Int J Cancer 1987;40: 469–473.

67   Mabuchi K, Bross DS, Kessler II: Risk factors for male breast cancer. J Natl Cancer Inst 1985;74: 371–375.

Katiyar/Mukhtar

68   Bueno DE, Mesquita HB, Maisonneuve P, Moerman CJ, et al: Lifetime consumption of alcoholic beverages, tea and coffee and exocrine carcinoma of the pancreas: A population-based case-control study in the Netherlands. Int J Cancer 1992;50:514–522.

69   Jain M, Howe GR, St Louis P, et al: Coffee and alcohol as determinants of risk of pancreas cancer: A case-control study from Toronto. Int J Cancer 1991;47:384–389.

70   Hiatt RA, Klatsky AL, Armstrong MA: Pancreatic cancer, blood glucose and beverage consumption. Int J Cancer 1988;41:794–797.

71   Mabuchi K, Bross DS, Kessler II: Epidemiology of cancer of the vulva. A case-control study. Cancer 1985;55:1843–1848.

72   MacMahon B, Yen S, Trichopoulos D, et al: Coffee and cancer of the pancreas. N Engl J Med 1981;304:630–633.

73   Mack TM, Yu MC, Hanisch R, et al: Pancreas cancer and smoking, beverage consumption, and past medical history. J Natl Cancer Inst 1986;76:49–60.

74   Kinlen LJ, McPherson K: Pancreas cancer and coffee and tea consumption: A case-control study. Br J Cancer 1984;49:93–96.

75   Lin TM, Chen KP, Lin CC, et al: Retrospective study on nasopharyngeal carcinomas. J Natl Cancer Inst 1973;51:1403–1408.

76   Henderson BE, Louie E, Soo Hoo Jing J, et al: Risk factors associated with nasopharyngeal carcinoma. N Engl J Med 1976;295:1101–1106.

77   Shanmugaratnam K, Tye CY, Goh EH, et al: Etiological factors on nasopharyngeal carcinoma: A hospital-based, retrospective, case-control, questionnaire study; in Ito Y (ed): Nasopharyngeal Carcinoma, Etiology and Control. Lyon, IARC, 1978, pp 199–212.

78   Mukhtar H, Wang ZY, Katiyar SK, et al: Tea components: Antimutagenic and anticarcinogenic effects. Prev Med 1992;21:351–360.

79   Mukhtar H, Katiyar SK, Agarwal R: Green tea and skin – Anticarcinogenic effects. J Invest Dermatol 1994;102:3–7.

80   Katiyar SK, Agarwal R, Mukhtar H: Green tea in chemoprevention of cancer. Comp Ther 1992; 18:3–8.

81   Wang ZY, Khan WA, Bickers DR, et al: Protection against polycyclic aromatic hydrocarbon-induced skin tumor initiation in mice by green tea polyphenols. Carcinogenesis 1989;10:411–415.

82   Katiyar SK, Agarwal R, Wang ZY, et al: (–)-Epigallocatechin-3-gallate in *Camellia sinensis* leaves from Himalayan region of Sikkim: Inhibitory effects against biochemical events and tumor initiation in SENCAR mouse skin. Nutr Cancer 1992;18:73–83.

83   Agarwal R, Mukhtar H: Cutaneous chemical carcinogenesis; in Mukhtar H (ed): Pharmacology of the Skin. Boca Raton, CRC Press, 1991, pp 371–387.

84   DiGiovanni J: Multistage carcinogenesis in mouse skin. Pharmacol Ther 1992;54:63–128.

85   Katiyar SK, Agarwal R, Wood GS, et al: Inhibition of 12-O-tetradecanoylphorbol-13-acetate-caused tumor promotion in 7,12-dimethylbenz[a]anthracene-initiated SENCAR mouse skin by a polyphenolic fraction isolated from green tea. Cancer Res 1992;52:6890–6897.

86   Huang M-T, Ho C-T, Wang ZY, et al: Inhibitory effect of topical application of a green tea polyphenol fraction on tumor initiation and promotion in mouse skin. Carcinogenesis 1992;13:947–954.

87   Yoshizawa S, Horiuchi T, Fujiki H, et al: Antitumor-promoting activity of (–)-epigallocatechin gallate, the main constituent of 'tannin' in green tea. Phytother Res 1987;1:44–47.

88   Katiyar SK, Agarwai R, Mukhtar H: Inhibition of both stage I and stage II skin tumor promotion in SENCAR mice by a polyphenolic fraction isolated from green tea: Inhibition depends on the duration of polyphenol treatment. Carcinogenesis 1993;14:2641–2643.

89   Athar M, Agarwal R, Wang ZY, et al: All trans-retionic acid protects against free radical generating compounds-mediated conversion of chemically- and ultraviolet B radiation-induced skin papillomas to carcinomas. Carcinogenesis 1991;12:2325–2329.

90   Katiyar SK, Agarwal R, Mukhtar H: Protection against malignant conversion of chemically induced benign skin papillomas to squamous cell carcinomas in SENCAR mice by a polyphenolic fraction isolated from green tea. Cancer Res 1993;53:5409–5412.

91   Elmets CA: Cutaneous photocarcinogenesis; in Mukhtar H (ed): Pharmacology of the Skin. Boca Raton, CRC Press, 1991, pp 389–416.

92 Wang ZY, Agarwal R, Bickers DR, et al: Protection against ultraviolet B radiation-induced photocar-cinogenesis in hairless mice by green tea polyphenols. Carcinogenesis 1991;12:1527–1530.

93 Wang ZY, Huang M-T, Ferraro T, et al: Inhibitory effect of green tea in the drinking water on tumorigenesis by ultraviolet light and 12-O-tetradecanoylphorbol-13-acetate in the skin of SKH-1 mice. Cancer Res 1992;52:1162–1170.

94 Wang ZY, Huang M-T, Lou Y-R, et al: Inhibitory effects of black tea, green tea, decaffeinated black tea, and decaffeinated green tea on ultraviolet B light-induced skin carcinogenesis in 7,12-dimethylbenz[a]anthracene-initiated SKH-1 mice. Cancer Res 1994;54:3428–3435.

95 Liu Q, Wang Y, Crist KA, et al: Analysis of p[53] and H-ras mutations in UV- and UV/green tea-induced tumorigenesis in the skin of SKH-1 mice. Proc Am Assoc Cancer Res 1995;36:591.

96 Wang ZY, Huang M-T, Ho C-T, et al: Inhibitory effect of green tea on the growth of established skin papillomas in mice. Cancer Res 1992;52:6657–6665.

97 Katiyar SK, Agarwal R, Zaim MT, et al: Protection against N-nitrosodiethylamine and benzo[a]pyr-ene-induced forestomach and lung tumorigenesis in A/J mice by green tea. Carcinogenesis 1993; 14:849–855.

98 Wang ZY, Agarwal R, Khan WA, et al: Protection against benzo[a]pyrene and N-nitrosodiethylam-ine-induced lung and forestomach tumorigenesis in A/J mice by water extracts of green tea and licorice. Carcinogenesis 1992;13:1491–1494.

99 Wang ZY, Hong JY, Huang M-T, et al: Inhibition of N-nitrosodiethylamine- and 4-(methylnitroesam-ino)-1-(3-pyridyl)-1-butanone-induced tumorigenesis in A/J mice by green tea and black tea. Cancer Res 1992;52:1943–1947.

100 Xu Y, Ho C-T, Amin SG, et al: Inhibition of tobacco-specific nitrosamine-induced lung tumorigenesis in A/J mice by green tea and its major polyphenol as antioxidants. Cancer Res 1992;52:3875–3879.

101 Katiyar SK, Agarwal R, Mukhtar H: Protective effects of green tea polyphenols administered by oral intubation against chemical carcinogen-induced forestomach and pulmonary neoplasia in A/J mice. Cancer Lett 1993;73:167–172.

102 Shi ST, Wang Z, Theresa JS, et al: Effect of green tea and black tea on 4-(methylnitrosamino)-1-(3-pyridyl)-1-butanone bioactivation, DNA methylation and lung tumorigenesis in A/J mice. Cancer Res 1994;54:4641–4647.

103 Wu RR, Lin YP, Chen HY: Effect of Fujian oolong tea, jasmine tea, green tea and tea standing overnight on urethan-induced lung neoplasia in mice. International Tea-Quality-Human Health Symposium (China), 1987, pp 118–119.

104 Chen JS: The effect of Chinese tea on the occurrence of esophageal tumors induced by N-nitrosome-thylbenzylamine in rats. Prev Med 1992;21:385–391.

105 Gao GD, Zhou LF, Qi G, et al: Initial study of antitumorigenesis of green tea: Animal test and flow cytometry. Tumor 1990;10:42–44.

106 Yang CS, Hong JY, Wang ZY: Inhibition of nitrosamine-induced tumorigenesis by diallyl sulfide and tea; in Waldron K (ed): Food and Cancer Prevention. Cambridge, Royal Society of Chemistry, 1992.

107 Fujita Y, Yamane T, Tanaka M, et al: Inhibitory effect of (−)-epigallocatechin gallate on carcinogen-esis with N-ethyl-N′-nitro-N-nitrosoguanidine in mouse duodenum. Jpn J Cancer Res 1989;80: 503–505.

108 Hirose M, Hoshiya T, Akagi K, et al: Effects of green tea catechins in rat multi-organ carcinogenesis model. Carcinogenesis 1993;14:1549–1553.

109 Yamane T, Hagiwara N, Tateishi M, et al: Inhibition of azoxymethane-induced colon carcinogenesis in rat by green tea polyphenol fraction. Jpn J Cancer Res 1991;82:1336–1339.

110 Narasiwa T, Fukaura Y: A very low dose of green tea polyphenols in drinking water prevents N-methyl-N-nitrosourea-induced colon carcinogenesis in F344 rats. Jpn J Cancer Res 1993;84: 1007–1009.

111 Chen ZY, Yan RQ, Qin GZ, et al: Effect of six edible plants on the development of aflatoxin B[1]-induced γ-glutamyltranspeptidase-positive hepatocyte foci in rats. Chung Hua Liu Tsa Chih (Chin J Cancer) 1987;9:109–111.

112 Li Y: Comparative study on the inhibitory effect of green tea, coffee and levamisole on the hepatocar-cinogenic action of diethylnitrosamine. Chung Hua Liu Tsa Chih (Chin J Cancer) 1991;13:193–195.

113 Nagabhushan M, Sarode AV, Nair J, et al: Mutagenicity and carcinogenicity of tea, *Camellia sinensis*. Indian J Exp Biol 1991;29:401–406.

114 Hara Y: Prophylactic function of tea polyphenols. 204th American Chemical Society National Meeting, Washington 1992.

115 Hirose M, Hoshiya T, Akagi K, et al: Inhibition of mammary gland carcinogenesis by green tea catechins and other naturally occurring antioxidants in female Sprague-Dawley rats pretreated with 7,12-dimethylbenz[*a*]anthracene. Cancer Lett 1994;83:149–156.116.

116 Sakamoto K, Reddy D, Hara Y, et al: Impact of green or black tea polyphenols on canine mammary tumor cells in culture. Proc Am Assoc Cancer Res 1995;36:595.

117 Harada N, Takabayashi F, Oguni I, et al: Anti-promotion effect of green tea extracts on pancreatic cancer in golden hamster induced by N-nitroso-bis(2-oxopropyl)amine. Proceedings of the International Symposium on Tea Science, (Japan), 1991.

118 Mohan RR, Khan SG, Agarwal R, et al: Testosterone induces ornithine decarboxylase activity and mRNA expression in human prostate carcinoma cell line LNCaP: Inhibition by green tea. Proc Am Assoc Cancer Res 1995;36:274.

119 Katiyar SK, Agarwal R, Ekker S, et al: Protection against 12-O-tetradecanoylphorbol-13-acetate-caused inflammation in SENCAR mouse ear skin by polyphenolic fraction isolated from green tea. Carcinogenesis 1993;14:361–365.

120 Agarwal R, Katiyar SK, Khan SG, et al: Protection against ultraviolet B radiation-induced effects in the skin of SKH-1 hairless mice by a polyphenolic fraction isolated from green tea. Photochem Photobiol 1993;58:695–700.

121 Katiyar SK, Agarwal R, Korman NJ, et al: Inhibition of tumor promoter-caused induction of interleukin-1-alpha, tumor necrosis factor-alpha, and ornithine decarboxylase gene expression in SENCAR mouse skin by tea polyphenols. Proc Am Assoc Cancer Res 1995;36:594.

122 Wang ZY, Cheng SJ, Zhou ZC, et al: Antimutagenic activity of green tea polyphenols. Mutat Res 1989;223:273–289.

123 Jain AK, Shimoi K, Nakamura Y, et al: Crude tea extracts decrease the mutagenic activity of N-methyl-N'-nitro-N-nitrosoguanidine in vitro and in intragastric tract of rats. Mutat Res 1989;210:1–8.

124 Kada T, Kaneko K, Matsuzaki S, et al: Detection and chemical identification of natural bio-antimutagens, a case of the green tea factor. Mutat Res 1985;150:127–132.

125 Shimo K, Nakamura Y, Tomita I, et al: The pyrogallol-related compounds reduced UV-induced mutations in *Escherichia coli* B/r WP_2. Mutat Res 1986;173:239–244.

126 Ito Y, Ohnishi S, Fujie K: Chromosome aberrations induced by aflatoxin B_1 in rat bone marrow cells in vivo and their suppression by green tea. Mutat Res 1989;222:253–261.

127 Cheng S, Lin P, Ding L, et al: Inhibition of green tea extract on mutagenicity and carcinogenicity. Proceedings of the International Symposium on Tea Science (Japan), 1991, pp 195–199.

128 Weisburger JH, Nagao M, Wakabayasi K, et al: Prevention of heterocyclic amine formation by tea and tea polyphenols. Cancer Lett 1994;83:143–147.

129 Conney AH: Induction of microsomal enzymes by foreign chemicals and carcinogenesis by polycyclic aromatic hydrocarbons. GHA Clowes Memorial Lecture. Cancer Res 1982;42:4875–4917.

130 Mukhtar H, Agarwal R, Bickers DR: Cutaneous metabolism of xenobiotics and steroid hormones; in Mukhtar H (ed): Pharmacology of the Skin. Boca Raton, CRC Press, 1991, pp 89–110.

131 Wang ZY, Das M, Bickers DR, et al: Interaction of epicatechins derived from green tea with rat hepatic cytochrome P_{450}. Drug Metab Dispos 1988;16:98–103.

132 Sohn OS, Surace A, Fiala ES, et al: Effects of green and black tea on hepatic xenobiotic metabolizing systems in the male F344 rat. Xenobiotica 1994;24:119–127.

133 Khan SG, Katiyar SK, Agarwal R, et al: Enhancement of antioxidant and phase II enzymes by oral feeding of green tea polyphenols in drinking water to SKH-1 hairless mice: Possible role in cancer chemoprevention. Cancer Res 1992;52:4050–4052.

134 Agarwal R, Mukhtar H: Oxidative stress in skin chemical carcinogenesis; in Fuchs J, Packer L (eds): Oxidative Stress in Dermatology. New York, Dekker, 1993, pp 207–241.

135 Agarwal R, Katiyar SK, Zaidi SIA, et al: Inhibition of tumor promoter-caused induction of ornithine decarboxylase activity in SENCAR mice by polyphenolic fraction isolated from green tea and its individual epicatechin derivatives. Cancer Res 1992;52:3582–3588.

136 Perchellet J, Perchellet EM: Antioxidants and multistage carcinogenesis in mouse skin. Free Radic Biol Med 1989;7:377–408.
137 Khan WA, Wang ZY, Athar M, et al: Inhibition of the skin tumorigenicity of (+)-7β,8α-dihydroxy-9α,10α-epoxy-7,8,9,10-tetrahydrobenzo[a]pyrene by tannic acid, green tea polyphenols and quarcetin in SENCAR mice. Cancer Lett 1988;42:7–12.
138 Katiyar SK, Agarwal R, Mukhtar H: Inhibition of spontaneous and photo-enhanced lipid peroxidation in mouse epidermal microsomes by epicatechin derivatives from green tea. Cancer Lett 1994; 79:61–66.
139 Bhimani R, Frenkel K: Suppression of H_2O_2 production and oxidative DNA damage in HeLa cells by (–)-epigallocatechin gallate. Proc Am Assoc Cancer Res 1991;32:126.
140 Laskin JD, Heck D, Laskin DL, et al: Inhibitory effects of a green tea polyphenol fraction on 12-O-tetradecanoylphorbol-13-acetate-induced hydrogen peroxide formation in mouse epidermis; in Huang MT, Ho CT, Lee CY (eds): Phenolic Compounds in Foods and Health. II. Antioxidant and Cancer Prevention, Washington, 1992, pp 308–314.
141 Cerruti PA: Mechanisms of action of oxidant carcinogens. Cancer Detect Prev 1989;14:281–284.

Dr. Hasan Mukhtar, Department of Dermatology, University Hospitals of Cleveland,
Case Western Reserve University, 2074 Abington Road, Cleveland, OH 44106 (USA)

Simopoulos, AP (ed): Metabolic Consequences of Changing Dietary Patterns.
World Rev Nutr Diet. Basel, Karger, 1996, vol 79, pp 185–221

....

Coffee and Cancer: A Review of Human and Animal Data

Astrid Nehlig[a], *Gérard Debry*[b]

[a] INSERM U398, Faculté de Médecine, Strasbourg, et
[b] Centre de Nutrition Humaine, Université de Nancy I, Nancy, France

Contents

Introduction

Extensive work has been performed to determine if coffee and caffeine possess genotoxic, mutagenic or carcinogenic potentials. In vitro studies, animal work, and epidemiological surveys have been undertaken in order to see if there is a correlation between the frequency of specific human cancers and coffee drinking. However, it must be noted that in the majority of animal studies the doses of coffee or caffeine administered are extremely high, sometimes reaching toxic levels. In experimental cancerology, such high doses are used to determine the margin of safety of the substance being tested. It must be proven that even very high doses of a given substance do not induce any genotoxic, mutagenic or carcinogenic effects before it can be guaranteed as safe for human consumption.

In the present review, after recalling data on coffee consumption, composition and caffeine metabolism, we will focus first on the mutagenic and antimutagenic effects of coffee both given alone or interacting with other mutagens. Thereafter, we will develop the possible carcinogenic effects of coffee in animals and humans.

Coffee Consumption

World coffee consumption is increasing. Analyzing the data from surveys carried out in the United States, Japan and Western Germany for the period of 1980–1991, it appears that the number of coffee drinkers has decreased by 2–5% in the three countries, while coffee consumption, in terms of number of cups/consumer/day has increased in each country [1–3]. In all three countries, coffee consumption decreased in the younger population, whereas soft drink consumption increased by 13.7% in that group in the United States [1]. In older groups, coffee consumption per capita is stable or increasing [1–3].

The methods of preparation of coffee as well as the size of the cups vary largely with the country. Indeed, coffee can be boiled, filtered, percolated or prepared as expresso, Greek/Turkish "mud" or soluble coffee [4, 5]. The extraction efficiency of caffeine differs for each type of preparation and ranges from 75 to 100% [5] whereas the size of the cup varies from 30 to 190 ml [4]. The content of caffeine per cup varies from 19 to 160 mg of caffeine according to the type of coffee, size of the cup, and country [4]. A mean size cup (150 ml) of caffeinated coffee contains in general about 90 mg of caffeine for brewed and filtered coffee and 63 mg of caffeine for soluble instant coffee [6]. The same volume of decaffeinated coffee contains 3 mg of caffeine, whereas the content of caffeine reaches 32–42 mg in 150 ml of tea and 16 mg in 150 ml of cola drinks [6]. The daily consumption of caffeine in the general population ranges from 202 to 283 mg of caffeine which represents 2.7–4.0 mg/kg/day in males and females 20–75 years old [6].

Composition of Coffee

The composition of coffee is quite complex and depends on the species and variety of green coffee, but also, for a same quality of coffee, on cultivation methods, maturation of the berries, and storage of the green beans. The technological procedures for preparation and industrial treatment of green beans as well as the ways of preparation of coffee modify the levels of its various constituents. Coffee represents a type of food whose range of products formed during industrial treatments is largest [7]. Indeed, because of the numerous different analytical procedures, there is no real consensus on the exact composition of coffee. The two most common types, *Coffea arabica* L. and *Coffea canephora,* variety *robusta* contain about 1.3–2.4% caffeine, 4.9–6.4% acids (chlorogenic, aliphatic and quinine), 33–37% polysaccharides, 10% proteins, 11–17% lipids, 23% caramelized products and 4.5% ashes [7–9]. More detailed information is available in the book of Clarke and Macrae [10] and those of Viani [9, 11, 12].

In addition to these various components, coffee can also contain contaminants either of exogenous or endogenous origin. Contaminants of exogenous origin are mainly pesticides, mycotoxins and paraffins. Pesticides and mycotoxins are destroyed by roasting and usually almost totally absent from coffee [13–16]. Paraffins can contaminate coffee beans during their storage in jute sacks. Paraffin concentrations of 100–150 mg/kg have been detected in roasted coffee beans [17].

Endogenous contaminants are formed during the various procedures of preparation and roasting of coffee. These are aromatic polycyclic hydrocarbons, heterocyclic amines, nitrosamines and a few other substances [7]. Aromatic polycyclic hydrocarbons are formed during roasting. Their amount in the different types of coffee is fairly constant (0.01–4.4 µg/kg) [12,16]. The most widely studied is 3,4-benzopyrene. Heterocyclic amines and nitrosamines have been detected in roasted and instant coffee [7, 18]. Free radicals have also been found in coffee [19] and hydrogen peroxide can be generated by oxygenation of coffee during the preparation procedure [7].

Metabolism of Caffeine

The metabolism of caffeine has been extensively reviewed [20–23]. The metabolic pathways of caffeine show multiple and separate demethylations, C-8 oxidation, and uracil formation in humans and rodents. The major metabolic difference between rodents and humans is that, in the rat, 40% of caffeine metabolites are trimethyl derivatives whereas they represent only 6% in humans [24, 25]. Humans are characterized by the quantitative importance of 3-methyl demethylation leading to the formation of paraxanthine. This first metabolic step represents 72–80% of caffeine metabolism. In the monkey, theophylline is the predominant metabolite of caffeine, whereas in the rat, caffeine metabolism leads to similar amounts of each dimethylxanthine [23, 25].

The half-life of caffeine ranges from 0.7 to 1.2 h in the rat and the mouse, 3 to 5 h in the monkey and from 2.5 to 6 h in humans [22, 26–28]. No difference in the metabolic fate of caffeine is observed between men and women [29, 30]. However, caffeine half-life is 25% longer (6.9 h) in the luteal phase of the menstrual cycle compared with the follicular phase (5.5 h) [31]. The use of oral contraceptives can double caffeine half-life [30, 32, 33]. The half-life of the methylxanthine is also considerably increased during pregnancy, averaging 7 h in mid-pregnancy and 10.5 h during the last trimester of pregnancy [34–38], but returns to normal values within a few weeks postpartum [35, 39].

Mean distribution space ranges from 0.5 to 0.8 liter/kg in newborn infants, adults and elderly subjects [23]. In different animal species, a similar distribution space of 0.8 liter/kg has been reported [40, 41]. These values are in agreement with the distribution of caffeine into the intracellular tissue water [42].

Finally, in comparing results of drug administration in both humans and animals, a correction factor for the dose must be applied, also called metabolic body weight ($=$ body weight$^{3/4}$) [43]. Indeed, dose equivalents based on metabolic body weight are substantially lower than those based on body weight: 20 mg/kg in the rat is equivalent to about 17 cups of coffee (at 100 mg/cup) in a 70-kg man on a body weight basis, but only to 4–6 cups when correction is made for differences in metabolic body weight [43].

Mutagenic and Antimutagenic Effects of Coffee

Many reviews have focused on the mutagenic effects of high doses of coffee and caffeine. These effects have been found in various biological systems such as bacteria and yeast, fungi, and in cultured mammalian cells [44–53].

In vitro Studies

Coffee and caffeine are mutagenic to bacteria and fungi. Coffee always induces mutations in *Salmonella typhimurium* TA 100 [54–56], TA 102 [54, 56–58], and TA 104 [56–58] which are quite sensitive to oxidizing mutagens, as well as in *Escherichia coli* WP2 uvrA/pKM101 and K12 [59–61]. All types of coffee, instant, caffeine-containing or decaffeinated and various blends have similar mutagenic effects [55, 56, 59]. Also, the mutagenic effect of coffee has been observed in various mammalian cells in culture, as among others hamster [62, 63] and rat fibroblasts [64], and human lymphocytes [63, 64]. However, the mutagenic effect of coffee appears only at a specific stage of mitosis [62, 65, 66] and also when cells are exposed to coffee in the absence of liver extracts.

Indeed, in bacteria as in mammalian cells in culture, the addition of liver extracts suppresses these chromosomal aberrations. It appears that certain enzymes found in liver extracts, such as glyoxalase I and II, in association with catalase and glutathione reductase, can inactivate to a certain extent the mutagenic effects of coffee [44, 54, 67]. This observation is of critical importance when evaluating the risk of mutagenicity in humans since substances which can be inactivated in this way during in vitro tests are usually non-carcinogenic in mammals [68].

In vivo Studies

Oral administration of large amounts of instant coffee (up to 3–6 g/kg) in mice that had previously received intravenous injections of coffee-sensitive bacteria (*S. typhimurium* TA 1537 or *E. coli* K-12) does not induce mutagenic effects [67]. Micronucleus tests, which detect induction of chromosomal aberrations that are valid predictors of carcinogenic effects demonstrate that force-feeding mice with large quantities of instant coffee, 0.5–3.0 g/kg/day for 5 consecutive days, induces no modification in chromosome structure [69, 70]. Sister chromatid exchange tests show that in hamsters exposed to single doses of 1.0–2.5 g/kg of instant coffee there is no deleterious effect on DNA structure [69]. Thus, coffee in the amounts usually consumed by man is not likely to induce any genetic mutations or chromosomal aberrations.

Interaction of Coffee and Caffeine with Other Mutagenic Substances

Coffee and caffeine cover a wide spectrum of genetic activity in various biological systems. They can potentiate or inhibit the effects of a great number of mutagenic agents [47,71,72].

Potentiating Mutagenic Effects of Coffee and Caffeine

In numerous cell lines, coffee and caffeine increase synergistically the cytotoxicity of X-rays [73–78], ultraviolet light [79–81], and chemotherapeutic agents [82–87]. Caffeine also increases the cytotoxicity of X-rays in mouse embryos at the one- or two-cell stage [88, 89]. The molecular mechanism of this synergistic action is not well understood. Caffeine accentuates the inhibition of replication initiation in damaged cells [83, 90], decreases the duration of phase G2 of mitosis in treated cells [78], increases chromosome damage [91, 92] and sister chromatid exchanges [93]. Caffeine potentiates chromosomal aberrations while not inducing them per se [94–96]. In fact, caffeine might block a repair process and thus increase the percentage of cell death without modifying error frequency in lesion repair [97].

Antimutagenic Effects of Coffee and Caffeine

Conversely, in various strains of microorganisms, coffee and caffeine inhibit the mutagenic effect of numerous factors, such as among others ultraviolet light [98,99], thymine deprivation in the culture medium [100], mitomycin C [101], nitroso derivatives [102–104], rubicin derivatives [105, 106] and benzopyrene [107]. In mice, coffee (225–1,125 mg/kg) similarly inhibits the mutagenic effect of various substances, such as mitomycin C, cyclophosphamide and procarbazine [108] and tetradecanoylphobol-13-acetate [109]. The effects vary in intensity as a function of the time at which the cells are exposed to coffee as compared to the acting time of the mutagenic agent [101]. Inhibitory action is maximal when caffeine is administered 2 h before the genotoxic agent; it is less marked when the two substances are given simultaneously. It is nil when the coffee is administered 2–4 h after the genotoxic agent [108]. The molecular mechanism of this antimutagenic effect of coffee is still unknown.

Coffee administered to mice at doses of 150 mg to 1 g/kg also inhibits the mutagenic effects of synthesized nitrosurea in bone marrow and in epithelial cells of the colon. Coffee inhibits nitrosation of urea in the stomachs of mice [110]. In microorganisms or in mammalian cells, the antimutagenic effects of instant coffee, either caffeine-containing or decaffeinated, and of brewed coffee are comparable [99,110].

In conclusion, it appears that coffee and caffeine have generally no mutagenic risk in mammals and humans, certainly because of the rapid metabolism of caffeine in mammals. However, in some situations with a reduced clearance of caffeine (liver disease, pregnancy), it has been suggested that caffeine together with exposure to other mutagenic agents could increase the generation of chromosomal aberrations, although the actual risk remains very slight [72]. On the other hand, the enhancement of chromosomal defects by caffeine could conceivably be beneficial in the treatment of cancer. Indeed, tumor cells could be killed by lower doses of X-rays and cytostatic agents when applied in conjunction with caffeine than when applied alone [72]. These aspects will be described in more detail in the following part of this review.

Possible Carcinogenic Effects of Coffee

The impact of daily consumption of coffee on tumorigenesis has been the subject of extensive research, both in animals and in man.

Animal Studies

The potential carcinogenic effects of coffee and caffeine in animals were reviewed in recent publications [111–114]. Würzner [112] points out that evaluation of the carcinogenic effects of a substance in treated animals must be based on four criteria: (1) higher incidence of dose-dependent tumors than that of the control group; (2) significantly earlier onset of dose-dependent tumors; (3) observation of unusual types of tumors, and (4) tendency toward metastasis and malignancy of tumors already observed in control animals.

Potential Carcinogenic Effects of Coffee and Caffeine

Chronic ingestion does not induce any abnormal formation of tumors or cancers in rats or mice [115–121]. This holds true whether coffee is brewed or instant, regular or decaffeinated, added to the animals' food or drinking water up to the equivalent of 60–80 cups of coffee per day in humans, over a period of 1 or 2 years, even during gestation [115]. Würzner et al. [120] observed even a decreased incidence of tumors in rats after chronic exposure to high concentrations of coffee. Caffeine added to the drinking water, to the food, or administered by gavage for 1–2 years at doses ranging from 0.1 to 2%, is no more an inducer of tumors in rats or mice than is coffee [119, 122–128].

Rare studies have demonstrated a carcinogenic effect of caffeine. Caffeine at doses of 0.05% in drinking water stimulates spontaneous mammary tumorigenesis in mice [129] and is able to accelerate pancreatic carcinogenesis in hamsters when administered during the postinitiation phase of the tumor [130]. Finally, pituitary adenomas were observed in female rats after 12 months of caffeine administration at doses of 2 g/l in drinking water [131].

Most studies indicate that coffee and caffeine do not have a carcinogenic effect in laboratory animals. In general, the tumors observed are those normally found in the studied species. Coffee and caffeine do not accelerate tumorigenesis nor do they increase the incidence of such tumors [132]. In a recent study, only two components of coffee, caffeic acid and catechol, which are both antioxidants, were incriminated as inducing agents of cancers of gastric epithelium in both male and female rats and mice [133].

Interaction with Other Carcinogenic Substances

Coffee and caffeine can modulate the effects of carcinogenic agents in animals [71, 108]. Thus, caffeine potentiates the carcinogenic effects of a number of chemical substances or physical inducers [134–140]. Caffeine can increase the incidence of mammary gland carcinogenesis induced by administration of 7,12-dimethylbenz[a]anthracene (DMBA) in rats. However, this increase is significant only when caffeine treatment begins 3 days after administration of the carcinogen, i.e., during the promotion phase of the tumor [141–144]. When caffeine is given during the initiation phase, i.e., before and during, or during carcinogen administration, formation of mammary gland tumors is significantly reduced [141–144]. Conversely, caffeine has no effect on intestinal carcinogenicity in rats [145], whereas it inhibits or delays development of breast cancer in rats [146, 147] or mice [148]. When caffeine is associated with a diet high in unsaturated fat, duration of tumor development is reduced considerably as compared to exposure to one of the two agents taken alone [143]. Coffee reduces also the incidence of tumors related to a high-fat diet [149, 150], or due to other carcinogenic agents [151–153].

Green coffee beans are rich in inducers of detoxification systems and/or activation of xenobiotics, particularly activity of glutathione S-transferase [112, 154, 155]. Among the inducers contained in green coffee beans are two diterpenes, kahweol and cafestol palmitate [156, 157] that increase sixfold glutathione S-transferase activity in liver and intestinal mucous membranes [155]. Although caffeine does not seem to be the causal factor in the antitumor effect of beverages with high levels of methylxanthines [145], it is able to increase hepatic activities of arylhydrocarbon hydroxylase, cytochrome P_{450}, glutathione S-transferase as well as hepatic concentration of reduced gluta-thione, that could explain its antitumor action [158] by inactivation of the carcinogenic oxygen free radicals [159]. Thus, green coffee inhibits DMCA-induced carcinogenesis in mice [154, 160], chlorogenic and caffeic acids inhibit carcinogenesis due to methylazoxy-methanol in hamsters [161], and kahweol and cafestol inhibit DMBA-induced carcinogenesis in hamsters [162]. Other phenolic acids found in coffee, such as caffeic and ellagic acid, reduce in vitro mutagenesis and in vivo carcinogenesis induced by benzopyrene in mice [163–165], DMBA-induced mutagenesis in rats [166], and nuclear aberrations in mice [167].

The effect of combining caffeine with other anticarcinogenic agents has also been studied in cultured cells of human osteosarcoma [168] and in patients with osteosarcoma [169], human bladder cancer cells in vitro [170], and in animal tumor models [171, 172]. Caffeine stimulates the tumor-inhibiting effect of several substances, such as cyclophosphamide, mitomycin C, adriamycin, cisplastin, bleomycin, pleomycin, thiothera and nitrosurea derivatives [168–172]. Therefore, these studies suggest that caffeine could be used to enhance the antineoplasic properties of medications in the treatment of cancer [168–172]. However, when administered in conjunction with chlorpromazine and nitrosu-rea, caffeine failed to improve treatment outcomes in humans with metastatic malignant melanoma [173]. Likewise, caffeine has no synergistic effect with two other antitumor agents, vincristine and methotrexate [168, 169].

Recent studies have suggested that caffeine or pentoxifylline may reduce or partially prevent late radiation injury in animals and humans [174–177]. In animals, the methylxanthine administration was initiated concurrent with radi-ation and was continued through the time at which late radiation injury was assessed, i.e., 30–40 weeks [175, 176]. In one human study, pentoxifylline was used as an interventional therapy for soft tissue ulceration or necrosis with an initiation at about 30 weeks after radiation [174]. In the most recent study, an increased caffeine intake at the time of radiotherapy is related to decreased incidence of severe late radiation injury in cervical cancer patients [177].

In summary, there are no clear-cut conclusions from these studies on the potential carcinogenic effects of coffee [114, 178–180]. In fact, according to conditions, coffee and caffeine either have no carcinogenic effect in animals, or they can induce tumors, potentiate or inhibit the carcinogenic effects of other substances, or they possess a tumor-inhibiting effect. Therefore, it is very difficult to draw conclusions from these studies on the potential effects of coffee and caffeine on human carcinogenesis. It is generally agreed that coffee and caffeine have very little carcinogenic effect in humans [53, 73, 112, 114]. In the rest of this review, we will discuss in detail the relationship between consumption of coffee and development of different cancers in humans.

Epidemiological Studies

Numerous epidemiological studies have focused on the relationship between coffee consumption and cancer incidence in humans. We will examine the results regarding cancers of the digestive system, the urinary system and the genital apparatus.

A recent study points out that the role of coffee and caffeine as causal agents of major diseases remains equivocal. Actually, many discrepancies in the results are due to imprecise measurements or to confounding factors. The only significant confounders in studies of the effects of coffee or caffeine consumption on health are sex and tobacco consumption. Other possible confounders are taken into account only if they are recognized to be risk factors for the disease being studied. For example, confounders in men would be level of fat in the diet, absorption of vitamin C and index of body mass; confounders in women include vitamins absorbed, consumption of alcohol, stress, and health status [181].

Cancers of the Digestive Tract

Recent reviews provided a detailed analysis of the effects of coffee on the incidence of various types of cancers of the digestive tract [113, 182–187].

Cancer of the Pancreas. In 1970, Stocks [188] demonstrated a positive correlation between coffee consumption and mortality due to pancreatic cancer in men across 20 countries. Then in 1981, the study of Lin and Kessler [189] and mainly that of MacMahon et al. [190] considered coffee consumption as a risk factor for pancreatic cancer. The possible relationship between coffee drinking and pancreatic cancer has since been the focus of numerous studies yielding equivocal and controversial results (table 1) with no clear conclusions

Table 1. Effect of coffee and tea consumption on pancreatic cancer: data from representative epidemiologic studies.

Authors and country	Cases, n	Sex	Beverage	Relative risk for coffee intake				
				0	1–2	3–4	5–7	>7
MacMahon et al., 1981 United States [190]	369	Both	TC	1	2.1	2.8*	3.2*	
Jick and Dinan, 1981 United States [193]	83	Both	TC	1	0.7		0.5	
Lin and Kessler, 1981 United States [218]	13	M	DC	1			1.6	
	15	F	DC	1			2.1	
Nomura et al., 1981 Hawaii [194]	28	M	TC	1	2.8	1.8		2.9
Goldstein, 1982 United States [196]	91	Both	TC	1	1.8	1.6		
Heuch et al., 1983 Norway [197]	3,146	M	TC	1	1.0	1.2	0.7	0.9
Wyndner et al., 1983 United States [199]	275	Both	TC	1	1.0	1.0		1.0
Kinlen and McPherson, 1984 UK [201]	216	Both	TC	1		0.9		
			T	1		2.3*	2.3*	2.6
Gold et al., 1985 United States [203]	201	M	TC	1	1.5	1.0	1.3	
		F	TC	1	1.2	1.6	2.9	
Mack et al., 1986 United States [206]	490	Both	TC	1		1.6	2.0	
			T	1		0.7	0.7	
	282	M	TC	1		1.5	2.9	
		M	T	1		1.1		
	208	F	TC	1		1.5	1.0	
		F	T	1		0.7		
Hsieh et al., 1986 United States [204]	172	Both	TC	1	1.4	1.2	2.0	1.5
	85	M	TC	1	1.1	1.0	2.4	1.3
	87	F	TC	1	1.3	1.0	2.2	1.4
Norell et al., 1986 Sweden [208]	99	Both	TC	1	1.6		1.0	
Wyndner et al., 1986 United States [209]	127	M	TC	1		0.7		
	111	F	TC	1	1.6	0.9		

Table 1 (Continued)

Authors and country	Cases, n	Sex	Beverage	Relative risk for coffee intake				
				0	1–2	3–4	5–7	>7
La Vecchia et al., 1987 Italy [211]	150	Both	CC	1	1.7	1.4	1.1	
			DC	1	0.9			
			T	1	0.8	1.1		
Raymond et al., 1987 Switzerland [212]	88	Both	TC	1	0.9		1.3	
			T	1	2.2*	1.0		
Falk et al., 1988 United States [213]	363	M	TC	1	0.7	0.5*	0.7	1.4
		F	TC	1	0.7	0.7	1.0	0.9
Hiatt et al, 1988 United States [215]	55	Both	TC	1	0.9		0.7	
Clavel et al., 1989 France [217]	98	M	TC	1	1.1	1.4	2.1	
	63	F	TC	1	3.9*	6.7*	9.6*	
Cuzick and Babiker, 1989 UK [219]	216	Both	TC	1	0.9	0.6	1.4	
			T	1		0.8	0.9	0.9
Olsen et al., 1989 United States [220]	212	Both	TC	1	0.5	0.7		0.6
Farrow and Davis, 1990 United States [221]	148	Both	TC	1	0.7	1.0		1.1
Ghadirian et al., 1991 Canada [227]	179	Both	TC	1	0.4	0.8	0.5	0.6
			CC	1	0.8	1.1	0.9	0.8
			DC	1	1.7	1.0	1.0	0.8
Jain et al., 1991 Canada [223]	249	Both	TC	1	0.9	0.9		0.9
Bueno de Mesquita et al, 1992 The Netherlands [224]	176	Both	TC	1	0.7	0.4	0.6	
			T	1	0.5	0.8	1.0	
Kalapothaki et al., 1993 Greece [229]	181	Both	TC	1	0.8	0.6	0.9	

Coffee and tea consumption are given in cups/day. M = Male; F = female; TC = total coffee intake; CC = caffeinated coffee; DC = decaffeinated coffee; T = tea.
  *p < 0.05.

[181–187, 191–232]. In some studies, the correlation between coffee consumption and pancreatic cancer is positive [190, 210–212, 228, 230], with a higher risk for decaffeinated coffee users [228]. However, often the correlation is not significant, limited to a specific daily intake [203, 204, 206, 211, 213, 218, 219] or to one sex [209, 213, 217]. In most studies, there is no correlation between consumption of coffee and cancer of the pancreas [193, 196–201, 205, 208, 214–216, 220–227, 229, 232]. Acccording to some recent studies, coffee drinkers would even be less exposed to cancer of the pancreas than nondrinkers [213, 224, 227]. Regarding tea consumption, in one study at all doses [201] and another one for 1–2 cups/day [212] there is a correlation between tea intake and cancer of the pancreas. In the other studies, tea has no consequence on pancreatic cancer [206, 211, 219, 224] or could even be somewhat protective [206, 224]. This inconsistency has been pointed out in a recent review [233]. Regarding the risk factors for pancreatic cancer related to the type of coffee consumed [234], studies on the role of decaffeinated coffee in the genesis of pancreatic cancer, though in limited number, showed either a negative association [186, 235] or an increased risk compared to regular coffee [228].

Even though ingestion of coffee cannot be considered a causal factor of pancreatic cancer, several authors have observed that this type of cancer induces an increase in fluid intake during the last 1–3 years of the disease. Before the final stage of the disease, there is no association between consumption of coffee and cancer of the pancreas [200–202]. The disparities among results obtained in various studies might be explained by differences in the beverage most frequently consumed in the country in which the study was performed, and by differences in the stage of the disease at the time of the study. A positive correlation between coffee consumption and pancreatic cancer in the terminal phase of the disease cannot be excluded.

There is a strong positive correlation between tobacco consumption and pancreatic cancer with an incidence twice as high for heavy smokers as for nonsmokers [213, 215, 216, 219, 221, 236–239]. Tobacco is strongly related to histological alterations of pancreatic cells, while consumption of coffee is not, according to a histopathological study in 611 human pancreases [240]. Therefore, consumption of coffee cannot be considered a cause of pancreatic cancer but the determining factors of this type of cancer remain unknown. The relationship between consumption of coffee or alcohol and type of occupation, diabetes mellitus, pancreatitis, and pancreatic cancer still remains uncertain. Actually, environmental and dietary factors are so numerous that it would be difficult to isolate the influence of one single factor such as absorption of alcohol, fatty foods, or fruits and vegetables. A recent epidemiological study of pancreatic cancer concluded that future research should be oriented towards possible links between cancer of the pancreas and dietary habits [182]. In fact, several studies demonstrate an increased risk in individuals who consume large quantities of charcoal-broiled meat and fatty foods [208, 216] and point to the protective role of consumption of fruits and vegetables against cancer of the pancreas [208, 212, 216].

In conclusion, most studies demonstrate that coffee consumption does not represent a significant risk factor for cancer of the pancreas. However, it is not possible to exclude completely a slight association between high coffee consumption and pancreatic cancer, but this association could reflect bias or confounding factors [186, 235]. In that respect, Bonelli et al. [231] concluded that the overall evidence so far clearly indicates that the effect of coffee consumption on pancreatic cancer risk, if any, is likely to be minimal and not worth the effort and cost required for a long-term cohort study.

Cancer of the Colon and Rectum. The relationship between consumption of coffee and the incidence of colorectal cancer has been the subject of numerous studies. However, a recent review [241] confirms the inconsistent results of epidemiologic studies. As detailed in table 2, according to the study, there is either a positive correlation [207, 226, 242–247], a negative correlation [205, 248–260] or no correlation at all [261–266] between coffee or tea consumption and frequency of colorectal cancer. One study shows a direct association between coffee consumption and cancer of the colon, but not of the rectum [207] whereas the reverse is true in another one [248]. Conversely, numerous authors have supported the hypothesis that coffee consumption could decrease the risk of colon cancer [248, 251, 256, 262, 267–269], particularly in cases of high consumption of coffee [248, 251, 256, 262]. In fact, coffee can decrease excretion of bile acids, of cholesterol or both, and increase plasma concentrations of cholesterol. Cholesterol and bile acids promote the development of cancer of the intestine in animals [253, 267, 268, 270, 271], while patients suffering from colon cancer excrete more fecal cholesterol than those in the control group [272, 273]. Therefore, coffee consumption might rather have a protective effect against this type of cancer [186, 235].

Gastric and Esophageal Cancer. Although little is known about the pharmacological effect of coffee on gastric mucous membranes, in particular about a possible increase in acid secretion, two European studies [205, 274] and one American study [275] suggest that there is no apparent correlation between consumption of coffee and gastric cancer. Only one study, performed in Italy [255], indicates an increased risk of gastric cancer in heavy coffee drinkers (>5 cups/day) compared to those with low or moderate consumptions. Even though coffee undoubtedly affects gastric acid secretion, it does not seem to play a determinant role in stomach carcinogenesis.

Table 2. Effect of coffee and tea consumption on cancer of the colon and rectum: data from representative epidemiologic studies

Authors and country	Cases, n	Sex	Site	Beverage	0–1	2–3	3–4	>5
Higginson, 1966 United States [252]	340	Both	Colorectum	TC	1	0.5		0.6
Haenszel et al., 1973 United States [251]	179	Both	Colorectum	TC	1		0.7	
Bjelke, 1974 Norway [267]	162	M	Colon	TC	1			0.6
Miller et al., 1983 Canada [264]	348	M	Colon	CB	1		0.9	
		F	Colon	CB	1		1.1	
	194	M	Rectum	CB	1		1.1	
		F	Rectum	CB	1		0.8	
Watanabe et al., 1984 Japan [259]	178	Both	Colon	TC	1		0.8	
	65	Both	Rectum	TC	1		0.7	
Snowdon and Philips, 1984 United States [226]	53	M	Colon	TC	1	3.5*		
	83	F	Colon	TC	1	1.9		
Philips and Snowdon, 1985 United States [244]	35	Both	Rectum	TC	1	1.4		
Tajima and Tominaga, 1985 Japan [265]	65	Both	Colon	TC	1	1.2		1.1
	51	Both	Rectum	TC	1	1.3		1.0
Heilbrun et al., 1986 Hawai [245]	152	M	Colon	T	1	1.0		
	76	M	Rectum	T	1	4.2*		
Jacobsen et al., 1986 Norway [205]	100	Both	Colon	TC	1			0.6
	64	Both	Rectum	TC	1			1.1
Macquart-Moulin et al., 1986 France [254]	399	Both	Colorectum	TC	1	0.6		0.6
Nomura et al., 1986 Hawai [207]	108	M	Colon	TC	1	1.2		1.3*
	60	M	Rectum	T	1	0.9		0.6*
Wu et al., 1987 United States [266]	58	M	Colorectum	TC	1	1.3		1.5
	68	F	Colorectum	TC	1	1.5		1.2
La Vecchia et al., 1988 Italy [247]	339	Both	Colon	TC	1		1.4	
	236	Both	Rectum	TC	1		1.5*	

Table 2 (Continued)

Authors and country	Cases, n	Sex	Site	Beverage	Relative risk for coffee intake			
					0–1	2–3	3–4	>5
Tuyns et al., 1988	453	Both	Colon	TC	1	0.9		0.6*
Belgium [257]	365	Both	Rectum	TC	1	0.9		0.7
Jarebinski et al., 1989	98	Both	Rectum	TC	1	1.0		0.8
Yugoslavia [263]								
La Vecchia et al., 1989	455	Both	Colon	TC	1	0.9		0.6*
Italy [255]	295	Both	Rectum	TC	1	0.9		0.7*
Lee et al., 1989	203	Both	Colorectum	TC	1	0.7		0.7
Singapore [258]								
Rosenberg et al., 1989	717	Both	Colon	TC	1	1.0		0.7*
United States [256]	538	Both	Rectum	TC	1	1.1		1.2
Benito et al., 1990	286	Both	Colorectum	TC	1	0.6		0.8
Spain [249]								
Slattery et al., 1990	112	M	Colon	TC	1	1.7		2.2*
United States [246]	119	F	Colon	TC	1	1.3		0.9
Olsen and Kronborg, 1993			Colorectum					
Denmark [261]	49	Both	Cancer	TC	1		1.8	1.1
				T	1		1.5	
	119	Both	Adenoma	TC	1		0.5*	0.3*
				T	1		1.3	
Baron et al., 1994	352	Both	Colon	TC	1	0.8	0.7	0.5
Sweden [260]				T	1	1.0		
	217	Both	Rectum	TC	1	1.2	1.1	0.9
				T	1	0.6		

Coffee and tea consumption are given in cups/day. M = Male; F = female; TC = total coffee intake; CB = caffeinated beverages including coffee, tea and cola drinks; T = tea.
*p < 0.05.

Regarding cancer of the esophagus, two European studies [207, 256] observed a very slight non significant increase in relative risk (1.2) in heavy coffee drinkers compared to those who drink small or moderate quantities, while one Brazilian study [276] showed no association between coffee and tea consumption and the risk for cancers of the upper aerodigestive tract. The other studies, in Iran [277], South America [278] and Puerto Rico [279], report increased incidence of esophageal cancer in subjects who drink very hot coffee, tea or maté as compared to those who drink the same beverages either luke-warm or cold. In those cases, it is the temperature of the beverage and not the coffee itself that would be responsible for lesions of the esophageal mucous membrane [277–279].

Cancers of the Urinary Tract

Cancers of the Kidneys and Urinary Tract. Etiology of cancer of the renal parenchyma and urinary tract is poorly understood. Some of the suspected risk factors are the use of analgesics and other medications, and consumption of animal protein, tobacco and coffee. Conclusions of epidemiological surveys on the relationship between coffee consumption and renal cancer are contra-dictory. Several studies, including one across 16 countries, show a positive correlation between the two parameters [280–282], but this correlation disap-pears once tobacco consumption is taken into account [282–286]. Three other studies report an association between consumption of coffee and cancer of renal cells; in two recent studies, the risk is apparently higher for those who consume more than 7 cups/day compared to those who consume small (<2 cups) or moderate (2–4 cups) amounts, but this correlation is not significant [287, 288]. In another study, the correlation is somewhat inconsistent in both sexes [289] and in the third, the correlation is barely significant only in the case of decaffeinated coffee [290]. Two more recent studies find either no association or a negative correlation between coffee consumption and cancer of the renal parenchyma [205, 291]. In conclusion, there does not appear to be a consistent association between coffee consumption and adenocarcinomas of the kidney and urinary tract.

Cancer of the Bladder. As detailed in table 3, numerous epidemiological studies have raised the possibility that coffee consumption could represent a risk factor for bladder cancer but unambiguous results still are not available [292–334]. Many investigations found no correlation at all between coffee drinking and bladder cancer [299, 301, 304, 307, 309, 314, 317, 318, 321, 322, 324, 328, 333]. Only a few studies performed on subjects of both sexes show a dose-response relationship [292, 293, 296, 302, 304, 332, 334]. This dose-response relationship is limited to male subjects in three studies [302, 303, 307]. Furthermore, the positive correlation between consumption of coffee and bladder cancer is often very slight [304, 306, 317, 327, 328]. The correlation between bladder cancer and the type of coffee is also not very clear. Most studies have observed a correlation with ground coffee and espresso but not with instant or decaffeinated coffee [302, 303, 309, 334], while Cartwright et al. [294] did not report any heterogeneity between instant and ground coffee. The relative risk also varies greatly among individuals [329] and does not seem at all related to the duration of coffee consumption [335], although a recent

Table 3. Effect of coffee and tea consumption on cancer of the bladder and lower urinary tract (LUT): data from representative epidemiologic studies

Authors and country	Cases, n	Sex	Site	Beverage	0–1	2–3	3–4	>5
Dunham et al., 1968 [299]	493	M	Bladder	TC	1	1.4	2.0	1.7
Fraumeni et al., 1971 United States [300]		F	Bladder	TC	1	0.7	0.4	0.3
Cole, 1971	345	M	Bladder	TC	1	1.3	1.2	1.3
United States [298]	100	F	Bladder	TC	1	1.6	3.8	2.2
Bross and Tiddings, 1973	360	M	Bladder	TC	1	1.3	1.5	1.6
United States [327]	120	F	Bladder	TC	1	0.9	1.0	0.8
Morgan and Jain, 1974	158	M	Bladder	TC	1	0.6	0.9	0.8
Canada [328]	74	F	Bladder	TC	1	1.1	1.3	
	232	Both	Bladder	T	1	0.5	1.1	1.0
Simon et al., 1975	135	F	LUT	TC	1	2.2	1.9	2.3
United States [323]	132	F	LUT	T	1	1.3	0.8	
Miller, 1977	400	M	Bladder	TC	1		1.3	
Canada [312]		M	Bladder	T	1	0.8		
	118	F	Bladder	TC	1		1.6	
		F	Bladder	T	1	1.7		
Wynder and Goldsmith, 1977	574	M	Bladder	TC	1	1.4	1.9	2.0
United States [326]	158	F	Bladder	TC	1	1.0	1.9	1.3
Miller et al., 1978	183	M	Bladder	T	1		1.1	
Canada [313]	72	F	Bladder	T	1		0.9	
Mettlin and Graham, 1979	429	M	Bladder	TC	1	1.4	2.1	1.7
United States [311]	100	F	Bladder	TC	1	0.9	1.4	1.0
Howe et al., 1980	480	M	Bladder	TC	1	1.6	1.3	1.5
Canada [304]				T	1	1.0		
	152	F	Bladder	TC	1	0.7	1.7	1.3
				T	1	0.5		
Cartwright et al., 1981	631	M	Bladder	TC	1		1.1	
UK [294]	210	F	Bladder	TC	1		0.8	
Morrison et al., 1982	587	M	LUT	TC	1	0.8	0.8	1.5
United States [317]		F	LUT	TC	1	0.7	0.8	0.9
Morrison et al., 1982	541	M	LUT	TC	1	1.0	0.9	
UK [317]		F	LUT	TC	1	1.4	1.2	

Table 3 (Continued)

Authors and country	Cases, n	Sex	Site	Beverage	Relative risk for coffee intake			
					0–1	2–3	3–4	>5
Morrison et al., 1982	289	M	LUT	TC	1	1.0	1.3	1.9
Japan [317]		F	LUT	TC	1	0.7		0.7
Hartge et al., 1983	397	M	Bladder	TC	1	1.0	1.1	1.4
United States [302]	198	M	Bladder	T	1	1.1	1.0	
	164	F	Bladder	TC	1	0.9	0.8	0.9
	56	F	Bladder	T	1	1.7	1.2	
Marrett et al., 1983	412	M	Bladder	TC	1	1.6*	2.0*	2.0*
United States [309]		F	Bladder	TC	1	1.3	1.2	1.0
Ohno et al., 1985	293	M	Bladder	TC	1	0.7	1.1	1.8
Japan [318]				T	1	1.0		
		F	Bladder	TC	1	0.7	0.7	
				T	1	0.6		
Rebelakos et al., 1985	300	Both	Bladder	TC	1	1.2	1.7*	2.7*
Greece [320]								
Claude et al., 1986	340	M	LUT	TC	1	1.4	1.4	2.3*
Germany [296]				T	1	1.0	1.5	1.9
	91	F	LUT	TC	1	1.3	1.9	2.2
				T	1	1.9	1.3	1.9
Jensen et al., 1986	371	Both	Bladder	TC	1	1.4	1.4	1.8
Denmark [306]				T	1	0.8	2.0*	1.5*
Kabat et al., 1986	76	M	Bladder	TC	1	0.9	1.4	0.5
Denmark [307]	76	F	Bladder	TC	1	1.5	0.8	2.4
Piper et al., 1986	173	F	Bladder	TC	1	0.9	1.9	2.1
United States [319]								
Bravo et al., 1987	406	M	Bladder	TC	1	2.0*	2.7*	
Spain [293]								
Iscovich et al., 1987	117	Both	Bladder	TC	1	1.1	4.4*	12.0*
Argentina [305]				T	1	1.4	1.4	
Ciccone and Vineis, 1988	512	M	Bladder	TC	1	0.8	1.1	0.8
Italy [295]	55	F	Bladder	TC	1	1.4	0.8	0.8
Risch et al., 1988	826	M	Bladder	TC	1	1.1	1.2	0.9
Canada [321]				T	1	1.0		
		F	Bladder	TC	1	1.0	1.9	1.1
				T	1	1.0		

Table 3 (Continued)

Authors and country	Cases, n	Sex	Site	Beverage	Relative risk for coffee intake			
					0–1	2–3	3–4	>5
Slattery et al., 1988 United States [324]	419	M	Bladder	TC T	1 1	1.2 1.1	1.1	1.6
La Vecchia et al., 1989 Italy [308]	161	Both	Bladder	TC T	1 1	2.0 0.8	1.6	
Clavel and Cordier, 1991 France [297]	588	M	Bladder	TC	1	1.2		1.5
Mills et al., 1991 United States [330]	52	Both	Bladder	TC	1	0.4	2.0	
Pujolar et al., 1993 Spain [333]	438 59	M F	Bladder Bladder	TC TC	1 1	0.9 1.1	1.0 0.7	

Coffee and tea consumption are given in cups/day. M = Male; F = female; TC = total coffee intake; T = tea.

*p < 0.05.

study reported a fourfold higher risk for bladder cancer in the population who started consuming coffee before the age of 11 compared to those who started after the age of 14. After 14 years, the age of onset of coffee consuming had no effect on the relative risk for bladder cancer [332].

Thus, the possible relationship between coffee consumption and bladder cancer has not been demonstrated [235]. Actually, consumption of tobacco would be a greater risk factor than coffee in the development of bladder cancer [296, 304, 307, 336], although the frequent association between tobacco and coffee often makes evaluation difficult [337]. On the other hand, some studies seem to indicate that the most exposed groups would be nonsmokers who drink large amounts of coffee, i.e., more than 7 cups/day [296, 302, 305]. This risk is associated with a caffeine clearance that is twice as slow in nonsmokers than in smokers [338, 339].

The overall results of these studies, at times seemingly contradictory and difficult to interpret, indicate that in the large sample of population studied a strong association between coffee consumption and bladder cancer can be excluded. However, the relative risk for bladder cancer tends to be higher in heavy coffee drinkers but this risk is not related to the dose or to the duration of exposure [235]. These data suggest that coffee is definitely not the causal factor for bladder cancer. The correlation observed between coffee drinking and this type of cancer could be related to confounding factors, especially tobacco, dietary habits and occupation. Indeed, a recent overview of studies on coffee consumption and bladder cancer taking into account smoking does not suggest a clinically important association between the regular consumption of coffee and the development of bladder cancer in both men and women [340].

Moreover, caffeine and the numerous other substances contained in coffee could have direct or indirect metabolic effects and modify concentrations of carcinogenic or anticarcinogenic substances in bladder epithelium [341]. Since most of these substances or their metabolites are excreted by the urinary tract, they come into contact with the mucous membrane of the bladder. Moreover, coffee could be associated with increased risk of bladder cancer because of chlorinated tap water. Therefore, inconsistencies in the studies could be due to geographic variability in risk associated with the tap water component [334].

In conclusion, the relative risk for bladder cancer tends to be higher in coffee drinkers than in nondrinkers, but the risk is neither dose- nor duration-related [235], except apparently for people starting coffee consumption very early in life [332]. Therefore, the data do not implicate coffee as an important risk factor for bladder carcinogenesis especially since long-term exposure to coffee in animals elicits no carcinogenic effect at the urinary tract level.

Cancers of the Genital Organs

Cancer of the Prostate. Based on three studies, there does not seem to be any correlation between consumption of coffee and prostate cancer [205, 207, 243].

Cancer of the Ovaries. A positive correlation has been observed in some studies between consumption of coffee and frequency of ovarian cancer [188, 210, 342–345], but there is no relation between the quantity of coffee absorbed and the degree of risk [342, 344, 345]. On the other hand, in many other studies, the correlation observed between the two parameters is not significant [346–353]. However, interpretation of the findings is not clear. A weak association between cancer of the vulva and cancer of the cervix and coffee consumption has been found in one study [186].

Breast Cancer. A recent review analyzed data reported in the literature on the association between coffee and caffeine consumption and development of breast cancer or benign cystic mastopathy [354]. Most epidemiological studies have not found a positive association between coffee consumption and the risk of breast cancer [148, 181, 191, 355–367]. Only one study found a postive correlation between coffee consumption and breast cancer in women before menopause. This risk is not dose-dependent and is not present after menopause [368, 369]. On the contrary, numerous studies found no association to a weak negative correlation between breast cancer and coffee consumption [358, 359, 362, 363, 367, 370].

A recent study demonstrated that in women suffering from breast cancer, consumption of coffee seemed associated with a propensity for the tumor to be more or less differentiated. The authors did not find any completely undifferentiated tumor in women who drank large quantities of coffee [371]. Therefore, coffee or caffeine could have antitumor effects. Caffeine can inhibit or delay mitosis in many kinds of cells, probably due to variations in cyclic AMP concentration that influence DNA synthesis and mitosis [53, 372]. However, coffee with or without caffeine, is more active than caffeine alone. These results suggest that other substances contained in coffee might influence tumor differentiation, either in synergy with caffeine or even alone [373].

In a recent study, the association between body weight and breast cancer in women who drink coffee was taken into account. In the group of thin women, the risk of breast cancer is reduced 50% when they drink at least 5 cups of coffee per day compared with those who drink 2 cups or less. In the group of heavier women, the reverse association is observed. Those who drink large quantities of coffee have twice the risk of developing breast cancer but this increase is not statistically significant [373].

Therefore, coffee does not seem to be an etiologic factor in the development of breast cancer. Actually, consumption of coffee could even be beneficial.

Fibrocystic Breast Disease. The marked clinical improvement noted in fibrocystic breast disease after reduction or cessation of methylxanthine consumption [374–377] suggested a possible association between coffee ingestion and this disease, which is considered a risk factor for breast cancer. However, results of the studies are inconsistent, perhaps due to diverse histological aspects of the disease, use of inappropriate control groups, and frequent absence of data on total methylxanthine intake [181, 378]. Since these works have been published, several recent studies have found no association between coffee consumption and frequency of fibrocystic breast disease [379–388], whereas others have observed a positive correlation [389–392]. Therefore, at the present time there is no proof that coffee could have a carcinogenic effect on pre-existing benign breast disease.

Other Cancers

The effects of coffee consumption on other types of cancer have also been explored. Most studies found no association between coffee consumption and cancer of the liver, of the extrahepatic bile duct and of the lung, Hodgkin's disease, non-Hodgkin's lymphomas, myeloid leukemia and malignant melanomas [352, 393]. However, two studies did demonstrate a correlation between coffee consumption and lung cancer [205, 394]. According to one of the studies, the relative risk of lung cancer is increased significantly in heavy coffee drinkers (>5 cups/day), after taking into account factors such as age, smoking, and rural or urban habitat. Moreover, coffee would act synergistically with tobacco in the mortality related to lung cancer [389]. Lastly, a marked negative association was observed between coffee consumption and nonmelanomatous skin cancer.

Conclusion

In conclusion, in the doses usually consumed by man, coffee does not have any potential genotoxic, mutagenic or carcinogenic effect [235, 395]. There is still some debate on the effect of coffee in the carcinogenesis of the pancreas, colon, bladder and urinary tract. Some more rigorous studies would be necessary to reach a clear understanding of the potential carcinogenic effect of lifetime exposure to coffee in humans. Some epidemiological and animal studies have even suggested that coffee could delay development of certain tumors. The potentiation of the antitumor effects of some anticancer chemotherapy medications with high doses of caffeine (near toxic level) could perhaps be applied in the treatment of cancer but only on the condition that the secondary neurotoxic effects of large doses of methylxanthines can be managed. Moreover, a recent hypothesis is that coffee, in itself, may not be a causal factor in bladder carcinogenesis or a protective factor in colon carcinogenesis. Its apparent activity would be mediated by the N-acetyltransferase phenotype of the subject inducing slow acetylators to drink more coffee than fast acetylators [396]. However, this hypothesis remains to be tested in epidemiological studies controlling both coffee consumption and the acetylation phenotype.

References

1   National Coffee Association of USA: Coffee Drinking Study 1991. New York, NCA of USA, 1991.
2   Nippon Research Center: A Basic Survey for Monitoring Trends in the Demand for Coffee, June 1991. Tokyo, All Japan Coffee Association, 1991.
3   International Coffee Organization (ICO), Federal Republic of Germany: Coffee Consumption Habits Trends Data 1980 to 1990. ICO, ED PC 97/91 (E), July 1991.
4   D'Amicis A, Viani R: The consumption of coffee; in Garattini S (ed): Coffee, Caffeine and Health. New York, Raven Press, 1993, pp 1–16.
5   Peters A: Brewing makes the difference. Proc 14th International Scientific Colloquium on Coffee, San Francisco 1991, pp 97–106.
6   Debry G: La consommation du café, in Debry G (ed): Le Café et la Santé. Paris, Libbey, 1993, pp 43–73.
7   Debry G: Composition du café; in Debry G (ed): Le Café et la Santé. Paris, Libbey, 1993, pp 75–104.
8   Clarke RJ: Coffee technology; in Herschdoefer SH (ed): Quality Control in the Food Industry, ed 2. London, Academic Press, 1987, vol 4, pp 161–191.
9   Viani R: Coffee, ed 2. Vevey, Nestec, 1985.
10 Clarke RJ, Macrae R: Coffee, vol 1: Chemistry. London, Elsevier Applied Science Publishers, 1985.

11   Viani R: Coffee, in Ullman's Encyclopaedia of Industrial Chemistry. Weinheim, VCH, 1986, vol A7, pp 315–319.

12   Viani R: The composition of coffee; in Garattini S (ed): Caffeine, Coffee and Health. New York, Raven Press, 1993, pp 17–41.

13   Cetinkaya M: Organophosphor- und Organochlorpestizidrückstünde in Rohkaffee. Dtsch Lebensm Rundsch 1988;84:189–190.

14   Cetinkaya M, Von Düszeln J, Thiemann W, et al: Untersuchung von Organochlor-Pestizidrück-ständen in Roh- und Röstkaffee und deren Abbauverhalten beim Röst-Prozess. Z Lebensm Unters Forsch 1984;179:5–8.

15   Micco C, Miraglia M, Brera C, et al: The effect of roasting on the fate of aflatoxin B_1 in artificially contaminated green coffee beans. Proc 14th International Scientific Colloquium on Coffee, San Francisco 1991, pp 183–189.

16   Strobel RGK: Allergens and mould toxin contaminants; in Clarke RJ, Macrae R (eds): Coffee, vol 3: Physiology. London, Elsevier Applied Science Publishers, 1985, pp 215–320.

17   Grob K, Lanfranchi M, Egli J, et al: Determination of food contamination by mineral oil from jute sacks using coupled LC-GC. J Assoc Off Anal Chem 1991;74:506–512.

18   Sen NP, Seaman SW, Weber D: Mass spectrometric confirmation of the presence of N-nitrosopyrroli-dine. J Assoc Off Anal Chem 1990;73:325–327.

19   Troup GJ, Hutton DR, Dobbie JL, et al: Free radicals in coffee but not in tea (letter). Med J Aust 1988;148:537–538.

20   Arnaud MJ: The metabolism of coffee constituents, in Clarke RJ, Macrae R (eds): Coffee, vol 3: Physiology. London, Elsevier Applied Science Publishers, 1988, pp 33–55.

21   Arnaud MJ: Products of metabolism of caffeine; in Dews PB (ed): Caffeine: Perspectives from Recent Research. Berlin, Springer, 1984, pp 3–38.

22   Arnaud MJ: The pharmacology of caffeine. Prog Drug Res 1987;31:273–313.

23   Arnaud MJ: Metabolism of caffeine and other components of coffee; in Garattini S (ed): Coffee, Caffeine and Health. New York, Raven Press, 1993, pp 43–94.

24   Arnaud MJ: Comparative metabolic disposition of [1-Me^{14}C] caffeine in rats, mice and Chinese hamsters. Drug Metab Dispos 1985;13:471–478.

25   Berthou F, Guillois B, Riche C, et al: Interspecies variations in caffeine metabolism related to cytochrome P_{450}1A enzymes. Xenobiotica 1992;22:671–680.

26   Blanchard J, Sawers SJA: The absolute bioavailability of caffeine in man. Eur J Clin Pharmacol 1983;24:93–98.

27   Bonati M, Latini R, Galetti F, et al: Caffeine disposition after oral doses. Clin Pharmacol Ther 1982;32:98–106.

28   Parsons WD, Neims AH: Effect of smoking on caffeine clearance. Clin Pharmacol 1978;24:40–43.

29   Neims AH, Bailey J, Aldridge A: Disposition of caffeine during and after pregnancy (abstract). Clin Res 1979;27:A236.

30   Patwardhan RV, Desmond PV, Johnson RF, et al: Impaired elimination of caffeine by oral contracep-tive steroids. J Lab Clin Med 1980;95:603–608.

31   Balogh A, Irmisch E, Klinger G, et al: Untersuchungen zur Elimination von Coffein und Metamizol im Menstruationszyklus der fertilen Frau. Zentralbl Gynäkol 1987;109:1135–1142.

32   Callahan MM, Robertson RS, Branfman AR, et al: Comparison of caffeine metabolism in three nonsmoking populations after oral administration of radiolabeled caffeine. Drug Metab Dispos 1983;11:211–217.

33   Abernethy A, Todd EL: Impairment of caffeine clearance by chronic use of low-dose estrogen-containing oral contraceptives. Eur J Clin Pharmacol 1985;28:425–428.

34   Aldridge A, Bailey J, Neims AH: The disposition of caffeine during and after pregnancy. Semin Perinatol 1981;5:310–318.

35   Brazier JL, Ritter J, Berland M, et al: Pharmacokinetics of caffeine during and after pregnancy. Dev Pharmacol Ther 1983;6:315–322.

36   Kling OR, Christensen DH: Caffeine elimination in late pregnancy. Fed Proc 1979;38:218–226.

37   Knutti R, Rothweiler H, Schlatter C: Effect of pregnancy on the pharmacokinetics of caffeine. Eur J Clin Pharmacol 1981;21:121–126.

38 Knutti R, Rothweiler H, Schlatter C: The effect of pregnancy on the pharmacokinetics of caffeine. Arch Toxicol 1982;5:187–192.

39 Parsons WD, Pelletier JG: Delayed elimination of caffeine by women in the last 2 weeks of pregnancy. Can Med Assoc J 1982;127:377–381.

40 Bonati M, Garattini S: Interspecies comparison of caffeine disposition; in Dews PB (ed): Caffeine: Perspectives from Recent Research. Berlin, Springer, 1984, pp 48–56.

41 Bonati M, Latini R, Tognoni G, et al: Interspecies comparison of in vivo caffeine pharmacokinetics in man, monkey, rabbit, rat, and mouse. Drug Metab Rev 1984/85;15:1355–1383.

42 Burg AW, Werner E: Tissue distribution of caffeine and its metabolites in the mouse. Biochem Pharmacol 1972;21:923–936.

43 Gilbert RM: Caffeine as a drug of abuse; in Gibbins RJ, Israel Y, Popham RE, et al (eds): Research Advances in Alcohol and Drug Problems. New York, Wiley, 1976, vol 3, pp 49–176.

44 Aeschbacher HU: Mutagenicity of coffee; in Clarke RJ, Macrae R (eds): Coffee, vol 3: Physiology. London, Elsevier Applied Science Publishers, 1988, pp 195–213.

45 Grice HC: Genotoxicity and carcinogenicity assessment of caffeine and theobromine. Food Chem Toxicol 1987;25:295–296.

46 Haynes RH, Collins JDB: The mutagenic potential of caffeine, in Dews PB (ed): Caffeine. Perspectives from Recent Research. Berlin, Springer, 1984, pp 221–238.

47 Kihlman BA: Caffeine and Chromosomes. Amsterdam, Elsevier, 1977.

48 LaChance MP: The pharmacology and toxicology of caffeine. J Food Saf 1982;4:71–112.

49 Nehlig A, Debry G: Potential genotoxic, mutagenic and antimutagenic effects of coffee: A review. Mutat Res 1994;317:145–162.

50 Rosenkranz HS, Ennever FK: Evaluation of the genotoxicity of theobromine and caffeine. Food Chem Toxicol 1987;25:247–251.

51 Rosenkranz HS, Ennever FK: Genotoxicity and carcinogenicity assesssment of caffeine and theobromine. Food Chem Toxicol 1987;25:795–796.

52 Tarka SM: The toxicology of cocoa and methylxanthines: A review of the literature. Crit Rev Toxicol 1982;9:275–312.

53 Timson J: Caffeine. Mutat Res 1977;47:1–52.

54 Friederrich U, Hann D, Albertini S, et al: Mutagenicity studies with coffee: The influence of different factors on the mutagenic activity in the Salmonella/mammalian microsome test. Mutat Res 1984; 156:39–52.

55 Albertini S, Friederrich U, Schlatter C, et al: The influence of roasting procedure on the formation of mutagenic compounds in coffee. Food Chem Toxicol 1985;23:593–597.

56 Shane BS, Troxclair AM, McMillin DJ, et al: Comparative mutagenicity of nine brands of coffee to Salmonella typhimurium TA100, TA102, and TA104. Environ Mol Mutagen 1988;11:195–206.

57 Aeschbacher HU, Meier H, Ruch E, et al: Risk evaluation of coffee based on in vitro and in vivo mutagenicity testing; in MacMahon B, Sugimura T (eds): Coffee and Health, Banbury Report 17. New York, CSH Press, 1984, pp 89–97.

58 Nagao M, Suwa Y, Yoshizumi H, et al: Mutagens in coffee, in MacMahon B, Sugimura T (eds): Coffee and Health, Banbury Report 17. New York, CSH Press, 1984, pp 69–77.

59 Kosugi A, Nagao M, Suwa Y, et al: Roasted coffee beans produced compounds that induce prophage in E. coli and are mutagenic in E. coli and S. typhimurium. Mutat Res 1983;116:179–184.

60 Pons FW, Müller P: Induction of frameshift mutations by caffeine in Escherichia coli K12. Mutagenesis 1990;5:173–177.

61 Selby CP, Sancar A: Molecular mechanisms of DNA repair inhibition by caffeine. Proc Natl Acad Sci USA 1990;87:3522–3525.

62 Okuda A, Kimura G: Elongation of G1 phase by transient exposure of rat 3Y1 fibroblasts to caffeine during the previous and present generations. J Cell Sci 1988;89:379–386.

63 Aeschbacher HU, Ruch E, Meier H, et al: Instant and brewed coffees in the in vitro human lymphocyte mutagenicity test. Food Chem Toxicol 1985;23:747–752.

64 Chen ATL, Reidy JA, Annest JL, et al: Increased chromosome fragility as a consequence of blood folate levels, smoking status, and coffee consumption. Environ Mol Mutagen 1989;13: 319–324.

65   Schlegel R, Pardee AB: Caffeine-induced uncoupling of mitosis from the completion of DNA replication in mammalian cells. Science 1986;232:1264–1266.

66   Downes CS, Musk SRR, Watson JV, et al: Caffeine overcomes a restriction point associated with DNA replication, but does not accelerate mitosis. J Cell Biol 1990;110:1855–1859.

67   Aeschbacher HU, Würzner HP: An evaluation of instant and regular coffee in the Ames *Salmonella* mutagenicity test. Toxicol Lett 1980;5:139–145.

68   De Flora S: Detoxification of genotoxic compounds as a threshold mechanism limiting their carcinogenicity. Toxicol Pathol 1984;12:337–343.

69   Aeschbacher HU, Meier H, Ruch E, et al: Investigation of coffee in sister chromatid exchange and micronucleus tests in vivo. Food Chem Toxicol 1984;22:803–807.

70   Shimizu M, Yano E: Mutagenicity of instant coffee and its interaction with dimethylnitrosamine in the micronucleus test. Mutat Res 1987;189:307–311.

71   Roberts JJ: Mechanism of potentiation by caffeine of genotoxic damage induced by physical and chemical agents: Possible relevance to carcinogenesis; in Dews PB (ed): Caffeine. Perspectives from Recent Research. Berlin, Springer, 1984, pp 239–253.

72   Kihlman BA, Andersson HC: Effects of caffeine on chromosomes in cells of higher organisms. Rev Environ Health 1987;7:279–382.

73   Kihlman BA, Hanson K, Palitti F, et al: Potentiation of induced chromatid-type aberrations by hydroxyurea and caffeine in G_2; in Natarajan AT, Obe G, Altmann G (eds): Progress in Mutation Research. Amsterdam, Elsevier, 1985, vol 4, pp 11–24.

74   Labanowska J, Beetham KL, Tolmach LJ: Caffeine-induced modulation of the lethal action of X-rays on Chinese hamster V79 cells. Radiat Res 1988;115:176–186.

75   Natarajan AT, Obe G, Dulout FN: The effect of caffeine post-treatment on X-ray-induced chromosomal aberrations in human blood lymphocytes in vitro. Hum Genet 1980;54:183–189.

76   Pincheira J, Lopez-Saez JF: Effects of caffeine and cycloheximide during G_2 prophase in control and X-ray-irradiated human lymphocytes. Mutat Res 1991;251:71–77.

77   Tanzarella C, De Salvia R, Degrassi F, et al: Effect of post-treatments with caffeine during G2 on the frequency of chromosome-type aberrations produced by X-rays in human lymphocytes during G_1 and G_0. Mutagenesis 1986;1:41–44.

78   Waldren CA, Rasko I: Caffeine enhancement of X-ray killing in cultured human and rodent cells. Radiat Res 1978;73:95–110.

79   Domon M, Rauth AM: Effects of caffeine on ultraviolet-irradiated mouse L cells. Radiat Res 1969; 39:207–221.

80   Fujiwara Y, Tatsumi M: Replicative bypass repair of UV damage to DNA of mammalian cells. Caffeine-sensitive and caffeine-resistant mechanisms. Mutat Res 1976;37:91–110.

81   Musk SRR, Downes CS, Johnson RT: Caffeine induces uncoordinated expression of cell cycle functions after ultraviolet irradiation. Accelerated cycle transit, sister chromatid exchanges and premature chromosome condensation in a transformed Indian muntjac cell line. J Cell Sci 1988;90:591–599.

82   Goth-Goldstein R: Cell killing by various nitrosoureas and the potentiating effect of caffeine. Mutat Res 1982;94:237–244.

83   Murname JP, Byfield JE, Ward JF, et al: Effects of methylated xanthines on mammalian cells treated with bifunctional alkylating agents. Nature 1980;285:326–329.

84   Fingert HJ, Kindy RL, Pardee AB: Enhanced lethality by methylxanthines in human bladder cancer cells treated with thio-TEPA. J Urol 1984;132:609–613.

85   Rose WC, Trader MW, Dykes DJ, et al: Therapeutic potentiation of nitrosoureas using chlorpromazine and caffeine in the treatment of murine tumors. Cancer Treat Rep 1978;62:2085–2093.

86   Toshimitsu A, Bodell WJ: Effect of caffeine on cytotoxicity and sister chromatid exchange induction in sensitive and resistant rat brain tumor cells treated with 1,3-bis(2-chloroethyl)-1-nitrosourea. Cancer Res 1987;47:5052–5058.

87   Ceccherini I, Loprieno N, Sbrana I: Caffeine post-treatment causes a shift in the chromosome aberration types induced by mitomycin C, suggesting a caffeine-sensitive mechanism of DNA repair in G_2. Mutagenesis 1988;3:39–44.

88   Müller WU: Toxicity of various combinations of X-rays, caffeine, and mercury in mouse embryos. Int J Radiat Biol 1989;56:315–323.

89 Müller WU, Streffer C, Wurm R: Supraadditive formation of micronuclei in preimplantation mouse embryos in vitro after combined treatment with X-rays and caffeine. Teratog Carcinog Mutagen 1985;5:123–131.

90 Painter RB: Effect of caffeine on DNA synthesis in irradiated and unirradiated mammalian cells. J Mol Biol 1980;143:289–301.

91 Brogger A: Caffeine-induced enhancement of chromosome damage in human lymphocytes treated with methylmethanesulphonate, mitomycin C, and X-rays. Mutat Res 1974;23:353–360.

92 Lau CC, Pardee AB: Mechanisms by which caffeine potentiates lethality of nitrogen mustard. Proc Natl Acad Sci USA 1982;79:2942–2946.

93 Fox M: A caffeine-insensitive error-prone repair process in V79 Chinese hamster cells? Mutat Res 1977;46:118–125.

94 Pellicia F, Rocchi A: The effect of caffeine on DAPI-inducible fragile sites. Mutat Res 1992;282: 43–48.

95 Yunis JJ, Soreng AL: Constitutive fragile sites and cancer. Science 1984;226:1199–1204.

96 Yunis JJ, Soreng AL, Bowe AE: Fragile sites are targets of diverse mutagens and carcinogens. Oncogene 1987;1:59–69.

97 Tatsumi K, Strauss BS: Accumulation of DNA growing points in caffeine-treated human lymphoblastoid cells. J Mol Biol 1979;135:435–449.

98 Williams PH, Clarke CH: Pre- and post-irradiation-effects upon lethality and reversion in *Salmonella typhimurium.* J Gen Microbiol 1971;68:199–205.

99 Witkin EM, Farquharson EL: Enhancement and diminution of ultraviolet light-initiated mutagenesis by post-treatment with caffeine in *Escherichia coli;* in Wolstenhome GEW, O'Connor M (eds): Mutation as Cellular Process. London, Churchill, 1969, pp 36–49.

100 Menningham HD, Pons FW: Mutation induction by thymine deprivation in *Escherichia coli* B/r. I. Influence of caffeine. Mutat Res 1979;60:13–23.

101 Kim J, Levin RE: Mechanism of caffeine repression of mitomycin C induced reversion in *Salmonella typhimurium* strain TA94. Microbios 1988;53:181–190.

102 Clarke CH: Repair systems and nitrous acid mutagenesis in *E. coli* B/r. Mutat Res 1970;9: 359–368.

103 Hava P, Hejlova A, Soskova L: Antimutagenic effects of caffeine during nitrosoguanidine-induced mutagenesis in *Salmonella typhimurium* cells and phages. Folia Microbiol 1978;23:45–54.

104 Levin RE: Influence of caffeine on mutations induced by nitrosoguanidine in *Salmonella typhimurium* tester strains. Environ Mutag 1982;4:689–694.

105 Maekawa I, Shibata H, Furusawa S, et al: Reduction of epirubicin cytotoxicity by caffeine in P388 leukemia. Res Commun Subst Abuse 1992;12:71–74.

106 Furusawa S, Fujimura T, Kawauchi H, et al: Reduction of cytotoxic effect of pirarubicin by caffeine in P388 leukemia cells. Res Commun Subst Abuse 1992;13:269–272.

107 Yamaguchi T, Iki M: Inhibitory effect of coffee extract against some mutagens. Agric Biol Chem 1986;50:2983–2988.

108 Abraham SK: Inhibition of in vivo genotoxicity by coffee. Food Chem Toxicol 1989;27:787–792.

109 Yasukawa K, Takido M, Takeuchi M, et al: Inhibitory effect of glycyrrhizin and caffeine on two-stage carcinogenesis in mice. Yakugaku Zasshi 1988;8:794–796.

110 Aeschbacher HU, Jaccaud E: Inhibition by coffee of nitrosurea-mediated DNA damage in mice. Food Chem Toxicol 1990;28:633–637.

111 Grice HC: The carcinogenic potential of caffeine; in Dews PB (ed): Caffeine. Perspectives from Recent Research. Berlin, Springer, 1984, pp 201–220.

112 Würzner HP: Animal feeding studies with coffee; in Clarke RJ, Macrae R (eds): Coffee, vol 3: Physiology. London, Elsevier Applied Science Publishers, 1988, pp 171–194.

113 James JE: Caffeine and cancer; in James JE (ed): Caffeine and Health. New York, Academic Press, 1991, pp 190–218.

114 Nehlig A, Debry G: Genotoxic, mutagenic and carcinogenic effects of coffee, in Debry G (ed): Coffee and Health. London, Libbey, 1994, pp 471–516.

115 Bauer AR Jr, Rank RK, Kerr R, et al: The effects of prolonged coffee intake on genetically identical mice. Life Sci 1977;21:63–70.

116 Palm PE, Arnold EP, Rachwall PC, et al: Evaluation of the teratogenic potential of fresh-brewed coffee and caffeine in the rat. Toxicol Appl Pharmacol 1978;44:1–16.

117 Palm PE, Arnold EP, Nick MS, et al: Two-year toxicity/carcinogenicity study of fresh-brewed coffee in rats initially exposed in utero. Toxicol Appl Pharmacol 1984;74:364–382.

118 Stalder R, Bexter A, Würzner HP, et al: A carcinogenicity study of instant coffee in Swiss mice. Food Chem Toxicol 1990;28:829–837.

119 Takayama S, Nagao M, Suwa Y, et al: Long-term carcinogenicity studies on caffeine, instant coffee, and methylglyoxal in rats; in MacMahon B, Sugimura T (eds): Coffee and Health, Banbury Report 17. New York, CSH Press, 1984, pp 99–104.

120 Würzner HP, Lindstron E, Vuataz L: A 2-year feeding study of instant coffees in rats. I. Body weight, food consumption, haematological parameters and plasma chemistry. Food Cosmet Toxicol 1977;15:7–16.

121 Zeitlin BR: Coffee and bladder cancer. Lancet 1972;i:1066.

122 Brune H, Deutsh-Wenzel R, Habs M, et al: Investigation of the tumorigenic response to benzo[a]pyrene in aqueous coffee solution applied orally to Sprague-Dawley rats. J Cancer Res Clin Oncol 1981;102:153–157.

123 Johansson SL: Carcinogenicity of analgesics: Long-term treatment of Sprague-Dawley rats with phenacetin, phenazone, caffeine and paracetamol (acetamidophen). Int J Cancer 1981;27: 521–529.

124 Macklin AW, Szot RJ: Eighteen-month oral study of aspirin, phenacetin and caffeine in C57BL/6 mice. Drug Chem Toxicol 1980;3/2:135–163.

125 Mohr U, Althoff J, Ketkar MB, et al: The influence of caffeine on tumour incidence in Sprague-Dawley rats. Food Chem Toxicol 1984;22:377–382.

126 National Cancer Institute: Bioassay of mixture of aspirin, phenacetin, and caffeine for possible carcinogenicity. NCI-CG-TR-67, 1978.

127 Takayama S, Kubawara N: Long-term study on the effect of caffeine in Wistar rats. Gann 1982; 73:365–371.

128 Thayer PS, Kensler CJ: Exposure of four generations of mice to caffeine in drinking water. Toxicol Appl Pharmacol 1973;25:169–179.

129 Nagasawa H, Konishi R: Stimulation by caffeine of spontaneous mammary tumorigenesis in mice. Eur J Cancer Clin Oncol 1988;24:803–805.

130 Nishikawa A, Furukawa F, Imizawa T, et al: Effects of caffeine, nicotine, ethanol and sodium selenite on pancreatic carcinogenesis in hamsters after initiation with N-nitrosobis(2-oxopropyl)amine. Carcinogenesis 1992;13:1379–1382.

131 Yamagami T, Handa H, Takeuchi J, et al: Rat pituitary adenoma and hyperplasia induced by caffeine administration. Surg Neurol 1983;20:323–331.

132 Grice HC: Genotoxicity and carcinogenicity assessments of caffeine and theobromine. Food Chem Toxicol 1987;25:795.

133 Hirose M, Fukushima S, Shirai T, et al: Stomach carcinogenicity of caffeic acid, sesamol and catechol in rats and mice. Jpn J Cancer Res 1990;81:207–212.

134 Beck SL, Urbano CM: Potentiating effect of caffeine on the teratogenicity of acetazolamide in C57BL/6J mice. Teratology 1991;44:241–250.

135 Donovan PJ, Dipaulo JA: Caffeine enhancement of chemical carcinogen-induced transformation of cultured Syrian hamster cells. Cancer Res 1974;34:2720–2727.

136 Hoshino H, Tanooka H: Caffeine enhances skin tumour induction in mice. Toxicol Lett 1979;4: 83–85.

137 Ledinko N, Evans M: Enhancement of adenovirus transformation of hamster cells by N-methyl-N-nitroguanidine, caffeine and hydroxylamine. Cancer Res 1973;33:2936–2938.

138 Raikow RB, Meredith RF, Brozovich BJ, et al: Potentiating effect of methyl methanesulphonate on Friend virus leukemogenesis. Proc Soc Exp Biol Med 1979;161:210–215.

139 Zamansky GB, Kleinman LF, Little JB, et al: The effect of caffeine on the ultraviolet light induction of SV40 from transformed hamster kidney cells. Virology 1976;73:468–475.

140 Minton JP, Abou-Issa H, Foecking MK, et al: Caffeine and unsaturated fat diet significantly promotes DMBA-induced breast cancer in rats. Cancer 1983;51:1249–1253.

141 Welszch CW, Scieszka KM, Senn ER, et al: Caffeine (1,3,7-trimethylxanthine), a temperate promoter of DMBA-induced rat mammary gland carcinogenesis. Int J Cancer 1983;32:479–484.

142 Welsch CW, Dehoog JV, O'Connor DH: Influence of caffeine and/or coffee consumption on the initiation and promotion phases of 7,12-dimethylbenz[a]anthracene-induced rat mammary gland tumorigenesis. Cancer Res 1988;48:2068–2073.

143 Welsch CW, Dehoog JV: Influence of caffeine consumption on 7,12-dimethylbenz[a]anthracene-induced mammary gland tumorigenesis in female rats fed a chemically defined diet containing standard and high levels of unsaturated fat. Cancer Res 1988;48:2074–2077.

144 Welsch CW, Dehoog JV, O'Connor DH: Influence of caffeine consumption on carcinomatous and normal mammary gland development in mice. Cancer Res 1988;48:2078–2082.

145 Balansky R, Blagoeva P, Mircheva Z, et al: Effect of metabolic inhibitors, methylxanthines, antioxidants, alkali metals, and corn oil on 1,2-dimethylhydrazine carcinogenicity in rats. Anticancer Res 1992;12:933–940.

146 Petrek JA, Sandberg WA, Cole MN, et al: The inhibitory effect of caffeine on hormone-induced rat breast cancer. Cancer 1985;56:1977–1981.

147 Wolfrom DM, Rao AR, Welsch CW: Caffeine inhibits development of benign mammary gland tumors in carcinogen-treated female Sprague-Dawley rats. Breast Cancer Res Treat 1991;19: 269–275.

148 Vanderploeg LC, Welsch CW: Inhibition by caffeine of ovarian hormone-induced mammary gland tumorigenesis in female GR mice. Cancer Lett 1991;56:245–250.

149 Woutersen RA, Van Gardener-Hoetmer A, Bax J, et al: Modulation of dietary fat-promoted pancreatic carcinogenesis in rats and hamsters by chronic coffee ingestion. Carcinogenesis 1989;10: 311–316.

150 Woutersen RA, Van Gardener-Hoetmer A, Bax J, et al: Modulation of putative preneoplastic foci of exocrine pancreas of rats and hamsters. Interaction of dietary fat and coffee. Dig Dis Sci 1989; 34:789–796.

151 Miller EG, Formby WA, Rivera-Hidalgo F, et al: Inhibition of hamster buccal pouch carcinogenesis by green coffee beans. Oral Surg Oral Med Oral Pathol 1988;65:745–749.

152 Nomura T: Diminution of tumorigenesis initiated by 4-nitroquinoline-1-oxide by post treatment with caffeine. Nature 1976;260:547–549.

153 Theiss JC, Shimkin MB: Inhibiting effect of caffeine on spontaneous and urethan-induced lung tumors in strain A mice. Cancer Res 1978;38:1757–1761.

154 Wattenberg LW: Inhibition of neoplasia by minor dietary constituents. Cancer Res 1983;43:2448s–2553s.

155 Sparnins VL, Lam LKT, Wattenberg LW: Effects of coffee on glutathione S-transferase in the metabolism of chemical carcinogens and other electrophilic agents. Adv Cancer Res 1979;29:175–274.

156 Lam LKT, Sparnins VL, Wattenberg LW: Isolation and identification of kahweol palmitate and cafestol palmitate as active constituents in green coffee beans that enhance glutathione S-transferase activity in the mouse. Cancer Res 1982;42:1193–1198.

157 Lam LKT, Sparnins VL, Wattenberg LW: Effects of derivatives of kahweol and cafestol on the activity of glutathione S-transferase in mice. J Med Chem 1987;30:1399–1403.

158 Gandhi RK, Khanduja KL: Action of caffeine in altering the carcinogen-activating and γ-detoxifying enzymes in mice. J Clin Biochem Nutr 1992;12:19–26.

159 Kappus H: Oxidative stress in chemical toxicology. Arch Toxicol 1987;60:144-149.

160 Abraham SK: Inhibitory effects of coffee on the genotoxicity of carcinogens in mice. Mutat Res 1991;262:109–114.

161 Mori H, Tanaka T, Shima H, et al: Inhibitory effect of chlorogenic acid on methylazoxy-methanol acetate induced carcinogenesis in the large intestine and liver of hamsters. Cancer Lett 1986;30: 49–54.

162 Miller EG, McWhorter K, Rivera-Hidalgo F, et al: Kahweol and cafestol: Inhibitors of hamster buccal pouch carcinogenesis. Nutr Cancer 1991;15:41–46.

163 Wood AW, Huang MT, Chang RL, et al: Inhibition of the mutagenicity of bay-region diol epoxides of polycyclic aromatic hydrocarbons by naturally occurring plant phenols: Exceptional activity of ellagic acid. Proc Natl Acad Sci USA 1982;79:5513–5517.

164 Lesca P: Protective effects of ellagic acid and other plant phenols on benzo[a]pyrene-induced neoplasia in mice. Carcinogenesis 1983;4:1651–1653.

165 Watyenberg LW, Coccia JB, Lam LKT: Inhibitory effects of phenolic compounds on benzo[a]pyrene-induced neoplasia. Cancer Res 1980;40:2820–2823.

166 Raj AS, Heddle JA, Newmark HL, et al: Caffeic acid as an inhibitor of DMBA-induced chromosomal breakage in mice assesssed by bone marrow micronucleus test. Mutat Res 1983;124:247–253.

167 Wargowich MJ, Eng VWS, Newmark HL: Inhibition by plant phenols of benzo[a]pyrene-induced nuclear aberrations in mammalian intestinal cells: A rapid in vivo assessment method. Food Chem Toxicol 1985;23:47–49.

168 Tomita K, Tsuchiya H: Caffeine enhancement of the effect of anticancer agents on human sarcoma cells. Jpn J Cancer Res 1989;80:83–88.

169 Tsuchiya H, Yasutake H, Yokogawa A, et al: Effect of chemotherapy combined with caffeine for osteosarcoma. J Cancer Res Clin Oncol 1992;118:567–569.

170 Fingert HJ, Kindy RL, Pardee AB: Enhanced lethality by methylxanthines in human bladder cancer cells treated with thiothera. J Urol 1984;132:609–613.

171 Allen TE, Aliano NA, Cowan RJ, et al: Amplification of the antitumor activity of pleomycins and bleomycins in rats and mice by caffeine. Cancer Res 1985;45:2516–2521.

172 Cohen MH: Enhancement of the antitumor effect of 1,3-bis(2-chloroethyl)-1-nitrosurea by various psychotropic drugs in combination with caffeine. J Pharmacol Exp Ther 1975;194:475–479.

173 Cohen MH, Scholenfeld D, Wolter J: Randomized trial of chlorpromazine, caffeine and methyl CCNU in disseminated melanoma. Cancer Treat Rep 1980;64:151–153.

174 Dion MW, Hussey DH, Doornbos JF, et al: Preliminary results of a pilot study of pentoxifylline in the treatment of late radiation soft tissue necrosis. Int J Radiat Oncol Biol Phys 1990;19:401–407.

175 Dion MW, Hussey DH, Osborne JW: The effect of pentoxifylline on early and late radiation injury following fractionated irradiation in C3H mice. Int J Radiat Oncol Biol Phys 1989;17:101–107.

176 Koh WJ, Stelzer KJ, Peterson LM, et al: Effect of pentoxifylline on radiation-induced lung and skin toxicity in rats. Int J Radiat Oncol Biol Phys 1994;29:312–317.

177 Stelzer KJ, Koh WJ, Kurtz H, et al: Caffeine consumption is associated with decreased severe late toxicity after radiation to the pelvis. Int J Radiat Oncol Biol Phys 1994;30:411–417.

178 Pozniak PC: The carcinogenicity of caffeine and coffee: A review. Am Diabet Assoc 1985;85:1127–1133.

179 Committee on Diet, Nutrition and Cancer. Assembly of Life Sciences, National Research Council: Diet, Nutrition and Cancer. Washington, National Academy Press, 1982.

180 Sandler RS: Diet and cancer: Food additives, coffee, and alcohol. Nutr Aliment Cancer 1983;4:273–279.

181 Schreiber GB, Robins M, Maffeo CE, et al: Confounders contributing to the reported associations of coffee or caffeine with disease. Prev Med 1988;17:295–309.

182 Binstock M, Krakow D, Stamler J, et al: Coffee and pancreatic cancer: An analysis of international mortality data. Am J Epidemiol 1983;118:630–640.

183 Boyle P, Hsieh CC, Maisonneuve P, et al: Epidemiology of pancreas cancer (1988). Int J Pancreatol 1989;5:327–346.

184 Boyle P, Maisonneuve P, Levi F, et al: Cancer patterns in Central Europe. Lung, stomach, colorectal, pancreas, breast and uterus; in Vital Statistics in Poland. Warsaw, Interpress, 1990.

185 La Vecchia C: Epidemiological evidence on coffee and digestive tract cancers: A review. Dig Dis 1990;8:281–286.

186 La Vecchia C: Coffee and cancer epidemiology; in Garattini S (ed): Caffeine, Coffee, and Health. New York, Raven Press, 1993, pp 379–398.

187 Sivak A: An evaluation of epidemiology studies of coffee consumption and cancer. Proc 14th International Scientific Colloquium on Coffee, San Francisco 1991, pp 31–40.

188 Stocks P: Cancer mortality in relation to national consumption of cigarettes, solid fuel, tea and coffee. Br J Cancer 1970;24:215–225.

189 Lin RS, Kessler II: A multifactorial model for pancreatic cancer in man. JAMA 1981;9:147–152.

190 MacMahon B, Yen S, Trichopoulos D, et al: Coffee and cancer of the pancreas. N Engl J Med 1981;304:630–633.

Coffee and Cancer

191 Pfeffer F, Rosas HA, Vargas F, et al: Tabaquismo, consumo de bebidas alcoholicas y café como factores asociados al desarrollo de cancer de pancreas. Rev Invest Clin 1989;41:205–208.

192 Feinstein AR, Horwitz RI, Spitzer WO, et al: Coffee and pancreatic cancer, the problems of etiologic science and epidemiologic case-control research. JAMA 1981;246:957–961.

193 Jick H, Dinan BJ: Coffee and pancreatic cancer. Lancet 1981;ii:92.

194 Nomura A, Stemmerman GN, Heilbrun LK: Coffee and pancreatic cancer. Lancet 1981;ii:415.

195 Bernada CC, MacMahon B, Yen S, et al: Coffee and pancreatic cancer. N Engl J Med 1982;315: 587–588.

196 Goldstein HR: No association found between coffee and cancer of the pancreas. N Engl J Med 1982;306:997.

197 Heuch I, Kvale G, Jacobsen BK, et al: Use of alcohol, tobacco and coffee, and risk of pancreatic cancer. Br J Cancer 1983;48:637–643.

198 Whittemore AS, Paffenbarger RS Jr, Anderson K, et al: Early precursors of pancreatic cancer in college men. J Chronic Dis 1983;36:251–256.

199 Wynder EL, Hall NEL, Polansky M: Epidemiology of coffee and pancreatic cancer. Cancer Res 1983;43:3900–3906.

200 Kinlen L, Goldblatt P, Fox J, et al: Coffee and pancreas cancer: Controversy in part explained? Lancet 1984;ii:282–283.

201 Kinlen LJ, McPherson K: Pancreas cancer and coffee and tea consumption: A case-control study. Br J Cancer 1984;49:93–96.

202 Nomura A, Heilbrun LK, Stemmermann GN: Coffee and pancreatic cancer. Lancet 1984;i: 917.

203 Gold EB, Gordis L, Diener MD, et al: Diet and other risk factors for cancer of the pancreas. Cancer 1985;55:460–467.

204 Hsieh CC, MacMahon B, Yen S, et al: Coffee and the pancreatic cancer. N Engl J Med 1986;315: 587–588.

205 Jacobsen BK, Bjelke E, Kvale G, et al: Coffee drinking, mortality, and cancer incidence: Results from a Norwegian prospective study. J Natl Cancer Inst 1986;76:823–831.

206 Mack TM, Yu MC, Hanisch R, et al: Pancreas cancer and smoking, beverage consumption, and past medical history. J Natl Cancer Inst 1986;76:49–60.

207 Nomura A, Heilbrun LK, Stemmermann GN: Prospective study of coffee consumption and the risk of cancer. J Natl Cancer Inst 1986;76:587–590.

208 Norell SE, Ahlbom A, Erwald R, et al: Diet and pancreatic cancer: A case-control study. Am J Epidemiol 1986;124:894–902.

209 Wynder EL, Dieck GS, Hall NEL: Case-control study of decaffeinated coffee consumption and pancreatic cancer. Cancer Res 1986;46:5360–5363.

210 Clavel F, Benhamou E, Tarayre M, et al: More on coffee and pancreatic cancer. N Engl J Med 1987;316:483–484.

211 La Vecchia C, Liati P, Decarli A, et al: Coffee consumption and risk of pancreatic cancer. Int J Cancer 1987;40:309–313.

212 Raymond L, Infante F, Tuyns AJ, et al: Alimentation et cancer du pancréas. Gastroentérol Clin Biol 1987;11:488–492.

213 Falk RT, Pickle LW, Fontham ET, et al: Life-style risk factors for pancreatic cancer in Louisiana: A case-control study. Am J Epidemiol 1988;128:324–336.

214 Gorham ED, Garland CF, Garland FC, et al: Coffee and pancreatic cancer in a rural California county. West J Med 1988;148:48–53.

215 Hiatt RA, Klatsky AL, Armstrong MA: Pancreatic cancer, blood glucose and beverage consumption. Int J Cancer 1988;41:794–797.

216 Mills PK, Beeson WL, Abbey DE, et al: Dietary habits and past medical history as related to fatal pancreas cancer risk among adventists. Cancer 1988;61:2578–2585.

217 Clavel F, Benhamou E, Auquier A, et al: Coffee, alcohol, smoking and cancer of the pancreas: A case-control study. Int J Cancer 1989;43:17–21.

218 Lin RS, Kessler II: A multifactorial model for pancreatic cancer in man. Epidemiologic evidence. JAMA 1981;245:147–152.

219 Cuzick J, Babiker AG: Pancreatic cancer, alcohol, diabetes mellitus and gall-bladder disease. Int J Cancer 1989;43:415–421.

220 Olsen GW, Mandel JS, Gibson RW, et al: A case-control study of pancreatic cancer and cigarettes, alcohol, coffee and diet. Am J Public Health 1989;79:1016–1019.

221 Farrow DC, Davis S: Risk of pancreatic cancer in relation to medical history and the use of tobacco, alcohol and coffee. Int J Cancer 1990;45:816–820.

222 Gordis L: Consumption of methylxanthine-containing beverages and risk of pancreatic cancer. Cancer Lett 1990;52:1–12.

223 Jain M, Howe GR, Louis PS, et al.: Coffee and alcohol as determinants of risk of pancreas cancer: A case-control study from Toronto. Int J Cancer 1991;47:384–389.

224 Bueno de Mesquita HB, Maisonneuve P, Moerman CJ, et al: Lifetime consumption of alcoholic beverages, tea and coffee and exocrine carcinoma of the pancreas: A population-based case-control study in the Netherlands. Int J Cancer 1992;50:514–522.

225 Severson RK, Davis S, Polissar L: Smoking, coffee and cancer of the pancreas. Br Med J 1982; 285:214.

226 Snowdon DA, Philips RL: Coffee consumption and risk of fatal cancers. Am J Public Health 1984; 74:820–823.

227 Ghadirian P, Simard A, Baillargeon J: Tobacco, alcohol, and coffee and cancer of the pancreas. A population-based, case-control study in Quebec, Canada. Cancer 1991;67:2664–2670.

228 Lyon JL, Mahoney AW, French TK, et al: Coffee consumption and the risk of cancer of the exocrine pancreas: A case-control study in a low-risk population. Epidemiology 1992;3:164–170.

229 Kalapothaki V, Tzonou A, Hsieh CC, et al: Tobacco, etanol, coffee, pancreatitis, diabetes mellitus, and cholelithiasis as risk factors for pancreatic carcinoma. Cancer Causes Control 1993;4: 375–382.

230 Farinati F, Della Libera G, Valiante F, et al: Coffee consumption and pancreatic cancer: A cancer-controlled case-control study. Eur J Gastroenterol Hepatol 1994;6:189–190.

231 Bonelli L, Sciarello S, Bruzzi P: Coffee consumption and pancreatic cancer: A cancer-controlled case-control study (reply). Eur J Gastroenterol Hepatol 1994;6:190–191.

232 Zatonski WA, Boyle P, Przewozniak K, et al: Cigarette smoking, alcohol, tea and coffee consumption and pancreas cancer risk: A case-control study from Opole, Poland. Int J Cancer 1993;53:601–607.

233 Yang CS, Wang ZY: Tea and cancer. J Natl Cancer Inst 1993;85:1038–1049.

234 Faivre J: Epidémiologie du cancer du pancréas. Quels facteurs de risque? Rev Prat 1989;74:107–112.

235 World Health Organization: IARC Monographs on the Evaluation of Carcinogenic Risks to Humans, vol 51: Coffee, Tea, Maté, Methylxanthines and Methylglyoxal. Lyon, International Agency for Research on Cancer, 1991.

236 Doll R, Peto R: Mortality in relation to smoking: 20 years' observations on male British doctors. Br Med J 1976;ii:1525–1536.

237 Hammond EC: Smoking in relation to the death rates of one million men and women. Natl Cancer Inst Monogr 1966;19:127–204.

238 Hirayama T: A large-scale cohort study on the relationship between diet and selected cancers of digestive organs; in Bruce WJ, Correa P, Lipkin M, et al (eds): Gastrointestinal Cancer: Endogenous Factors, Banbury Report 7. New York, CSH Press, 1981, pp 407–426.

239 Kahn HA: The Dorn study of smoking and mortality among US veterans. Natl Cancer Inst Monogr 1966;19:1–125.

240 Auerbach O, Garfinkel L: Histologic changes in pancreas in relation to smoking and coffee-drinking habits. Dig Dis Sci 1986;31:1014–1020.

241 Rosenberg L: Coffee and tea consumption in relation to the risk of large bowel cancer: A review of epidemiological studies. Cancer Lett 1990;52:163–171.

242 Graham S, Dayal H, Swanson M, et al: Diet in the epidemiology of cancer of colon and rectum. J Natl Cancer Inst 1978;61:709–714.

243 Philips RL, Snowdon DA: Association of meat and coffee use with cancers of the large bowel, breast and prostate among Seventh-Day Adventists: Preliminary results. Cancer Res 1983;43:2403S–2408S.

244 Philips RL, Snowdon DA: Dietary relationships with fatal colorectal cancer among Seventh-Day Adventists. J Natl Cancer Inst 1985;74:307–317.

245 Heilbrun LK, Nomura A, Stemmermann GN: Black tea consumption and cancer risk: A prospective study. Br J Cancer 1986;54:677–683.

246 Slattery ML, West DW, Robinson LM: Tobacco, alcohol, coffee, and caffeine as risk factors for colon cancer in a low-risk population. Epidemiology 1990;1:141–145.

247 La Vecchia C, Negri E, Decarli A, et al: A case-control study of diet and colorectal cancer in northern Italy. Int J Cancer 1988;41:492–498.

248 Abu-Zeid HA, Choi NW, Hsu P: Factors associated with risk of cancer of the colon and rectum (abstract). Am J Epidemiol 1981;114:442.

249 Benito E, Obrador A, Stiggelbout A, et al: A population-based case-control study of colorectal cancer in Majorca. I. Dietary factors. Int J Cancer 1990;45:69–76.

250 Bjelke E: Epidemiological studies of cancer of the stomach, colon, and rectum with special emphasis on the role of diet. Ann Arbor, University Microfilms, 1973, vol 2–4.

251 Haenszel W, Berg JW, Segi M, et al: Large bowel cancer in Hawaiian Japanese. J Natl Cancer Inst 1973;51:1765–1779.

252 Higgisson J: Etiological factors in gastrointestinal cancer in man. J Natl Cancer Inst 1966;37:527–545.

253 La Vecchia C: Epidemiological evidence on coffee and digestive tract cancers: A review. Dig Dis 1990;8:281–286.

254 Macquart-Moulin G, Roboli E, Cornee J, et al.: Case-control study on colorectal cancer and diet in Marseille. Int J Cancer 1986;38:183–191.

255 La Vecchia C, Ferraroni M, Negri E, et al: Coffee consumption and digestive tract cancers. Cancer Res 1989;49:1049–1051.

256 Rosenberg L, Werler MM, Palmer JR, et al: The risks of cancers of the colon and rectum in relation to coffee consumption. Am J Epidemiol 1989;130:895–903.

257 Tuyns A, Kaaks R, Haelterman M: Colorectal cancer and the consumption of foods: A case-control study in Belgium. Nutr Cancer 1988;11:189–204.

258 Lee HP, Gourley L, Duffy S, et al: Colorectal cancer and diet in an Asian population – A case-control study among Singapore Chinese. Int J Cancer 1989;43:1007–1016.

259 Watanabe Y, Tada M, Kawamoto K, et al: A case-control study of cancer of the rectum and the colon. Nippon Shokakibyo Gakkai Zasshi 1984;81:185–193.

260 Baron JA, Gerhardsson de Verdier M, Ekbom A: Coffee, tea, tobacco, and cancer of the large bowel. Cancer Epidemiol Biomark Prev 1994;5:566–570.

261 Olsen J, Kronborg O: Coffee, tobacco and alcohol as risk factors for cancer and adenoma of the large intestine. Int J Epidemiol 1993;22:398–402.

262 Dales LG, Friedman GD, Ury HK, et al: A case-control study of relationships of diet and other traits to colorectal cancer in American blacks. Am J Epidemiol 1979;109:132–144.

263 Jarebinski M, Adanja B, Vlajinac H: Case-control study of relationship of some biosocial correlates to rectal cancer patients in Belgrade, Yugoslavia. Neoplasma 1989;36:369–374.

264 Miller AB, Howe GR, Jain M, et al: Food items and food groups as risk factors in a case-control study of diet and colorectal cancer. Int J Cancer 1983;32:155–161.

265 Tajima K, Tominaga S: Dietary habits and gastro-intestinal cancers: A comparative case-control study of stomach and large intestinal cancers in Nagoya, Japan. Jpn J Cancer Res 1985;76:705–716.

266 Wu AH, Paganini-Hill A, Ross RK, et al: Alcohol, physical activity and other risk factors for colorectal cancer: A prospective study. Br J Cancer 1987;55:687–694.

267 Bjelke E: Colon cancer and blood-cholesterol. Lancet 1974;i:1116-1117.

268 Jacobsen BK, Thelle DS: Coffee, cholesterol and colon cancer: Is there a link? Br Med J 1987;294:4–5.

269 Lowenfelds AB: Is increased cholesterol excretion the link between serum cholesterol and colon cancer? Nutr Cancer 1983;4:280–284.

270 Broitman SA: Cholesterol excretion and colon cancer. Cancer Res 1981;41:3738–3740.

271 Cruse P, Lewin M, Clark CG: Dietary cholesterol is co-carcinogenic for human colon cancer. Lancet 1979;i:752–755.

272 Reddy BS, Wynder EL: Metabolic epidemiology of colon cancer: Fecal bile acids and neutral sterols in colon cancer patients and patients with adenomatous polyps. Cancer 1977;39:2533–2539.

273 Lipkin M, Reddy BS, Weisburger J, et al: Non-degradation of fecal cholesterol in subjects at high risk for cancer of the large intestine. J Clin Invest 1981;67:304–307.

274 Trichopoulos D, Ouranos G, Day NE, et al: Diet and cancer of the stomach: A case-control study in Greece. Int J Cancer 1985;36:291–297.

275 Graham S, Schotz W, Partino P: Alimentary factors in the epidemiology of gastric cancer. Cancer 1972;30:927–938.

276 Pintos J, Franco EL, Oliveira BV, et al: Maté, coffee, and tea consumption and risk of cancers of the upper aerodigestive tract in Southern Brazil. Epidemiology 1994;5:583–590.

277 Ghadarian P: Thermal irritation and oesophagal cancer in Northern Iran. Cancer 1987;60:1909–1914.

278 Victora CG, Munoz N, Day NE, et al: Hot beverages and oesophagal cancer in Southern Brazil: A case-control study. Int J Cancer 1987;39:710–716.

279 Martinez I: Cancer in the oesophagus in Puerto Rico. Mortality and incidence analysis 1950-1961. Cancer 1964;17:1279–1288.

280 Armstrong B, Doll R: Environmental factors and cancer incidence and mortality in different countries with special responses to dietary practices. Int J Cancer 1975;15:617–631.

281 Schmauz R, Cole P: Epidemiology of cancer of the renal pelvis and ureter. J Natl Cancer Inst 1974;52:1431–1434.

282 Shennan DH: Renal carcinoma and coffee consumption in 16 countries. Br J Cancer 1973;28:473–476.

283 Armstrong B, Garrod A, Doll R: A retrospective study of renal cancer with special reference to coffee and animal protein consumption. Br J Cancer 1976;33:127–136.

284 McLaughlin JK, Blot WJ, Mandel JS, et al: Etiology of cancer of the renal pelvis. J Natl Cancer Inst 1983;71:287–291.

285 McLaughlin JK, Mandel JS, Blot WJ, et al: A population-based case-control study of renal carcinoma. J Natl Cancer Inst 1984;72:275–284.

286 Wynder EL, Mabuchi K, Whitmore WF: Epidemiology of adenocarcinoma of the kidney. J Natl Cancer Inst 1974;53:1619–1634.

287 Ross RK, Paganini-Hill A, Landolph J, et al: Analgesics, cigarette smoking, and other risk factors for cancer of the renal pelvis and ureter. Cancer Res 1989;49:1045–1048.

288 Maclure M, Willet W: A case-control study of diet and risk of renal adenocarcinoma. Epidemiology 1990;1:430–440.

289 Yu MC, Mack TM, Hanish R, et al.: Cigarette smoking, obesity, diuretic use, and coffee consumption as risk factors for renal cell carcinoma. J Natl Cancer Inst 1986;77:351–356.

290 Goodman MT, Morgenstern H, Wynder EL: A case-control study of factors affecting the development of renal cell cancer. Am J Epidemiol 1986;124:926–941.

291 McCredie M, Ford JM, Stewart JH: Risk factors for cancer of the renal parenchyma. Int J Cancer 1988;42:13–16.

292 Bravo P, Del Rey J, Sanchez J, et al: Caféy analgésicos como factores de riesgo del cancer de vejiga. Arch Esp Urol 1986;39:337–341.

293 Bravo P, Del Rey J, Conde M: Risk factors of bladder cancer in Spain. Neoplasma 1987;35:633–637.

294 Cartwright RA, Adib R, Glashan R, et al: The epidemiology of bladder cancer in West Yorkshire. A preliminary report on non-occupational aetiologies. Carcinogenesis 1981;2:343–347.

295 Ciccone G, Vineis P: Coffee drinking and bladder cancer. Cancer Lett 1988;41:45–52.

296 Claude J, Kunze E, Frenzel-Beyme R, et al: Life-style and occupational risk factors in cancer of the lower urinary tract. Am J Epidemiol 1986;124:578–589.

297 Clavel J, Cordier S: Coffee consumption and bladder cancer risk. Int J Cancer 1991;47:207–212.

298 Cole P: Coffee drinking and cancer of the lower urinary tract. Lancet 1971;i:1335–1337.

299 Dunham LJ, Rabson AS, Stewart HL, et al: Rates, interview and pathology study of cancer of the urinary bladder in New Orleans, Louisiana. J Natl Cancer Inst 1968;41:683–709.

300 Fraumeni JF, Scotto J, Dunham LF: Coffee drinking and bladder cancer. Lancet 1971;ii:1204.

301 Gonzales CA, Lopez-Abente G, Errezola M, et al: Occupation, tobacco use, coffee, and bladder cancer in the county of Mataro (Spain). Cancer 1985;55:2031–2034.

302 Hartge P, Hoover R, West DW, et al: Coffee drinking and risk of bladder cancer. J Natl Cancer Inst 1983;70:1021–1026.

303 Hopkins J: Coffee drinking and bladder cancer. Food Chem Toxicol 1984;22:481–495.

304 Howe GR, Burch JD, Miller AB, et al: Tobacco use, occupation, coffee, various nutrients and bladder cancer. J Natl Cancer Inst 1980;64:701–713.

305 Iscovich J, Castelletto R, Esteve J, et al: Tobacco smoking, occupational exposure and bladder cancer in Argentina. Int J Cancer 1987;40:734–740.

306 Jensen OM, Wahrendorf J, Knudsen JB, et al: The Copenhagen case-control study of bladder cancer. II. Effect of coffee and other beverages. Int J Cancer 1986;37:651–657.

307 Kabat GC, Dieck GS, Wynder EL: Bladder cancer in non smokers. Cancer 1986;57:362–367.

308 La Vecchia C, Negri E, Decarli A, et al: Dietary factors in the risk of bladder cancer. Nutr Cancer 1989;12:93–101.

309 Marrett LD, Walter SD, Meigs W: Coffee drinking and bladder cancer in Connecticut. Am J Epidemiol 1983;177:113–127.

310 Matanoski GM, Elliott EA: Bladder cancer epidemiology. Epidemiol Rev 1981;3:203–229.

311 Mettlin C, Graham S: Dietary risk factors in human bladder cancer. Am J Epidemiol 1979;110:255–263.

312 Miller AB: The etiology of bladder cancer from the epidemiological viewpoint. Cancer Res 1977;40:1246–1268.

313 Miller CT, Neutel CI, Nair RC, et al: Relative importance of risk factors in cancer carcinogenesis. J Chronic Dis 1978;31:51–56.

314 Mommsen S, Aagard J, Sell A: A case-control study of female bladder cancer. Eur J Cancer Clin Oncol 1983;19:725–729.

315 Morrison AS: Geographic and time trends of coffee imports and bladder cancer. Eur J Cancer 1978;14:51–54.

316 Morrison AS: Advances in the etiology of urothelial cancer. Urol Clin North Am 1984;11:557–566.

317 Morrison AS, Buring JE, Verhoek WG, et al: Coffee drinking and cancer of the lower urinary tract. J Natl Cancer Inst 1982;68:91–94.

318 Ohno Y, Aoki K, Obata K, et al.: Case-control study of urinary bladder cancer in Metropolitan Nagoya. Cancer Inst Monogr 1985;69:229–243.

319 Piper JM, Matanoski GM, Tonascia J: Bladder cancer in young women. Am J Epidemiol 1986;123:1033–1042.

320 Rebelakos A, Trichopoulos D, Tzonou A, et al: Tobacco smoking, coffee drinking, and occupation as risk factors for bladder cancer in Greece. J Natl Cancer Inst 1985;75:455–461.

321 Risch HA, Burch JD, Miller AB, et al.: Dietary factors and the incidence of cancer of the urinary bladder. Am J Epidemiol 1988;127:1179–1191.

322 Savitz DA, Baron AE: Estimating and correcting for confounder misclassification. Am J Epidemiol 1989;129:1062–1071.

323 Simon D, Yen S, Cole P: Coffee drinking and cancer of the lower urinary tract. J Natl Cancer Inst 1975;54:587–591.

324 Slattery ML, West DW, Robison LM: Fluid intake and bladder cancer in Utah. Int J Cancer 1988;42:17–22.

325 Weinberg DM, Ross RK, Mack TM, et al: Bladder cancer etiology. A different perspective. Cancer 1983;51:675–680.

326 Wynder EL, Goldsmith R: The epidemiology of bladder cancer. A second look. Cancer 1977;40:1246–1268.

327 Bross DJ, Tiddings J: Another look at coffee drinking and cancer of the urinary bladder. Prev Med 1973;2:455–461.

328 Morgan RW, Jain MG: Bladder cancer: Smoking, beverages and artificial sweteners. Can Med Assoc J 1974;111:1067–1070.

329 Najem GR, Louria DB, Seebode JJ, et al: Life time occupation, smoking, caffeine, saccharine, hair dyes and bladder carcinogenesis. Int J Epidemiol 1982;11:212–217.

330 Mills PK, Beeson WL, Phillips RL, et al: Bladder cancer in a low risk population. Results from the Adventist health study. Am J Epidemiol 1991;133:230–239.

331 D'Avanzo B, La Vecchia C, Franceshi S, Negri E, et al: Coffee consumption and bladder cancer risk. Eur J Cancer 1992;28:1480–1484.

332 Gremy F, Momas I, Daures JP: Nouveaux aperçus sur les facteurs de risque du cancer de la vessie. Une enquête épidémiologique cas-témoins dans le département de l'Hérault. Bull Acad Natl Méd 1993;17:47–62.

333 Pujolar AE, Gonzalez CA, Lopez-Abente G, et al: Bladder cancer and coffee consumption in smokers and non-smokers in Spain. Int J Epidemiol 1993;22:38–44.

334 Vena JE, Freundenheim J, Graham S, et al.: Coffee, cigarette smoking, and bladder cancer in Western New York. Ann Epidemiol 1993;3:586–591.

335 Sullivan JW: Epidemiologic survey of bladder cancer in Greater New Orleans. J Urol 1982;128: 281–283.

336 D'Avanzo B, La Vecchia C, Franceschi S, et al: Coffee consumption and bladder cancer risk. Eur J Cancer 1992;28A:1480–1484.

337 Dannelli F, La Rosa F, Saltalamacchia G, et al: Tobacco smoking, coffee, cocoa and tea consumption in relation to mortality from urinary bladder cancer in Italy. Eur J Epidemiol 1989;5:392–397.

338 Morrison AS: Control of cigarette smoking in evaluating the association of coffee drinking and bladder cancer; in MacMahon B, Sugimura T (eds): Coffee and Health, Banbury Report 17. New York, CSH Press, 1984, pp 127–136.

339 Benowitz NL, Hall SM, Modin G: Persistent increase in caffeine concentrations in people who stop smoking. Br Med J 1989;298:1075–1076.

340 Viscoli CM, Lachs MS, Horwitz RI: Bladder cancer and coffee drinking: A summary of case-control research. Lancet 1993;341:1432–1437.

341 Campbell ME, Spielberg SP, Kalow W: A urinary metabolite ratio that reflects systemic caffeine clearance. Clin Pharmacol Ther 1987;42:157–165.

342 Hartge P, Lesher LP, McGowan L, et al: Coffee and ovarian cancer. Int J Cancer 1982;30: 531–532.

343 La Vecchia C, Franceschi S, Decarti A, et al: Coffee drinking and risk of epithelial ovarian cancer. Int J Cancer 1984;33:559–562.

344 Trichopoulos D, Papapostolou M, Polychronopoulou A: Coffee and ovarian cancer. Int J Cancer 1981;28:691–693.

345 Whittemore AS, Wu ML, Paffenbarger RS Jr, et al: Personal and environmental characteristics related to epithelial ovarian cancer. II. Exposures to talcum powder, tobacco, alcohol, and coffee. Am J Epidemiol 1988;128:1228–1240.

346 Byers T, Marshall J, Grahams S, et al: A case-control study of dietary and non-dietary factors in ovarian cancer. J Natl Cancer Inst 1983;71:681–686.

347 Cramer DW, Welch WR, Hutchinson GB, et al: Dietary animal fat in relation to ovarian cancer risk. Obstet Gynecol 1984;63:833–838.

348 Miller DR, Rosenberg L, Helmrich SP, et al: Ovarian cancer and coffee drinking, in MacMahon B, Sugimura T (eds): Coffee and Health, Banbury Report 17. New York, CSH Press, 1984, pp 157–165.

349 Miller DR, Rosenberg L, Kaufmann DW, et al: Epithelial ovarian cancer and coffee drinking. Int J Epidemiol 1987;16:13–17.

350 Snowdon DA, Philips RL: The relationship between fatal ovarian cancer and diet and reproductive factors. Am J Epidemiol 1983;118:439.

351 Trichopoulos D, Tzonou A, Polychronopoulou A, et al: A case-control investigation of a possible association between coffee consumption and ovarian cancer in Greece, in MacMahon B, Sugimura T (eds): Coffee and Health, Banbury Report 17. New York, CSH Press, 1984, pp 149–155.

352 Tzonou A, Day NE, Trichopoulos D, et al: The epidemiology of ovarian cancer in Greece: A case-control study. Eur J Cancer Clin Oncol 1984;20:1045–1052.

353 Polychronopoulou A, Tzonou A, Hsieh CC, et al: Reproductive variables, tobacco, ethanol, coffee and somatometry as risk factors for ovarian cancer. Int J Cancer 1993;55:402–407.

354 Wolfrom D, Welsch CW: Caffeine and the development of normal, benign and carcinomatous human breast tissues: A relationship? J Med 1990;21:225–250.

355 Cremer SBL, Lucker TPC, Katan MB: Coffee and health. 3. Effects on foetal growth and development and on breast tumors. Voeding 1988;49:106–110.

356 La Vecchia C, Talamini R, Decarli A, et al: Coffee consumption and the risk of breast cancer. Surgery 1986;100:477–481.

357 Lawson DH, Jick H, Rothman KJ: Coffee and tea consumption and breast disease. Surgery 1981; 90:801–803.

358 Lê M: Coffee consumption, benign breast disease and breast cancer. Am J Epidemiol 1985;122:721.

359 Lê MG, Hill C, Kramar A, et al.: Alcoholic beverages consumption and breast cancer in a French case-control. Am J Epidemiol 1984;120:350–357.

360 Lubin JH, Burns PE, Blot WJ, et al: Dietary factors and breast cancer risk. Int J Cancer 1981;28: 685–689.

361 Lubin F, Ron E, Wax Y, et al: Coffee and methylxanthines in benign and malignant breast disease, in MacMahon B, Sugimura T (eds): Coffee and Health, Banbury Report 17. New York, CSH Press, 1984, pp 177–187.

362 Lubin F, Ron E, Wax Y, et al: Coffee and methylxanthines and breast cancer, a case-control study. J Natl Cancer Inst 1985;74:569–573.

363 Mansel RE, Webster DJ, Burr M, et al: Is there a relationship between coffee consumption and breast disease (abstract). Br J Surg 1982;69:295.

364 Phelps HM, Phelps CE: Caffeine ingestion and breast cancer. A negative correlation. Cancer 1988; 61:1051–1054.

365 Rosenberg L, Miller DR, Helmrich SP, et al: Breast cancer and coffee drinking, in MacMahon B, Sugimura T (eds): Coffee and Health, Banbury Report 17. New York, CSH Press, 1984, pp 189–203.

366 Rosenberg L, Miller DR, Helmrich SP, et al: Breast cancer and the consumption of coffee. Am J Epidemiol 1985;122:391–399.

367 Schairer C, Brinton LA, Hoover RN: Methylxanthines and breast cancer. Int J Cancer 1987;40: 469–473.

368 Rohan TE, McMichael AJ: Methylxanthines and breast cancer. Int J Cancer 1988;41:390–393.

369 Folsom AR, McKenzie DR, Bisgard KM, et al: No association between caffeine intake and post-menopausal cancer incidence in the Iowa women's health study. Am J Epidemiol 1993;138:380–383.

370 Smith SJ, Deacon JM, Chilvers CED, et al: Alcohol, smoking, passive smoking and caffeine in relation to breast cancer risk in young women. Br J Cancer 1994;70:112–119.

371 Pozner J, Papatestas AE, Fagerstrom R, et al: Association of tumor differentiation with caffeine and coffee intake in women with breast cancer. Surgery 1986;100:482–488.

372 Graham TM: Surface membrane enzymes in neoplasia, in Hynes RO (ed): Surfaces of Normal and Malignant Cells. New York, Wiley, 1979, pp 199–246.

373 Vatten LJ, Solvoll K, Loken B: Coffee consumption and the risk of breast cancer. A prospective study of 14,593 Norwegian women. Br J Cancer 1990;62:267–270.

374 Minton JP, Foecking MK, Webster DJT, et al: Caffeine, cyclic nucleotides, and breast disease. Surgery 1979;86:105–111.

375 Minton JP, Abou-Issa H, Reiches N, et al: Clinical and biochemical studies on methylxanthine-related fibrocystic disease. Surgery 1981;90:299–304.

376 Brooks PG, Gart S, Heldfond AJ, et al: Measuring the effect of caffeine restriction on fibrocystic breast disease. J Reprod Med 1981;26:279–282.

377 Ernster VL, Mason L, Goodson WH, et al: Effects of caffeine-free diet on benign breast disease: A randomized trial. Surgery 1991;1:263–267.

378 Schreiber GB, Maffeo CE, Robins M, et al: Measurement of coffee and caffeine intake: Implications for epidemiologic research. Prev Med 1988;17:280–294.

379 Allen SS, Froberg DG: The effect of decreased caffeine consumption on benign proliferative breast disease: A randomized clinical trial. Surgery 1987;101:720–730.

380 Heyden S, Fodor JG: Coffee consumption and fibrocystic breasts: An unlikely association. Can J Surg 1986;29:208–211.

381 Heyden S, Muhlbaier LH: Prospective study of 'fibrocystic breast disease' and caffeine consumption. Surgery 1984;96:479–484.

382 Lawson DH, Jick H, Rothman KJ: Coffee and tea consumption and breast disease. Surgery 1981; 90:801–803.

383 Levinson W, Dunn PM: Non-association of caffeine and fibrocystic bresat disease. Arch Intern Med 1986;146:1773–1775.
384 Lubin F, Ron E, Wax Y, et al.: A case-control study of caffeine and methylxanthines in benign breast disease. JAMA 1985;253:2388–2392.
385 Marshall J, Graham S, Swanson M: Caffeine consumption and benign breast disease. A case-control comparison. Am J Public Health 1982;72:610–612.
386 Parazzini F, La Vecchia C, Riundi R, et al: Methylxanthine, alcohol-free diet and fibrocystic breast disease: A factorial clinical trial. Surgery 1986;99:576–581.
387 Rohan TE, Cook MG, McMichael AJ: Methylxanthines and benign proliferative epithelial disorders of the breast in women. Int J Epidemiol 1989;18:626–633.
388 Schairer C, Brinton LA, Hoover RN: Methylxanthines and benign breast disease. Am J Epidemiol 1986;124:603–611.
389 Boyle CA, Borkowitz GS, Livolsi VA, et al: Caffeine consumption and fibrocystic breast disease: A case-control epidemiologic study. J Natl Cancer Inst 1984;72:1015-1019.
390 Hindi-Alexander MC, Zielezny MA, Montes N, et al: Theophylline and fibrocystic breast disease. J Allergy Clin Immunol 1985;75:709–715.
391 La Vecchia C, Franceschi S, Parazzini F, et al: Benign breast disease and consumption of beverages containing methylxanthine. J Natl Cancer Inst 1985;74:995–1000.
392 Odenheimer DJ, Zunzunegui MV, King MC, et al: Risk factors for benign breast disease. A case-control study of discordant twins. Am J Epidemiol 1984;120:565–571.
393 Yen S, Chung-Cheng H, MacMahon B: Extrahepatic bile duct cancer and smoking, beverage consumption, past medical history, and oral-contraceptive use. Cancer 1987;59:2112–2116.
394 Gibson R, Schuman L, Bjelke E: A prospective study of coffee consumption and mortality from cancer (abstract). Am J Epidemiol 1985;122:520.
395 Jensen H, Madsen JL: Diet and cancer. Review of the literature. Acta Med Scand 1988;223:293–304.
396 Vineis P: Hypothesis: Coffee consumption, N-acetyltransferase phenotype, and cancer. J Natl Cancer Inst 1993;85:1004–1005.

Astrid Nehlig, PhD, INSERM U398, Faculté de Médecine, 11, rue Humann,
F–67085 Strasbourg Cedex (France)

Subject Index

CONTE

Introduction

INTRODUCTION

From the international superstar to the local hero, the powerful manager to the humble roadie, the global television show to the rough gig at the corner pub, punk rock to folk rock, acid jazz to trad jazz, Bach to Mozart and Chopin to Brahms, writing the Number One hit to creating the jingle of the century and dealing with the media along the way – these are only some aspects of the world of contemporary music!

This myriad of structures and organisations is daunting to the inexperienced but an authoritative book at an advanced level has at last arrived. The *Essential Guide to Music* informs and educates on all areas of music which fall into eight broad categories: popular music, the development of forms and styles, performing music, musical equipment and technology, recording music, the music business and the law, music and the media and employment in the music industry.

The book is aimed at students and other adult readers with a deep interest in the music business. It is written in an informative magazine style and includes black and white photographs, diagrams and statistics. Each chapter is self-contained, enabling study of specialist areas. The order of individual topics, however, presents an excellent study plan.

Student tasks are set to ensure deeper understanding of the key points, and many of these are of a practical and creative nature. For example, the tasks in the chapter on media and music include interviewing music business personnel and undertaking research by reading, listening to and viewing music media products. Likewise, the chapter on recording music will require students to utilise music technology to a high level. At every turn students are encouraged to evaluate each activity constructively, allowing preparation for real-life situations.

Most of all, the book is to enable further knowledge and enjoyment of the most exciting business in the world.

Tudor Morris and Wendy Munro

The Publishers would like to acknowledge the following photographic agencies:

Lebrecht: 7, 12, 18, 23, 27, 35 (bottom), 40, 42, 43, 45, 49, 51, 52, 59, 64, 67, 68, 82, 194; **Redferns:** 5, 10, 15, 19, 33, 123, 132, 148, 192, 195; **LFI:** 2, 133; **AKG:** 54, 56, 59; **PA News:** 29; **Corbis:** 35 (top); **Soundcraft:** 143; **Sally and Richard Greenhill:** 198. Thanks to Graham Metcalf for diagrams.